Exercise and Sports Science: Advanced Concepts and Practices

Exercise and Sports Science: Advanced Concepts and Practices

Edited by Albert Plummer

SYRAWOOD
PUBLISHING HOUSE
New York

Published by Syrawood Publishing House,
750 Third Avenue, 9th Floor,
New York, NY 10017, USA
www.syrawoodpublishinghouse.com

Exercise and Sports Science: Advanced Concepts and Practices
Edited by Albert Plummer

International Standard Book Number: 978-1-68286-734-1 (Hardback)

Cataloging-in-Publication Data

Exercise and sports science : advanced concepts and practices / edited by Albert Plummer.
p. cm.
Includes bibliographical references and index.
ISBN 978-1-68286-734-1
1. Exercise. 2. Sports sciences. 3. Sports. 4. Physical education and training.
I. Plummer, Albert.
GV481 .E94 2019
613.7--dc23

Printed in China.

TABLE OF CONTENTS

PREFACE

Exercise is a physical activity that enhances physical fitness, and maintains overall health and wellness. It is essential for the prevention of aging, strengthening of muscles, honing athletic skills and maintenance of weight. Physical exercises are classified into the three types- aerobic exercise, anaerobic exercise and flexibility exercises. Exercises are also targeted at increasing accuracy, agility, power and speed. The study of how sports and exercise promote health and performance of the human body is under the domain of sports and exercise science. It integrates areas of physiology, anatomy, psychology, biomechanics and biokinetics. This book is a compilation of chapters that discuss the most vital concepts and emerging trends in the field of exercise and sports science. Selected concepts that redefine this field have been presented in this book. A number of latest researches have been included to keep the readers up-to-date with the global concepts in this area of study.

Various studies have approached the subject by analyzing it with a single perspective, but the present book provides diverse methodologies and techniques to address this field. This book contains theories and applications needed for understanding the subject from different perspectives. The aim is to keep the readers informed about the progresses in the field; therefore, the contributions were carefully examined to compile novel researches by specialists from across the globe.

Indeed, the job of the editor is the most crucial and challenging in compiling all chapters into a single book. In the end, I would extend my sincere thanks to the chapter authors for their profound work. I am also thankful for the support provided by my family and colleagues during the compilation of this book.

Editor

1

"Athletic Identity Measurement Scale": Translation, Adaptation and Validation for Brazil

Walan Robert da Silva
Universidade do Estado de Santa Catarina, Florianópolis, SC, Brasil

Elisa Pinheiro Ferrari
Thiago Emannuel Medeiros
Universidade do Estado de Santa Catarina, Florianópolis, SC, Brasil

Kamyla Thais Dias de Freitas
Universidade do Estado de Santa Catarina, Florianópolis, SC, Brasil

Claudio Marcelo Tkac
Pontifícia Universidade Católica do Paraná, Curitiba, PR, Brasil

Fernando Luiz Cardoso
Universidade do Estado de Santa Catarina, Florianópolis, SC, Brasil

Abstract—The aim of this study was to translate, adapt and validate the version of the Athletic Identity Measurement Scale (AIMS) for Brazilian Portuguese. The methodological procedures were conducted according to international recommendations: translation, back-translation, review by a board of experts, empirical fieldwork testing and inferential statistical analyses. The psychometric properties were evaluated by applying the translated scale to 127 university students. Reproducibility was assessed through stability and homogeneity assessment. Validity was assessed by comparing the scores obtained from the athletes and university students. The results showed good internal consistency ($\alpha = 0.78$), when item 3 was removed and the Cronbach's alpha value increased to 0.82. Through factor analysis, we verified that the items had loadings in two domains. Intra-class correlation coefficient for test and retest was 0.91. Comparison between athletes and university students showed good discriminant validity. According the cultural adaptation process the adapted instrument has excellent psychometric properties and is reliable for the Brazilian culture.

Keywords: translating, reproducibility of results, athletic performance.

Introduction

Identity study has been intriguing psychologists for over a century, and although it has many definitions (Brewer, Raalte & Linder, 1993; Lamont-Mills & Christensen, 2006; Wiechman & William, 1997), practically all of them share the core assumption that the subject's identity acts as one of the main determinants of internal behavior. According to Cieslak (2004), individuals define their identity through social living. Thus, athlete-subjects will define their identity through experienced sporting interactions (Wiechman & Williams, 1997) and this mutual interaction between the athlete and the sporting situation called the attention of the scientific community for the study of athletic identity (AI).

AI may be understood as how athlete-subjects, who practice a sport in a systematic and professional way, build the notion of themselves, in relation to the emotions of their interpersonal living and their interactions resulting from sporting practices (Brewer *et al.*, 1993). Studies regarding this subject have shown that this is a social construct, clearly influenced by friends, family, colleagues, trainers, and the sporting context. This interaction allows the athletes to form identities that enable them, to distinguish themselves from others and, simultaneously giving them a feeling of belonging to a defined group (Anderson & Coleman, 2008). In addition, influencing experiences, relationships and their involvement with the sporting activity (Cornelius, 1995; Lau, Cheung & Randsdell, 2007; Lau, Fox & Cheung, 2004, Anderson, Mâsse, Zhang, Coleman& Chang, 2009).

With that in mind, many authors have been trying to develop an AI concept since the 90s (Brewer *et al.*, 1993; Horton & Mack, 2000; Hurst, Hale, Smith & Collins, 2000; Martin, Mushet & Smith, 1995; Smith, Hale & Collins, 1998). Accordingly, Brewer *et al.* (1993) proposed an instrument for its evaluation, the Athletic Identity Measurement Scale (AIMS), which many national and international studies have broadly used (Martin *et al.*, 1995; Murphy, Petitpas & Brewer, 1996; Grove, Lavallee & Gordon, 1997; Martin, Eklund & Mushett,1997; Tasiemski, Kennedy, Gardner & Blaikley, 2004; Grove, Fish & Eklund, 2004; Lamont-Mills &Christensen, 2006; Brewer, Cornelius, Stephan & Van Raalte,2010), including its translation and adaptation to many countries (Harris & Watson, 2011; Schmid & Seiler, 2003; Hale, James &

Stambulova, 1999; Hin &Anderson, 2008) to evaluate AI in different sports.

According to previous studies, we did not find the existence of a national instrument to evaluate AI, as well as the translation, adaptation and validation of the AIMS for the Brazilian population. The validation of the instrument for Brazil will bring another tool to help in assessing the identity of our current athletes, as well as to examine the athletic identity of young people interested in starting a life in sports. Therefore, the objective of this study was to translate, adapt and validate the version of the AIMS for Brazilian Portuguese that have been used informally inside the country.

Methods

AIMS is an instrument developed by Brewer *et al.* (1993) aiming to evaluate the levels of AI. It is composed of 7 items, subdivided in to three subscales or dimensions: social identity (items 1, 2 and 3), exclusivity (items 4, 5) and negative affectivity (items 6, 7), with a 7-point Likert scale as answer format, varying from 1 (completely disagree) to 7 (agree), resulting in a total AI score, with a sum of the answers given by the participant, 7 points being the minimum score and 49 the highest. Higher score means stronger AI".

For the process of translation and empirical and analytical testing of the instrument, the methodological steps presented in Figure 1 and described in the topics below were conducted. We accepted the theoretical construct built by the authors, with focus on translation and empirical and analytical testing of the instrument in Portuguese.

Translation and cross-cultural adaptation

To ensure the quality of the adaptation, this study followed the essential steps recommended by specialized literature (Hutchinson, Bentzen & Konig-Zanhn, 1996; Guillemin, Bombardier & Beaton 1993; Alexandre & Guirardello, 2002). These steps are described below.

First two independent sworn translators, whose first language was Portuguese, translated the AIMS. Therefore, we obtained two different versions of the scale: T1 and T2. After this stage, there was a meeting with both translators and the principal investigators, which defined a consensual T1+2 version in Brazilian Portuguese.

The T1+2 version was handed to a third sworn translator, whose first language was English, and who was fluent in Portuguese and did not know the original instrument. The questionnaire T1+2 was translated to English (back-translation). The original version and the back-translation were then compared in a meeting between the last translator and the principal investigator, who established a consensual Portuguese version named T3.

Cultural adaptation

After the translation, the clarity and reliability of T3 were tested on 90 athletes selected by convenience taking into consideration the inclusion criteria, training in a systematic way, participating in high performance competitions, training in a systematic way at least for 1 year and training at least 3 times a week from the cities of Curitiba and Guarapuava, Paraná, of whom 74 were men and 16 were women, distributed across the following sports: 43 soccer, 34 swimming and 13 indoor soccer athletes. They answered both versions, T3 and T1+2, to assess the level of agreement between versions and the clarity of all questions in both versions.

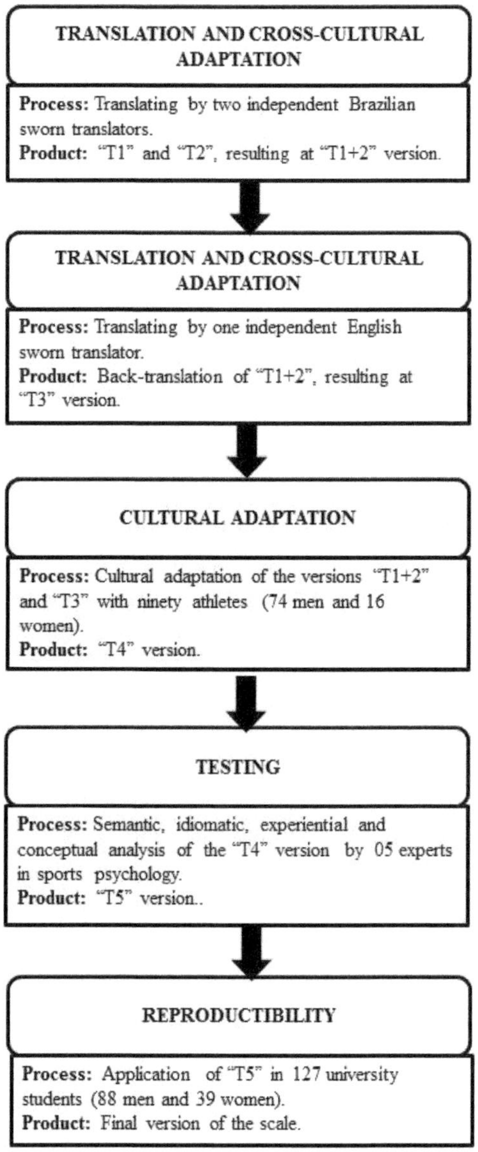

Figure 1. Methodological steps for translating, adapting and validating the AIMS.

In the first round, 45 research subjects received the T3 version of the instrument, and the other 45 received the T1+2 version. After an interval between 14 and 21 days, the scale was re-applied, with the subjects who answered T1+2 answering T3 and, conversely, the opposite also happened.

The respondents were instructed to answer the instrument normally, in addition to rating each item with a grade that represented its level of clarity, with "0" for very unclear and "10" for very clear, and giving suggestions for relevant changes. The level of clarity of the items was obtained through their mean grades, from the rating parameters proposed by Melo (2002): from 0 to 4, the question is confusing; from 5 to 7, the question is unclear; and from 8 to 10, the question is very clear. In the case of scores under 8, the corresponding items were reassessed by the researchers according to comments and suggestions by participants during the assessment. At the end of this step, we developed a new version of the instrument, version T4. We collected individual data, such as age, gender and sport practiced, along with the questionnaire.

For the last empirical procedure, the T4 version was sent to a board with five experts in physical education and five experts in sports psychology, who assessed equivalence in four areas: semantic, idiomatic, experiential and conceptual. After this assessment, the board identified and debated discrepancies. A report was produced and a final version was validated and approved, version T5.

In order to verify the scale's reproducibility and the validity of the construct proposed by the authors of the final version (T5), a second group of participants, selected by convenience taking into consideration the criteria, not being a professional athlete, composed of 127 university students from the physical education course – 88 men and 39 women, with a average age of 21.6 (±3.35) answered the final version of the instrument. The protocol for scale application was similar to the one used in the first gathering and the interval for reapplying the test was 14 days.

Reproducibility was verified through test and retest of the instrument, and discriminant validity was verified by comparing score means obtained from athletes and non-athletes, physical education students, for each item that composes the scale.

Statistical analysis

Data was categorized with Microsoft Excel® and analyzed using the Statistical Package for the Social Sciences (SPSS)®, version 20.0. We used descriptive statistics to describe participants. The analysis of the data distribution was verified through performing Kolmogorov-Smirnov normality, test Cronbach's Alpha was used to verify internal consistency, considering as minimum acceptable value 0.70 (Oviedo & Campo-Arias, 2005).

We assessed the construct's validity through exploratory factor analysis with Varimax rotation, which identifies common components in a large number of variables, a minimum acceptable load 0.50 was considered (Hair, Black, Babin, Anderson & Tatham, 2006).

This assessment makes it possible to determine how the scale is related to the theoretical concepts that support it. Test-retest reliability was tested using the intraclass correlation coefficient, paired t-test was used to compare the averages between the test and retest, and agreement was tested through Kappa index. Reference values for this analysis were: <0.40, weak correlation; 0.40 to 0.60, moderate correlation; 0.60 to 0.80, good to substantial correlation; >0.80, almost perfect or very good correlation (Fayers & Machin, 2007). The difference between results obtained from the two types of population was calculated using Student's t-test for independent samples. The level of significance adopted for all statistical tests was 5%.

The research was conducted within the standards established by the Declaration of Helsinki and approved by the Human Research Ethics Committee, according to Resolution CNS 196/96 under the protocol number: 275.381/2013.

Results

The results present data regarding dimensionality, internal consistency, reproducibility and sensitivity of the AIMS. We evaluated 217 individuals, 90 athletes and 127 non-athletes, Physical Education students corresponding to 100% participation. Factor analysis did not confirm the three dimensions of the AIMS – social identity, exclusivity and negative affectivity as proposed by the author. As shown inTable 1, the items analyzed had loadings in only two domains, "social identity/exclusivity" and negative affectivity, with a percentage of explanation of 46.99% for the first domain and 18.45% for the second.

Table 2 shows total Cronbach's alpha values, which indicate internal consistency, and the AIMS's alpha values if the shown item were to be removed from the scale. Each item was removed from the scale to verify changes in the scale's total alpha values. However, the highest value of Cronbach's alpha was observed after the removal of item 3.

Table 1. Exploratory factor analysis of the AIMS.

	Factor loading	
Items of the AIMS	**1st domain**	**2nd domain**
I consider myself an athlete.	0.77	
I have many goals related to sport.	0.76	
Most of my friends are athletes.	0.56	
Sport is the most important part of my life.	0.80	
I spend more time thinking about sport than anything else.	0.79	
I feel bad about myself when I do poorly in sport.		0.81
I would be very depressed if I were injured and could not compete in sport.		0.77
Percentage of explanation	46.99%	18.45%

Table 2. Total value and change in total Cronbach's alpha value after the exclusion of an AIMS item.

Scale items	**Changed α value**
Total value of the scale	0.78
If item 01 is excluded	0.74
If item 02 is excluded	0.72
If item 03 is excluded	0.82
If item 04 is excluded	0.75
If item 05 is excluded	0.72
If item 06 is excluded	0.79
If item 07 is excluded	0.76

α: Cronbach's alpha.

Table 3 shows values regarding the Kappa index, agreement percentage and the p-value of the paired t-test by performing test-retest. Furthermore, we call attention to the fact that the interclass correlation coefficient was 0.91 (data not presented).

Regarding discriminant validity in Table 4, we present the values of the comparison between scores referring to the AIMS items answered by the athletes and university students. According to presented data, athletes show higher values than university students ($p<0.05$), showing that the instrument can discriminate the aforementioned construct.

Table 3. Agreement of athletic identity measurements between test and retest of the 127 physical education students.

Scale items	Kappa	%A	p-value
I consider myself an athlete.	0.67	83.0%	0.001
I have many goals related to sport.	0.69	84.0%	0.001
Most of my friends are athletes.	0.61	85.0%	0.001
Sport is the most important part of my life.	0.60	82.0%	0.001
I spend more time thinking about sport than anything else.	0.57	80.0%	0.028
I feel bad about myself when I do poorly in sport.	0.60	80.0%	0.001
I would be very depressed if I were injured and could not compete in sport.	0.60	76.0%	0.001

%A: percentage of agreement. p- value of the test Kappa.

Table 4. Comparison between athletes and university students, according to the AIMS items.

AIMS items	Athlete Mean (SD) (n=90)	Non-athlete Mean (SD) (n=127)	T	p-value
I consider myself an athlete.	6.38 (0.97)	3.49 (2.15)	-11.92	0.001
I have many goals related to sport.	6.17 (1.24)	4.54 (2.26)	-6.22	0.001
Most of my friends are athletes.	5.54 (1.42)	3.00 (1.59)	-12.13	0.001
Sport is the most important part of my life.	5.94 (1.34)	4.11 (5.10)	-7.28	0.001
I spend more time thinking about sport than anything else.	5.48 (1.39)	3.74 (2.18)	-6.66	0.001
I feel bad about myself when I do poorly in sport.	6.20 (1.27)	4.75 (2.10)	-5.83	0.001
I would be very depressed if I were injured and could not compete in sport.	6.24 (1.44)	5.17 (2.25)	-4.00	0.001
Total identity	41.95 (5.90)	28.78 (11.80)	-9.73	0.001

SD: standard deviation; T: Student's t-test value.

Discussion

Cross-cultural adaptation is a necessary process when using instruments that were originally built in other languages and contexts, especially when it comes to psychological aspects and the cultural diversity of humans. After performing the steps recommended in the literature (Hutchinson *et al.*, 1996; Guillemin *et al.*, 1993; Alexandre & Guirardello, 2002), we obtained a Brazilian Portuguese version of the AIMS that was properly translated and adjusted to the local context. The availability of this instrument may encourage its use in studies regarding the relationship between AI and the behavior of athletes and sports practitioners.

The results obtained in the validation process of the AIMS-Brazil showed that the items referring to AI's assessment have sufficient validity and reliability to be used in other studies on the subject in Brazil. All of the seven items that compose the scale have factor loadings that justify their place in the scale, according to previously established criteria (Oviedo & Campo-Arias, 2005). The validated AIMS-Brazil met Likert's assumptions with acceptable Cronbach's alpha values, confirming a high internal consistency in the scale. Other studies that tested psychometric characteristics of the AIMS also found the internal consistency acceptable to high (Hale *et al.*, 1999; Hin & Anderseon, 2008; Schmid & Seiler, 2003). Despite small changes in the total value of Cronbach's alpha, when item 3 was removed the Cronbach's alpha value increased to 0.82, suggesting to the authors that the item 3 was not important for the scale, and its presence was not necessary in this context.

In terms of dimensionality, the AIMS-Brazil items had loadings in only two different factors, disproving the tri-dimensionality proposed by the authors, which may suggest isomorphism problems among the items created to represent each dimension in this population. Unfortunately, we did not find references to the dimensionality testing originally proposed in the AIMS in literature, which did not allow a comparison between results.

The instrument's reproducibility through the test-retest procedure was observed through Kappa coefficient and t-test for paired samples. In general, all items presented Kappa coefficients over 0.05, representing percentages of over 70.0% of answer agreement between test and retest. These values confirmed the investigation conducted by Schmid and Seiler (2003), which found high Kappa coefficient values in the AIMS validation for the German population. Furthermore, the means of the scores obtained in the first application and in the second do not show significant differences, showing that the items of the scale, as well as the instrument in general, offer good reliability, enabling us to assume a stability of the scale over time.

Another aspect observed by this study is discriminant validity. When we compared athletes and non-athletes differences about the AI was observed, indicating the ability of the instrument to discriminate between athletes and university students in all items, which presented significant differences among the average scores of answers given by both types of participants. This indicates that athletes have higher AI than other individuals, in this case, university students. This has also been highlighted in other international studies, which describe AI as a predictor of sporting orientation and participation (Lau *et al.*, 2007; Lau *et al.*, 2004; Anderson *et al.*, 2009).

As the limitation of this study highlights, the lack of comparison between athletes, ex athletes and non-athletes, it doesn't allow identifying if the instrument discriminates athletic identity of these three types of people. New research on the validation of the "Athletic Identity Measurement Scale" can test the variation of "Athletic Identity" between athletes and ex-athletes in order to verify the influence of aging process on this personality trait.

Conclusions

In conclusion, the Brazilian Portuguese version of the AIMS in the seven-item composition showed good psychometric performance when examined from a sample of athletes and physical education students from two municipalities of the state of Paraná, in southern Brazil.

The instrument presented satisfactory attributes of internal consistency, test-retest reliability, and discriminant validity. It is important to highlight the fact that we could not identify, in the Brazilian context, another specific instrument that assesses AI characteristics related to sporting orientation. Therefore, this instrument's availability may favor the development and effectiveness of psychological interventions related to sports. Furthermore, we also highlight the fact that even though the scale was developed for the North American population, the results found with its application confirm its effectiveness and reliability for use among Brazilians. However, some regional and sociocultural aspects must be analyzed with greater insight in order for the scale to be as extensive as it intends. Therefore, we suggest the development of further investigations nationwide in order to answer these questions – such as the proposed tri-dimensionality – in addition to including other age groups besides the ones investigated in this study.

References

Alexandre, N.M.C.,& Guirardello, E.de B. (2002). Adaptación cultural de instrumentos utilizados en salud ocupacional. *Revista Panamericana de Salud Publica. 11*(2), 109-111.

Anderson, C.B.,&Coleman, K,J. (2008).Adaptation and validation of the athletic identity questionnaire adolescent for Use with children. *Journal of Physical Activity & Health.5*(4), 539-558.

Anderson, C.B., Mâsse, L., Zhang, H., Coleman, K.J.,& Chang, S. (2009). Contribution of athletic identity to child and adolescent physical activity. *American Journal of Preventive Medicine. 37*(3), 220-226.

Brewer, B., Van Raalte, J.L.,&Linder, D.E. (1993). Athletic identity: Hercules' muscles or Achilles heel?. *International Journal of Sport Psychology.24*(2), 237-254.

Brewer, B., Cornelius, A.E., Stephan, Y.,&Van Raalte, J.L. (2010). Self-protective changes in athletic identity following anterior ligament reconstruction. *Psychology of Sport & Exercise. 11*(1), 1-5.

Cieslak, T.J. (2004). Describing and measuring the athletic identity construct scale development and validation. Tese de doutorado, Pós-Graduação em Filosofia. Universidade do Estado de Ohio, U.S. A.

Cornelius, A.E. (1995). The relationship between athletic identity, peer and faculty socialization, and college student development. *Journal of College Student Development. 36*(6), 560-573.

Fayers, P.,&Machin, D. (2007).*Quality of life: assessment, analysis and interpretation.* (2a ed.). New York: John Wiley & Sons.

Grove, R., Lavallee, D.,&Gordo, S. (1997).Coping with retirement from sport: the influence of athletic identity. *Journal of Applied Sport Psychology.9*(2), 191–203.

Grove, J.R., Fish, M.,& Eklund, R.C. (2004). Changes in athletic identity following team selection: Selfprotection versus self-enhancement. *Journal of Applied Sport Psychology.16*(1), 75-81.

Guillemim, F., Bombardier, C.,&Beaton, D. (1993). Cross-cultural adaptation of health-related quality of life measures: literature review and proposed guidelines. *Journal of Clinical Epidemiology. 46*(12), 1417-32.

Hair, Jr., Black, W.C., Babin, B.J., Anderson, R.E & Tatham, R.L. (2006). *Multivariate Data Analysis.* (6ª ed.). Upper Saddle River, NJ: Pearson Prentice Hall.

Hale, B.D., James, B.,&Stambulova, N.B. (1999). Determining the dimensionality of athletic identity: A herculean cross-cultural undertaking. *International Journal of Sport Psychology. 30*(1), 83-100.

Harris, B.S., &Watson, J. C. (2011). Assessing youth sport burnout: A self-determination identity theorydevelopment perspective. *Journal of Clinical Sport Psychology. 5*(2), 117-133.

Hin, Y.L.,&Andersen, M.B. (2008). Athletic identity in China: Examining the AIMS in a Hong Kong sample. *International Journal of sport & Exercise Psychology. 6*(2), 176-188.

Horton, R.S.,&Mack, D.E. (2000). Athletic identity in marathon runners: Functional focus or dysfunctional commitment ?. *Journal of sport Behavior. 23*(2), 101-119.

Hurst, R., Hale, B., Smith, D.,&Collins, Dave (2000). Exercise dependence, social physique anxiety, and social support in experienced and inexperienced bodybuilders and weightlifters. *British Journal of Sports Medicine. 34*(6), 431- 435.

Hutchinson,A., Bentzen, N.,& Konig-Zanhn, C. (1996) Crosscultural health-outcome assessment: a user's guide. The Netherlands: ERGHO; 1996.

Lamont-Mills, A., & Christensen, S.A. (2006). Athletic identity and its relationship to sport participation levels. *Journal of Science and Medicine in Sport. 9*(6), 472-478.

Lau, P.W.C., Cheung, M.W.L.,&Ransdell, L. (2007). Sport identity and sport participation: A cultural comparison between collective and individualistic societies. *International Journal of Sport & Exercise Psychology. 5*(1), 66-81.

Lau, P.W.C., Fox, K.R.,&Cheung, M.W.L. (2004). Psychosocial and socio-environmental correlates of sport identity and sport participation in secondary-age children. *European Journal of Sport Science. 4*(3), 1-21.

Martin, J.J., Mushett, C.A.,&Smith, K.L. (1995) Athletic identity and sport orientation of adolescent swimmers with disabilities. *Adapted Physical Activity Quarterly. 12*(2), 113-123.

Martin, J.J., Eklund, R.C.,&Mushett, C.A. (1997). Factor structure of the athletic identity measurement scale with athletes with disabilities. *Adapted Physical Activity Quarterly. 14*(1), 74-82.

Melo, S.I.L. (2002). Apostila do processo de validação de instrumentos de medida. Florianópolis: UDESC.

Murphy, G.M., Petitpas, A,J., & Brewer, B (1996). Identity foreclosure, athletic identity, and career maturity in intercollegiate athletes. *Sport Psychologist. 10*(3), 239-346.

Oviedo, H.C., Campo-Arias, A. (2005). Aproximación al uso del coeficiente alfa de Cronbach, *Revista Colombiana de Psiquiatría. 34*(4), 572-580.

Schmidt, J., & Seiler, R. (2003) Identity in high-performance sport: Psychometric investigations with a German Language adaptation of the Athletic Identity Measurement Scale(AIMS-D). *Diagnostica, 49*(4), 176-183.

Smith, D., Hale, B.,&Collin, S.D. (1998). Measurement of exercise dependence in bodybuilders. *Journal of Sports Medicine and Physical Fitness. 38*(1), 66-74.

Tasiemski, T., Kennedy, P., Gardner, B.P., &Blaikley, R.A. (2004). Athletic identity and sports participation in people with spinal cord injury. *Adapted Physical Activity Quarterly. 21*(4), 364-378.

Wiechman, S.A., &Williams, J. (1997). Relation of athletic identity to injury and mood disturbance. *Journal of Sport Behavior. 20*(2), 199-231.

Authors' note

Walan Robert da Silva and Kamyla Thais Dias de Freitas are affliated with the Graduate Program in Human Movement Sciences, State University of Santa Catarina, UDESC/ Gender Lab, Sexuality and Embodiment, LAGESC, Florianopolis- SC, Brazil.

Claudio Marcelo Tkac are affliated with the Pontifical Catholic University of Paraná, Health and Biosciences School, Graduation Course in Physical Education/ Research Group about Motor Behavior, GECOM, Curitiba-PR, Brazil.

Elisa Pinheiro Ferrari, Thiago Emannuel Medeiros, Fernando Luiz Cardoso are affliated with the Graduate Program in Human Movement Sciences, State University of Santa Catarina, UDESC/ Gender Lab, Sexuality and Embodiment, LAGESC, Florianopolis- SC, Brazil.

Corresponding author:

Elisa Pinheiro Ferrari
Rua: Paschoal Simone, 358, Coqueiros, Florianópolis, 88080-350, Santa Catarina, Brasil.
Email: elisaferrari_@hotmail.com

2

Perception of effort monitors internal load during compounded circuit training

Alessandra de Azevedo
Universidade Positivo, Curitiba, PR, Brasil

Lorena Fernanda de Matos
Universidade Federal do Paraná, Curitiba, PR, Brasil

Fábio Yuzo Nakamura
Universidade Estadual de Londrina, Londrina, PR, Brasil

Gleber Pereira
Universidade Federal do Paraná, Curitiba, PR, Brasil

Abstract—The aim of this study was to determine if rating of perceived exertion (RPE) could be used to monitor the internal load during compounded circuit training (CCT) sessions in women. Thirteen young adults women performed three sessions of CCT varying the intensity according to participants' maximum heart rate (50, 70 and 90%HR_{max}). Throughout the main part of CCT (35min), HR and RPE were measured. Both variables were significantly different among the exercise intensities. However, HR and RPE were not correlated. Probably because HR at the end of exercise was similar to the beginning at 90% and 70% of HR_{max} intensities, and lower than the beginning instant at 50% of HR_{max} intensity, whereas RPE increased from the beginning instant to the end of exercise for all intensities. Therefore, RPE is suitable to monitor the internal load during CCT sessions in women due to its possibility to detect the (in)tolerance to exercise, despite of the lack of correlation with HR.

Keywords: rating of perceived exertion, circuit weight training, heart rate.

Introduction

The circuit-weight training method, characterized by alternating exercises between upper- and lower-body segments performed at stations, has been widely used in fitness-related practice settings (Aniceto *et al.*, 2015). The physiological strain can be increased alternating strength and aerobic exercises, which maximizes the time-efficiency while addressing several aspects of physical fitness (Skidmore, Jones, Blegen, & Matthews, 2012). Such combination has been defined as compounded circuit training (CCT) (Monteiro *et al.*, 2008).

The CCT has been shown to be an adequate training strategy to produce cardiovascular improvements and greater energy expenditure for both men and women (Monteiro *et al.*, 2008). However, monitoring exercise intensity during the CCT has been neglected, in spite of its key role on modulating training adaptations, by controlling the workload during the sessions. Heart rate (HR) has been frequently used to quantify the physiological exercise intensity in high-intensity interval training (Ciolac *et al.*, 2014; Green *et al.*, 2006) and circuit-weight training (Skidmore *et al.*, 2012). On the other hand, perception of effort has been suggested to easily monitor exercise intensity in circuit-weight training (Skidmore *et al.*, 2012) and high-intensity interval training (Ciolac *et al.*, 2014; Green *et al.*, 2006). Thus, it would be useful to determine if perception of effort can also be used to monitor the internal load (physiological/perceptual strain) during CCT sessions.

The perception of effort, defined as the conscious sensation of how hard, heavy, and strenuous a physical task is (Goldstein, 2009; Marcora, 2010) and measured through the rating of perceived exertion (RPE) scale (Borg, 2000), has presented good correlation with physiological variables (e.g., HR, oxygen consumption and blood lactate concentration) in incremental exercise (Borg, Gunnar; Ljunggren, Gunilla; Ceci, 1985; Psycharakis, 2011; Wolff, René, & Faculté, 2003). However, such a relationship can be inflated by the corollary increase in both physiological response and perception of effort during incremental protocols. Nevertheless, it is hypothesized that RPE and HR would be significantly correlated during CCT sessions performed at different intensities. Thus, RPE could be a useful tool to monitor the internal load during CCT sessions, since it has been applied at a number of gyms specifically designed for women. Therefore, the aim of this study was to determine if RPE could be used to monitor the internal load during CCT sessions in women.

Materials and methods

Participants

Thirteen physically active young healthy women (24.8 ± 3.6 years, 64.0 ± 7.0 kg, 170 ± 10 cm, 23.0 ± 3.0 kg/m²) agreed to participate in this study. The Ethics Committee of the University approved the experimental procedures of this study (CAEE 45901015.0.0000.0093). The participants received information about the study and signed a consent form before starting the procedures.

Experimental procedures

The participants performed three sessions of CCT at different intensities, 50%, 70% and 90% of their maximum heart rate (HR_{max} = 220 – age), on different days. These intensities were based on a previous familiarization session with the experimental procedures, which also was used as a pilot study. All sessions were separated by six days, always performed at the same period and by the same researcher. During the whole experimental period, it was requested that the participants maintain their physical and dietary habits, and to avoid strenuous exercise 48h before each session. The participants were divided into four groups. Each group had its training intensity order randomly assigned. The training sessions consisted of 5 min warming up, 35 min as the main part performing the CCT, and 5 min of relaxation. During the main part, HR and RPE were measured every 5 min. A portable device (Electro FT1, Polar, Kempele, Finland) was used to monitor the HR. The 6-20 Borg scale was used to monitor the perception of effort (Borg, 2000). All the participants were familiar with the CCT and RPE scale.

However, to avoid misinterpretation to report perception of effort, before every session, the participants received the following instructions to use the RPE scale: "During the exercise, we want to evaluate your perception of effort. It depends on how difficult, heavy and hard is for you to exercise your legs or arms, how difficult it is to breathe, and general feeling of strain for the exercise. It does not depend on pain and burning sensation in your muscles of legs or arms. Look at this scale, where 6 means "no effort, at rest" and 20 means "maximal exertion". A score of nine corresponds to a "very light" exercise for a person which is like walking slowly at your own pace for a few minutes. A score of thirteen is an exercise "somewhat hard" but it still feels good to keep going. A score of seventeen or "very hard" is a very vigorous exercise, in which person can still perform it, but he/she really has to struggle and feeling of much difficulty and tired. A score of nineteen is an "exhaustive" exercise, being the most intense workout ever experienced. Try to evaluate your exertion feelings as honestly as possible, without thinking about the workload (e.g., heart rate, speed, power, intensity level of the exercise machine). It is important to rate your own feelings of effort, not how it compares to others. Any questions?"

Compounded circuit training

The training sessions consisted of alternating weight and aerobic exercises, controlled by time, and varying active and passive resting periods between exercise sets (Table 1). The first exercise intensity of CCT was based on a familiarization session.

Table 1. Exercises performed during the compounding circuit training sessions at different intensities.

50% HRmax Protocol **6 exercises** **Total Time: 35 minutes**	**70% HRmax Protocol** **6 exercises** **Total Time: 35 minutes**	**90% HRmax Protocol** **6 exercises** **Total Time: 35 minutes**
1. Bent Over Rows with bag (3kg) + Unilateral Skipping (2x20s + 2 min)	1. Agility Ladder + TRX Bent Over Rows + Jackknife Abdominal (3x45s + 20s + 20s)	1. Olympic Lifting with weight bar (8kg) (2 x 1min30s + 30s passive rest)
2. Push Ups Inclined + Squat + Walk (3x20s + 30s + 1min30s)	2. Agility Ladder + Zig-Zag run (2x45s + 45s)	2. Olympic Lifting with weight bar (8kg) + Stationary Run (3x40s + 40s)
3. Unilateral Skipping + Quick walk (4x30s + 15s)	3. TRX Push Ups + Lunge Step + Agility Ladder (3x30s + 30s + 1 lap in agility ladder)	3. Arm swing combined with Stationary Sprint Run + walk (4x20s + 10s)
4. Lunge + Bent Over Rows unilateral with halter (1kg) (3x20s + 20s + 1min passive rest)	4. Skipping + Agility Ladder (2x50s + 50s)	4. Skipping followed by stationary sprint + Bicycle Crunch Abdominal. (3x30s + 30s)
5. Stationary Run + Sit Up Abdominal (4x40s + 20s)	5. Push Ups In Agility Ladder + TRX Single Leg Squat (2x1 lap in agility ladder + 40s)	5. Deadlift combined with Skipping + Bicycle Crunch Abdominal. (3x 30s + 10s)
6. Hip Lifting with bag (3kg) + Oblique Abdominal (3x20s + 20s)	6. Stationary Run + Walk (4x30s + 15s)	6. Plank Abdominal + Reverse Plank (3x40s + 20s; 1min passive rest).

Statistical Analysis

The estimated power for comparisons of heart rate and perceived exertion was 0.94 for the number of participants in the present study. Data normality and homogeneity of variance were verified through Shapiro-Wilk and Levene tests, respectively. Then, two-way repeated measures ANOVA was run to determine differences between intensity (50, 70 and 90% HR_{max}) and time (5, 10, 15, 20, 25, 30, 35 min) for the dependent variables. Bonferroni post hoc test was used for multiple comparison purpose. The relationship between heart rate and perceived exertion at different intensities was checked using Pearson's correlation coefficient. The level of significance was $p < 0.05$.

Results

There was interaction between intensity and time for both HR (p=0.002) and RPE (p=0.003). Moreover, the HR was significantly different among the intensities at iso-time (same instant) (Figure 1, upper panel). The RPE was also significantly different among the intensities at iso-time (Figure 1, lower panel). However, HR and RPE presented different patterns over the time (Figure 1).

There was no correlation between heart rate and perceived exertion at different exercise intensities [50% (r= -0.11; p=0.31), 70% (r= -0.01; p=0.9) and 90% HR_{max} (r=0.15; p=0.14)].

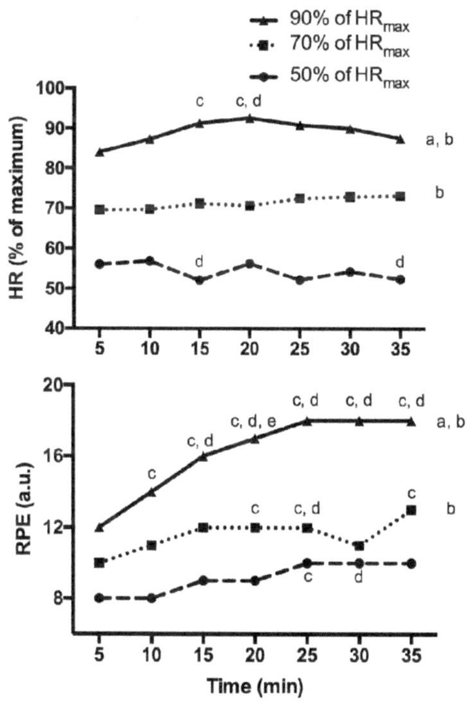

Figure 1. Mean and standard deviation of heart rate (HR) (upper panel) and rating of perceived exertion (RPE) (lower panel) at different instants during different compounding circuit training sessions based on maximum HR. For both HR and RPE variables: 90% of HR_{max} exercise intensity was significantly different from 70% and 50% of HR_{max} exercise intensities at iso-time (same instant) for the whole session; 70% of HR_{max} exercise intensity was significantly different from 50% of HR_{max} exercise intensity at isotime for the whole session. [a]Significantly different from 5 min at the same intensity; [b]Significantly different from 10 min at the same intensity. [c]Significantly different from 15 min at the same intensity.

Discussion

The aim of this study was to determine if perception of effort could be used to monitor the training load during CCT sessions performed at different intensities in women. Both variables - HR and RPE - were different among the CCT intensities, in which they were greater in sessions with higher exercise intensities. However, these variables presented different temporal pattern throughout the sessions, being not significantly correlated in any of the exercise sessions.

HR and RPE were greater during the sessions performed with higher exercise intensity. Such response is based on the manipulation of intensity through the active resting intervals between sets and multi-joint exercises performed at 70% and 90% of HR_{max}, requiring greater physiological demand (Ciolac *et al.*, 2014; Polito, 2015). However, HR and RPE were not significantly correlated at different exercise intensities during the CCT sessions. Previous studies have reported relationship between these variables during incremental workload exercise and during high-intensity interval training (Borg, *et al.* 1985; Psycharakis, 2011; Wolff *et al.*, 2003). On the other hand, previous study has shown different temporal pattern of HR and RPE changes during CCT (Skidmore *et al.*, 2012). Similarly, in the present study, the overall RPE increase occurred from the middle to the end of exercise session for all intensities. In contrast, HR at the end of exercise was similar to the beginning instant at 90% and 70% of HR_{max}, or at the end of exercise HR was lower than the beginning instant at 50% of HR_{max}.

It has been shown that HR is a relatively poor indicator of exercise intensity during intermittent training (Foster, *et al.*, 2001). The RPE has increased during the exercise even when physiological variables have been stabilized (Pires *et al.*, 2011). Moreover, it has been reported that previous mental fatigue has increased RPE, whereas neither HR nor oxygen consumption have changed (Marcora, Staiano, & Manning, 2009). The lack of correlation between HR and RPE, in these studies and in the present, can be explained based on the Psychobiological model, which postulates that perception of effort is the conscious awareness of the central motor command sent to the active muscles, independent of peripheral afferent feedback signals (Marcora, 2009; Smirmaul, Dantas, Nakamura, & Pereira, 2013). Therefore, as RPE is generated independently from other physiological responses (e.g., HR and oxygen consumption), it can be used not only to monitor exercise intensity, but also to detect the (in) tolerance to exercise (Rodríguez-Marroyo, Villa, García-López, & Foster, 2012). In fact, RPE has been shown to be more sensitive to the accumulated fatigue caused by prolonged multiple-day cycling race than HR (Rodríguez-Marroyo *et al.*, 2012).

Based on these arguments, RPE can be useful to monitor the training load during CCT sessions for women, although there was no correlation between HR and RPE. From a practical point of view, practitioners are suggested to use RPE scale during CCT sessions, since exercise (in)tolerance (i.e., task disengagement) is much more related to RPE than to other physiological variables, such as HR. Thus, to maintain a target level of RPE during each CCT, the HR can be even reduced over the exercise session. Future studies are needed to address the training effects of CCT guided by RPE.

Conclusion

Although there was no correlation between HR and RPE, it can be suggested that RPE can be useful to monitor the training load during CCT sessions for women, since it presents the possibility to detect the (in)tolerance to exercise. Empirically, healthy women can feel difficulty to maintain the exercise intensity during CCT, despite of HR stabilization throughout the session.

References

Aniceto, R.R., Ritti-Dias, R.M., dos Prazeres, T.M.P., Farah, B.Q., de Lima, F.F.M., & do Prado, W.L. (2015). Rating of perceived exertion during circuit weight training. *Journal of Strength and Conditioning Research*, (MAY), 1. http://doi.org/10.1519/JSC.0000000000000998

Borg, G. a. (2000). *Escalas de Borg para a dor eo esforço.*

Borg, G.; Ljunggren, G.; Ceci, R. (1985). The increase of perceived exertion, aches and pain in the legs, heart rate and blood lactate during exercise on a bicycle ergometere. *European Journal of Applied Physiology and Occupational Physiology*, *54*(4), 343–349.

Ciolac, E., Mantuani, S., Neiva, C., Veradi, C., Pêssoa-Filho, D., & Pimenta, L. (2014). Rating of perceived exertion as a tool for prescribing and self regulating interval training: a pilot study. *Biology of Sport*, *32*(2), 103–108. http://doi.org/10.5604/20831862.1134312

Foster, C, Florhaug, J.A., Franklin, J., Gottschall, L., Hrovatin, L.A., Parker, S., Doleshal, P., and Dodge, C. (2001). A New approach to monitoring exercise training. *J Strength Cond Res*, *15*, 109–115.

Goldstein, E. B. (2009). *Encyclopedia of perception*. Los Angeles.

Green, J.M., Mclester, J.R., Crews, T.R., Wickwire, P.J., Pritchett, R.C., & Lomax, R.G. (2006). RPE Association with Lactate and Heart Rate during High-Intensity Interval Cycling. *Medicine & Science in Sports & Exercise*, *38*(1), 167–172. http://doi.org/10.1249/01.mss.0000180359.98241.a2

Marcora, S. (2010). Afferent Feedback From Fatigued Locomotor Muscles Is Not an Important Determinant of Endurance Exercise Performance. *Journal of Applied Physiology*, *108*(2), 454–456. http://doi.org/10.1152/japplphysiol.00976.2009a

Marcora, S.M. (2009). Perception of effort during exercise is independent of afferent feedback from skeletal muscles, heart, and lungs. *Journal of Applied Phyiology*, *106*, 2060–2062. http://doi.org/10.1152/japplphysiol.90378.2008

Marcora, S.M., Staiano, W., & Manning, V. (2009). Mental fatigue impairs physical performance in humans. *Journal of Applied Physiology*, *106*(3), 857–864. http://doi.org/10.1152/japplphysiol.91324.2008

Monteiro, a G., Alveno, D. a, Prado, M., Monteiro, G. a, Ugrinowitsch, C., Aoki, M. S., & Piçarro, I. C. (2008). Acute physiological responses to different circuit training protocols. *The Journal of Sports Medicine and Physical Fitness*, *48*(4), 438–42. Retrieved from http://www.ncbi.nlm.nih.gov/pubmed/18997645

Pires, F.O., Lima-Silva, A.E., Bertuzzi, R., Casarini, D.H., Kiss, M.A., Lambert, M.I., & Noakes, T.D. (2011). The influence of peripheral afferent signals on the rating of perceived exertion and time to exhaustion during exercise at different intensities, *48*, 1284–1290.

Polito, M. (2015). Arterial E Duplo- -Produto Ao Exercício Contra-Resistência : Uma Revisão Da Literatura, (October).

Rodríguez-Marroyo, J.A., Villa, G., García-López, J., & Foster, C. (2012). Comparison of Heart Rate and Session Rating of Perceived Exertion Methods of Defining Exercise Load in Cyclists. *Journal of Strength and Conditioning Research*, *26*(8), 2249–2257. http://doi.org/10.1519/JSC.0b013e31823a4233

Skidmore, B.L., Jones, M.T., Blegen, M., & Matthews, T.D. (2012). Acute effects of three different circuit weight training protocols on blood lactate, heart rate, and rating of perceived exertion in recreationally active women. *Journal of Sports Science and Medicine*, *11*(4), 660–668.

Smirmaul, B.P.C., Dantas, J.L., Nakamura, F.Y., & Pereira, G. (2013). The psychobiological model : a new explanation to intensity regulation and (in)tolerance in endurance exercise. *Revista Brasileira de Educação Física E Esporte*, *27*(2), 333–340. http://doi.org/10.1590/S1807-55092013005000008

Psycharakis S.G.(2011). A longitudinal analysis on the validity and reliability of ratings of perceived exertion for elite swimmers. *Strength And Conditioning*, (6), 420–426.

Wolff, M., René, U., & Faculté, D. (2003). Reliability of Rating Scales of Perceived Exertion and Heart Rate During Progressive and Maximal Constant Load Exercises Till Exhaustion in Physical Education Students. *International Journal of Sports Medicine*, *24*(4), 285–290. http://doi.org/10.1055/s-2003-39502

Authors' note

Alessandra de Azevedo is affiliated with the Positivo University, Curitiba, PR, Brazil.

Lorena Fernanda de Matos is affiliated with the Physical Education Department, Federal University of Parana, Curitiba, PR, Brazil.

Fábio Yuzo Nakamura is affiliated with the Physical Education Department, State University of Londrina, Londrina, PR, Brazil.

Gleber Pereira is affiliated with the Positivo University, Curitiba, PR, Brazil and Physical Education Department, Federal University of Parana, Curitiba, PR, Brazil.

Corresponding author

Gleber Pereira
Universidade Federal do Paraná, Departamento de Educação Física, Rua Coração de Maria, 92 -BR 116 km 95, Jardim Botânico, Curitiba, Paraná, 80215-370, Brazil.
Email: gleber.pereira@gmail.com

3

Heart rate as an indicator for exercise prescription for normal, overweight, and obese adolescents

Kamilla Bolonha Gomes
Anselmo José Perez
Luciana Carletti
Universidade Federal do Espírito Santo, Vitória, ES, Brasil

Adilson Marques
Universidade de Lisboa, Portugal

Abstract—This study aimed to investigate the relationship between heart rate (HR) predicted and VO_2max using a CPET (cardiopulmonary exercise testing) among normal weight, overweight, and obese adolescents. The sample comprised 299 adolescents (142 boys), from Vitória (ES, Brazil), aged 10-14 years (12.6±1.4). Adolescents were classified into normal weight (n=236), overweight (n=34), and obese (n=29). Adolescents were subjected to a CPET ramp protocol on a treadmill. It was observed that the reserve heart rate (HRres) was similar to the maximum recommended oxygen uptake (VO_2) for the maintenance and improvement of cardiorespiratory fitness. It was also observed that HRres can be used to control the intensity of exercise sessions in physical education classes independent of weight status. In conclusion, the relationship between the HR and VO_2 for adolescents is linear, allowing the level of intensity to be determined by the HRres proportion related with the correspondent %VO_2max levels of intensity, according to BMI-for-age categories.

Keywords: cardiorespiratory fitness, adolescent, exercise

Introduction

Youth physical activity participation and physical fitness are associated with a number of health benefits: improvement in bone mineral density, aerobic fitness, muscular strength, endurance, cardiovascular risk factors, and mental health (Janssen & Leblanc, 2010). Moreover, physical fitness is one of the most important health status markers that predicts cardiovascular disease and mortality (Ortega, Ruiz, Castillo, & Sjostrom, 2008), mainly among overweight and obese individuals (Cobayashi, Oliveira., Escrivão, Silveira, & Taddei, 2010; Rodrigues, Perez, Carletti, Bissolli, & Abreu, 2007). In children and adolescents, physical fitness is associated with improved health-related biomarkers that may further influence young adulthood health (Foley, Quinn, Dwyer, Venn, & Jones, 2008; Simmons, Griffin, Steele, Wareham, & Ekelund, 2008).

As the health of young people is gaining attention, due to the global epidemic of obesity during childhood (Onis, Blossner, & Borghi, 2010), physical activity recommendations have been highlighted (World Health Organization, 2010) to prevent health problems (Garcia-Hermoso, Saavedra, Escalante, Sanchez-Lopez, & Martinez-Vizcaino, 2014; Prado *et al.*, 2014), improve health (Ortega *et al.*, 2008), and increase physical fitness levels (Strong *et al.*, 2005). Thus, safe and effective exercise prescription for young people is a growing concern because it is important that the exercise be at the appropriate frequency, duration and intensity.

Regardless of age, the intensity of physical activity is usually defined in terms of percentages of maximal oxygen uptake (%VO_2max), maximal heart rate (%HRmax) and reserve heart rate (%HRres), or as a multiple of resting metabolic rate (1 MET) (Garber *et al.*, 2011). Although the %VO_2max is the gold standard to determine exercise intensity, its measurement is still costly and and not easily available since a cardiopulmonary exercise testing (CPET) is required. These difficulties make the HR a an alternative option to measure exercise intensity. There is a linear relationship between VO_2max and HRmax at submaximal exercise intensities (Garber *et al.*, 2011).

The American College of Sports Medicine has recommended that the appropriate exercise intensity for improving cardiorespiratory fitness for adults is 50–85% of VO_2max, 60–90% of age-predicted HRmax (American College of Sports Medicine, 2013). The equivalency between HR and VO_2 is based on the fact that %VO_2max or %VO_2res equals the same %HRmax or %HRres. This was demonstrated by Swain and Leutholtz (1997), who observed that HRres was equivalent to VO_2res. In fact, the relationship between VO_2 and HR during rest and exercise is well documented for adults (Cunha, Midgley, Monteiro, & Farinatti, 2010; Swain & Franklin, 2002; Swain & Leutholtz, 1997; Swain, Leutholtz, King, Haas, & Branch, 1998), and extensively used for exercise prescription (ACSM, 2013). Nonetheless, there is limited research and evidence regarding the relationship between VO_2 and HR in children and adolescents (Ekelund *et al.*, 2001; Hui & Chan, 2006). Children and adolescents are physiologically different from adults and the association between VO_2 and HR might not be similar to the association known in adults, as observed by Hui and Chan (2006). Furthermore, there is no evidence of the influence of BMI categories on children and adolescents physical performance.

Establishing an objective criterion to prescribe children and adolescents exercise has practical implications for their health promotion. Exercise intensity recommended for children and adolescents needs further evaluation. Therefore, this study aimed to investigate and determine the relationship between HR predicted and VO_2max using a CPET among normal weight, overweight, and obese adolescents.

Methods

Participants

The present study used data of students from public and private schools in the 7 regions of Vitória municipality (ES, Brazil), aged 10-14 years (12.6±1.4). Data from a proportionate stratified random sample of students were collected as previously reported (Rodrigues, Perez, Carletti, Bissoli & Abreu, 2006), taking into account the location and number of students, by gender, in each school. All students from 10 to 14 years of age with a health status that allowed participation in physical education classes were eligible. Data from 380 (177 boys, 203 girls) out of 27491 students were collected. Of these 380 participants, 299 (142 boys, 157 girls) attended all inclusion criteria of CPET protocol. During physical education classes students were taken to the laboratory by social worker, or were accompanied by their parents. In the laboratory they were received by the research team conducting the CPET. Prior to testing, the participants and their guardians were informed about the objectives of the study, procedures, benefits, and probable risks of the investigation. Written informed consent was then obtained from the guardians. The Faculdade Salesiana de Vitória (ES, Brazil) Ethics Committee approved the study protocol, and the study was conducted according to ethical standards in sport and exercise science research (Harriss & Atkinson, 2013).

Experimental design:

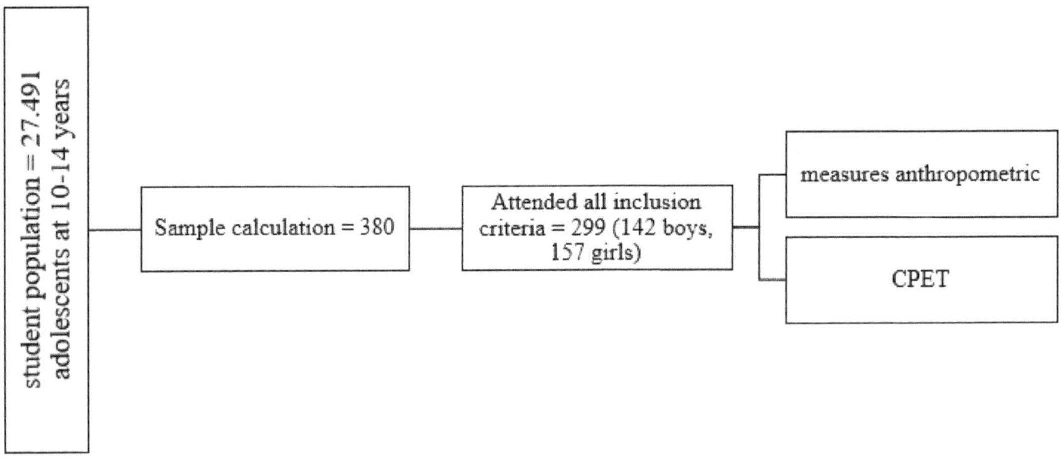

Measures Anthropometric

To assess weight status, participants were weighed to the nearest 0.1 kg wearing minimal clothes and without shoes, using an electronic scale (Welmy, model RW200; São Paulo, BR). Height was measured with a stadiometer to the nearest 0.1 cm. Body mass index was then calculated based on mass (kilograms) divided by height (square meters). Participants were classified into normal weight (NW, percentile < 85, n = 236), overweight (OW, percentile > 85 ≤ 97, n = 34), and obese (OB, percentile > 97, n = 29) categories according to age- and gender-specific cut-off points proposed by World Health Organization (Onis *et al.*, 2010).

Cardiopulmonary exercise testing protocol

Prior to CPET, participants were instructed on exercise testing procedures: how to walk and run on a treadmill, and then engaged in a standardized 2 minutes warm-up period. Participants walked and ran on a calibrated motor-driven treadmill (Inbrasport Super ATL, RGS, Brazil), according to an incremental exercise protocol (Rodrigues, Perez, Carletti, Bissoli, & Abreu, 2006). The test protocol started at 5 km/h with an inclination of 0.0%. The treadmill was then increased to the participants' comfortable running speed, to a maximum of 12 km/h; the inclination was raised until 12% was reached as described previously (Rodrigues, Bissoli, Pires, & Abreu, 2004) using an individualized protocol (Karila, de Blic, Waernessyckle,

Benoist, & Scheinmann, 2001). VO_2 and carbon dioxide (V_{CO2}) output were measured using a breath-by-breath analyser (CPX/D system; Medical Graphics Corporation, St Paul, MN, USA). The system also provided information about pulmonary ventilation, ventilator equivalent of oxygen, and respiratory exchange ratio. The equipment was calibrated before each participant's test, and parts of bare skin in contact with the equipment were sanitised before use. To consider whether the VO_2max was reached, at least three of the following criteria were observed (Karila *et al.*, 2001): 1) failure to maintain the required speed; 2) respiratory exchange ratio > 1.0; 3) HR within 5 beats/min of the age-predicted HRmax; 4) VO_2 max > 85% of predicted. Resting HR (HRresting) determination was obtained from a resting 12-lead electrocardiogram (ECG) (CardioPerfect RMD) connected to the equipment (CPX/D system; Medical Graphics Corporation, St Paul, MN, USA). Participants remained in the supine position for approximately five minutes, and the minimum HR was registered (HRresting). The test was performed at least 2 hours after the last meal. The lab temperature was maintained between 20 and 23 degrees Celsius, and there was equipment and pharmaceuticals for unforeseen cases with the participants.

Data analysis

HRres was obtained from the subtraction of HRmax measured in the CPET by HRresting (HRmax - HRresting). The HRres was then multiplied by the percentages 50, 60, 70, 80, and 90. From the values of HRmax, the predicted HR was calculated by the simple method (%HRmax): HRmax measure multiplied by the same percentage of HRres. These predicted values were then compared with the experimental results from CPET in the percentages of 50, 60, 70, 80 and 90 of VO_2max. Descriptive statistics were calculated (means, standard deviation) for all variables. Variables were examined for normality and homoscedasticity with Kolmogorov–Smirnov and Levene's tests. One-way ANOVA followed by Tukey's post hoc test, and student's t-test, were used to assess the differences among BMI categories and between sexes. The Pearson correlation was used to verify the relationship between absolute HR (measured and predicted) values in percentages of VO_2max in the three groups of adolescents. All statistical analyses were performed using SigmaStat 3.5. A value of $p < 0.05$ was considered significant.

Results

Characteristics of the participants according BMI categories are presented in Table 1.

The measured and predicted HR (beat.min^{-1}) results in different percentages of VO_2max intensity are presented in Table 2. For the three BMI categories, in both sexes, HR assessed by the simple method (% HRmax) was significantly lower than the HRres and HR measured during the CPET in all percentages of VO_2 analysed. The average HRresting used to compute HRres was 76±9 beats/min and 82±10 beats/min ($p < 0.05$) for NW, 78±9 beats/min and 83 ± 11 beats/min for OW, 86±14 beats/min and 90±11 beats/min for OB participants. Significant differences between OB participants and the other BMI categories (NW and OW) were observed. For HRmax in the CPET there were no significant differences among BMI categories (NW = 199±8 beats/min, OW = 200±8 beats/min, OB = 199±9 beats/min).

The correlation between measured HR *vs.* predicted method HRres, and HR *vs.* predicted simple method (%HRmax), in normal weight, overweight, and obese adolescents, are shown in Figures 1, 2 and 3. There was a high correlation among measured HR in all percentiles of VO_2max (50, 60, 70, 80 and 90%) with method HRres and %HRmax. This occurred for the three groups in both sexes. The medium and strong correlation values range from 0.50 to 0.80 of the three groups: normal weight, overweight and obesity, involving all percentages studied.

For the VO_2max directly measured in the CPET among NW participants, boys had significantly higher values than girls (48.2±7.2 vs 39.1±6.0 ml.kg/min; $p = 0.001$). For OW, boys also had a significantly higher value for VO_2max than girls (41.1±6.5 *vs* 35.3±5.1 ml.kg/min; $p = 0.006$). Nonetheless, among OB participants there was no significant difference between boys and girls (33.4±5.6 *vs* 32.1±4.4 ml.kg/min; p = 0.539).

Results of the %HR for percentages of VO_2max are presented in Table 3. For all levels of VO_2max intensity, gender, and BMI categories, no significant differences were observed.

For HRres, results are shown in Table 4. It is possible to observe that OB boys and girls had significantly higher percentages of HRres than NW boys and girls for all %VO_2max levels of intensity. Comparing boys and girls, differences between sexes were only observed for the NW, girls had lowers HRres for all %VO_2max levels of intensity.

Table 1. Anthropometric characteristics of participants aged 10-14 years.

	NW (n = 236)	OW (n = 34)	OB (n = 29)
Age	12.7±1.4	12.5±1.5	12.4±1.2
Weight (kg)	40.6±9	54.2±10*	65.8±12.5†#
Height (m)	1.52±0.11	1.55±0.1	1.57±0.09†
BMI (kg/m²)	17.5±2.0	22.5±1.7*	26.5±3.4†#

$p < 0.05$: *NW vs. OW; †NW vs. OB; #OW vs. OB.
NW, normal weight; OW, overweight; OB, obese; BMI, body mass index
Tests by ANOVA followed by Tukey's post hoc test.

Tables 2. HR (beats/min) values according percentages of VO_2max in normal weight, overweight, and obese adolescents

%VO2m-ax.		NW			OW			OB		
		Measured	Predicted		Measured	Predicted		Measured	Predicted	
		HR	HRres	Simple Method (%HRmax)	HR	HRres	Simple Method (%HR-max)	HR	HRres	Simple Method (%HRmax)
50	Boys	144±10*†	137±7#	99±4	144±9*	139±6#	100±4	143±12*	143±11#	99±5
	Girls	144±10*	140±7#	100±4	146±9*	141±8#	99±4	147±11*	144±7#	100±4
60	Boys	156±10*†	150±7#	119±5	156±9*	151±6#	120±4	155±12*	154±10#	119±6
	Girls	156±11*	152±7#	119±5	158±10*	153±8#	119±5	158±11*	155±7#	119±5
70	Boys	166±14*†	162±7#	139±6	170±8*†	163±6#	140±5	167±12*	165±10#	139±7
	Girls	167±11*	164±7#	139±6	170±10*	164±8#	139±6	170±10*	166±7#	139±6
80	Boys	179±12*†	174±7#	159±7	181±8*†	176±6#	160±6	179±13*	176±10#	159±8
	Girls	179±12	176±7#	159±6	182±11*	176±8#	159±7	182±11*	177±8#	159±7
90	Boys	191±14*†	186±8#	178±8	193±8*†	188±7#	180±7	191±14*	188±10	179±9
	Girls	191±13*	187±8#	179±7	195±11*	187±9	179±8	194±10*	188±8#	179±8

$p < 0.05$: * HR vs. Simple method HRmax; † HR vs. Simple method HRres; # HRres vs. Simple method HRmax
NW, normal weight; OW, overweight; OB, obese; BMI, body mass; HR, heart rate; HRres, reserve heart rate; HRmax, maximum heart rate.
Tested by ANOVA followed by Tukey's post hoc test

Tables 3. Percentages of measured HR according to percentages of VO_2max in normal weight, overweight, and obese adolescents.

%VO_2max		NW (%)	OW (%)	OB (%)
50%	Boys	72.6±4.6	72.0±3.0	71.7±4.0
	Girls	72.5±4.7	73.4±2.6	73.7±4.2
60%	Boys	78.5±4.3	78.2±2.7	77.8±3.6
	Girls	78.3±4.4	79.5±2.8	79.4±3.5
70%	Boys	84.4±4.4	84.8±2.2	83.8±3.7
	Girls	84.1±4.4	85.5±2.4	85.6±3.0
80%	Boys	90.3±4.8	90.7±2.2	90.1±4.0
	Girls	89.9±4.8	91.4±2.6	91.4±2.8
90%	Boys	96.3±5.5	96.7±2.5	95.8±4.2
	Girls	95.7±5.2	98.0±2.9	97.3±2.9

NW, normal weight; OW, overweight; OB, obese
Tested by ANOVA.

Table 4. HRres according to percentages of VO_2max in normal weight, overweight, and obese adolescents.

%VO_2max		NW (%)	OW (%)	OB (%)
50%	Boys	69.3±2.4	69.5±2.5	71.7±3.1*#
	Girls	70.5±2.4**	70.8±2.5	72.5±2.9*
60%	Boys	75.4±1.9	75.6±2.0	77.4±2.5*#
	Girls	76.4±1.9**	76.7±2.0	78.0±2.3*
70%	Boys	81.6±1.5	81.7±1.5	83.0±1.9*#
	Girls	82.3±1.4**	82.5±1.5	83.5±1.7*
80%	Boys	87.7±1.0	87.8±1.0	88.7±1.3*#
	Girls	88.2±1.0**	88.3±1.0	89.0±1.2*
90%	Boys	93.9±0.5	93.9±0.5	94.3±0.6*#
	Girls	94.1±0.5**	94.2±0.5	94.5±0.6*

$p < 0.05$: *NW vs. OB; † NW vs. OW; # OW vs. OB; **boys vs. girls.
NW, normal weight; OW, overweight; OB, obese
ANOVA followed by Tukey's post hoc test was used to test differences among BMI categories.
Student t-test was used to test differences between sexes.

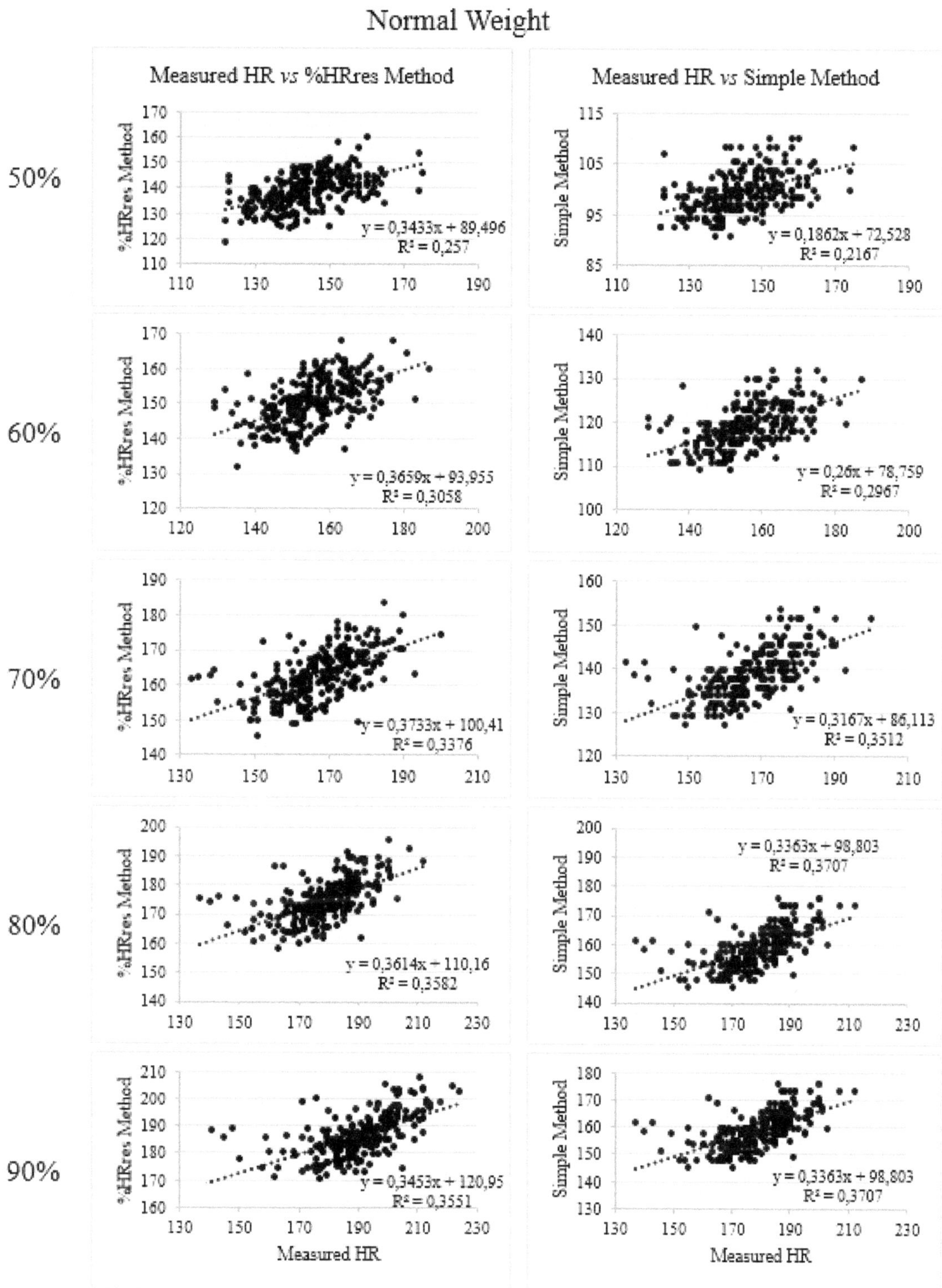

Figure 1. Correlation between measured HR *vs.* predicted %HRres method and measured HR *vs* predicted simple method (HRmax) in normal weight for both sexes together.

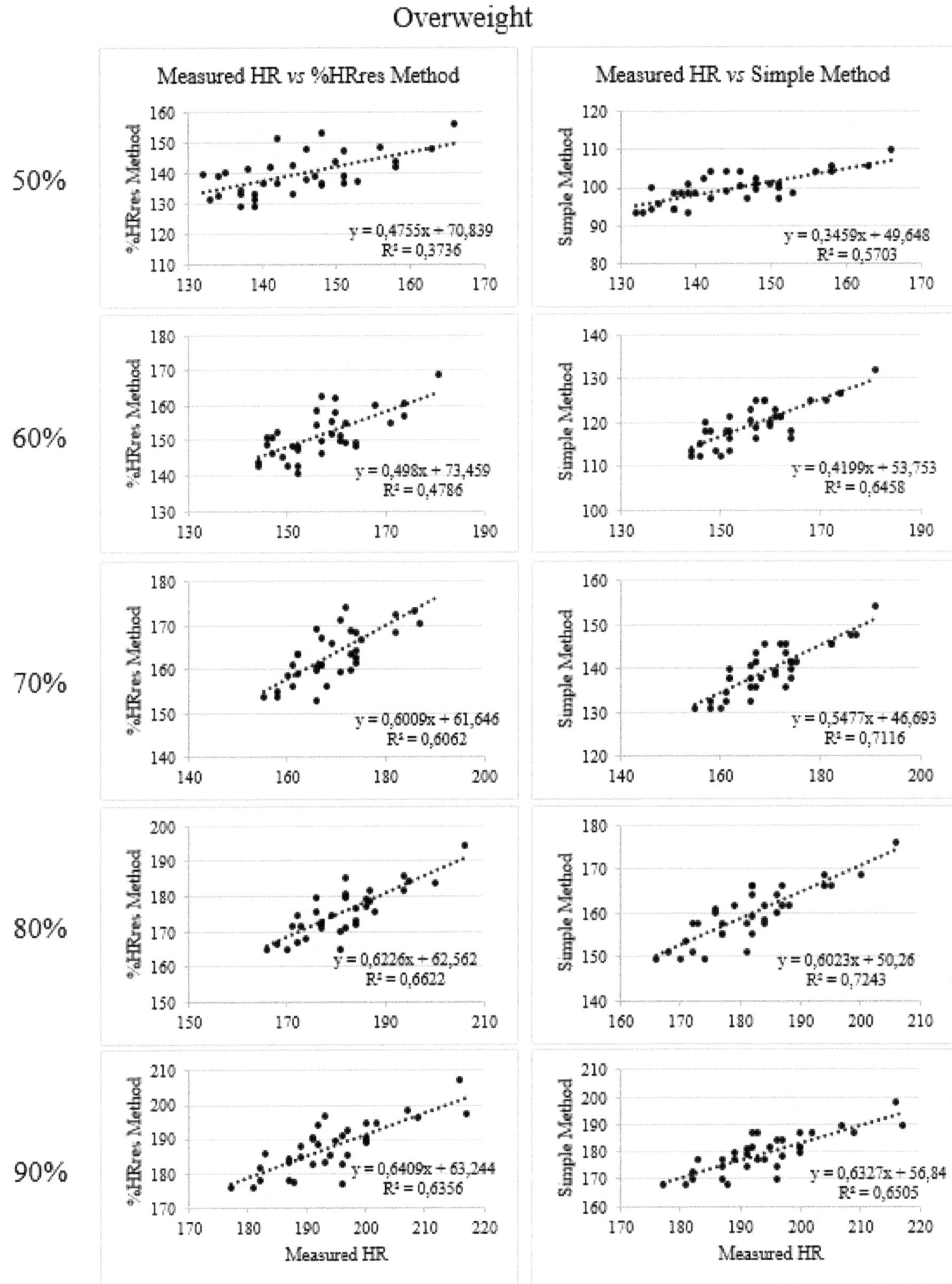

Figure 2. Correlation between measured HR *vs.* predicted %HRres method and measured HR *vs* predicted simple method (HRmax) in overweight in both sexes together.

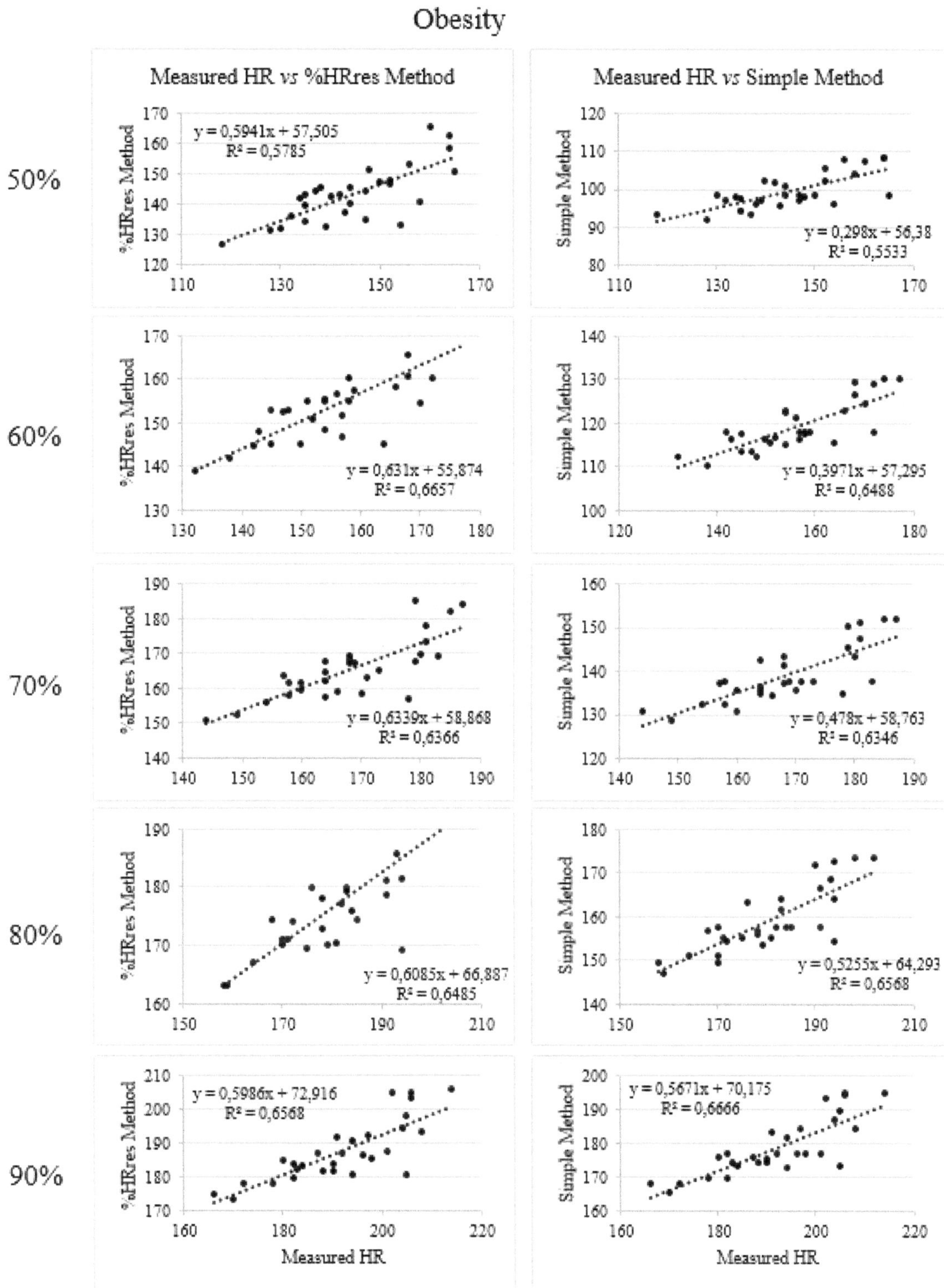

Figure 3. Correlation between measured HR *vs.* predicted %HRres method and measured HR *vs* predicted simple method (HRmax) in obesity in both genders together.

Discussion

It was observed that HRres were similar to the maximum recommended VO_2 for the maintenance and improvement of cardiorespiratory fitness for children and adolescents aged 10-14 years old. It was also observed that HRres can be used to control the intensity of exercise sessions in physical education classes for normal weight, overweight, and obese adolescents. This is considered a relatively inexpensive and easy way to allow teachers to know the higher %HRres necessary for obese adolescents.

For adults, the cardiorespiratory exercise recommendation is already defined (Cunha *et al.*, 2010; Garber *et al.*, 2011). To our knowledge there is no data for adolescents. Even though the values presented in this study are not in accordance with previous studies (Ekelund *et al.*, 2001; Hui & Chan, 2006), a similar linear relationship between the HR and VO_2 during CPET was observed, approving the use of HR as a valid parameter to estimate intensity in adolescents' physical activity. The differences between the studies can be explained by the characteristics of the sample (e.g. age average, weight, height) and the values of HRresting. For example, for the present study the HR used for the HRres calculation was the lowest registered by the ECG, after a 5-minute of resting, and not a baseline heart rate (registered when waking up).

According to Epstein *et al.* (2001), HRresting changes with age and FCmax is close to 200 beats/min during adolescence, showing consistency with the results found for HRmax in the three BMI categories. Despite not being an objective of this study (comparing these variables between ages of 10 to 14 years), it is worth emphasizing that HRres takes into consideration changes in HRresting and HRmax. This reinforces the importance of performing the CPET to identify the maximum measured HR in effort. Epstein *et al.* (2001) stated that the ACSM recommendations for adolescents may differ from the adult population with respect to intensity, duration/amount. This supports the need to understand the most suitable level of exercise intensity for adolescents. It is important to mention that the studies previously referred to are based on normal weight adolescents, since studies with overweight adolescents are scarce (Ekelund *et al.*, 2001; Hui & Chan, 2006).

In obese adults, the study performed by Pinet, Prud'homme, Gallant and Boulay (2008) suggests the use of HRres when it is not possible to assess oxygen consumption. This information is important because CPET method is not easily accessible to all populations, and has high costs of implementation, leaving HR as a valid and relatively simple variable which can be easily measured at a low cost. Thus, our findings suggest applying different recommendations of exercise for adolescents with distinct BMI categories, using the HRmax scale in CPET.

Even though we have identified correlation of medium intensity and good coefficient of correlation between HR predictive methods (HRres and HRmax), the values found in the %HRmax underestimate the amounts measured. Consequently, whether these results are to be used for exercise prescription, we would be underestimating the intensity of the effort, which is not in accordance with the ACSM recommendations (ACSM, 2013). However, these results differ when equations are used to predict HRmax (Cunha *et al.*, 2010) as previously demonstrated by Caputo, Cozzensa da Silva and Rombaldi (2012), in which the authors recommend avoiding the equations because they restrict the HRmax. So far, there is no appropriate formula for this estimation. Therefore, by choosing to use equations to calculate HRmax, and %HRmax, there is a risk of erroneous conclusions regarding the level of intensity to apply when prescribing exercise.

Using the data collected in this study, it is possible to identify more precisely, and at a low cost, benefits for adolescents, considering the relationship between the HRres and the length of the aerobic activity ($\geq$ 30 minutes per session, above 50%HRres) suggested in exercise programs (Epstein *et al.*, 2001), and the importance of using percentages (Ekelund *et al.*, 2001). In addition, the sample size and the techniques used in this study ensure the importance of the measure of the HRres.

In summary, it was observed that the relationship between the HR and VO_2 in CPET for adolescents aged 10-14 years is linear, for both sexes, allowing the level of intensity to be determined by the HRres proportion related with the correspondent $\%VO_2max$ levels of intensity according to BMI-for-age categories. HRres might be the most suitable parameter to prescribe exercises for adolescents, particularly overweight ones, because it is closer to the VO_2max intensity analysed, determining the appropriate aerobic stimuli to allow better performance of the cardiovascular system within this specific population.

Some limitations warrant mention when interpreting the findings from this study. Biological maturation was not assessed; the process of growth and development might influence the findings. The combination of sample size in general and the overweight and obese adolescents in particular may limit generalization of the results. Keeping all adolescents engaged and motivated during the tests, despite the instructors' efforts, was also one of the constraints identified during this study.

References

ACSM. (2013). *ACSM's guidelines for exercise testing and prescription.* Baltimore: Lippincott Williams & Wilkins.

Caputo, E., Cozzensa da Silva, M., & Rombaldi, A. (2012). Comparação da frequência cardíaca máxima obtida por diferentes métodos. *Revista de Educação Física/UEM, 23*(2), 277-284.

Cobayashi, F., Oliveira., F., Escrivão, M., Silveira, D., & Taddei, J. (2010). Obesidade e fatores de risco cardiovascular em adolescentes de escolas públicas. *Arquivos Brasileiros de Cardiologia, 95*(2), 200-206.

Cunha, F.A., Midgley, A.W., Monteiro, W.D., & Farinatti, P.T. (2010). Influence of cardiopulmonary exercise testing protocol and resting VO(2) assessment on %HR(max), %HRR, %VO(2max) and %VO(2)R relationships. *International Journal of Sports Medicine, 31*(5), 319-326.

Ekelund, U., Poortvliet, E., Yngve, A., Hurtig-Wennlov, A., Nilsson, A., & Sjostrom, M. (2001). Heart rate as an indicator of the intensity of physical activity in human adolescents. *European Journal of Applied Physiology, 85*(3-4), 244-249.

Epstein, L.H., Paluch, R.A., Kalakanis, L.E., Goldfield, G.S., Cerny, F.J., & Roemmich, J.N. (2001). How much activity do youth get? A quantitative review of heart-rate measured activity. *Pediatrics, 108*(3).

Foley, S., Quinn, S., Dwyer, T., Venn, A., & Jones, G. (2008). Measures of childhood fitness and body mass index are associated with bone mass in adulthood: a 20-year prospective study. *Journal of Bone and Mineral Research, 23*(7), 994-1001.

Garber, C.E., Blissmer, B., Deschenes, M.R., Franklin, B.A., Lamonte, M.J., Lee, I.M., Nieman, D.C., Swain, D.P. (2011). American College of Sports Medicine position stand. Quantity and quality of exercise for developing and maintaining cardiorespiratory, musculoskeletal, and neuromotor fitness in apparently healthy adults: guidance for prescribing exercise. *Medicine and Science in Sports and Exercise, 43*(7), 1334-1359.

Garcia-Hermoso, A., Saavedra, J.M., Escalante, Y., Sanchez-Lopez, M., & Martinez-Vizcaino, V. (2014). Endocrinology and Adolescence: aerobic exercise reduces insulin resistance markers in obese youth: a meta-analysis of randomized controlled trials. *European Journal of Endocrinology / European Federation of Endocrine Societies, 171*(4), R163-171.

Harriss, D.J., & Atkinson, G. (2013). Ethical standards in sport and exercise science research: 2014 update. *International Journal of Sports Medicine, 34*(12), 1025-1028.

Hui, S.S.C., & Chan, J.W.S. (2006). The relationship between heart rate reserve and oxygen uptake reserve in children and adolescents. *Research Quarterly for Exercise and Sport, 77*(1), 41-49.

Janssen, I., & Leblanc, A.G. (2010). Systematic review of the health benefits of physical activity and fitness in school-aged children and youth. *Int J Behav Nutr Phys Act, 7*, 40.

Karila, C., de Blic, J., Waernessyckle, S., Benoist, M.R., & Scheinmann, P. (2001). Cardiopulmonary exercise testing in children: an individualized protocol for workload increase. *Chest, 120*(1), 81-87.

Onis, M., Blossner, M., & Borghi, E. (2010). Global prevalence and trends of overweight and obesity among preschool children. *American Journal of Clinical Nutrition, 92*(5), 1257-1264.

Ortega, F.B., Ruiz, J.R., Castillo, M.J., & Sjostrom, M. (2008). Physical fitness in childhood and adolescence: a powerful marker of health. *International Journal of Obesity, 32*(1), 1-11.

Pinet, B.M., Prud'homme, D., Gallant, C.A., & Boulay, P. (2008). Exercise intensity prescription in obese individuals. *Obesity, 16*(9), 2088-2095.

Prado, W.L., Balagopal, P.B., Lofrano-Prado, M.C., Oyama, L.M., Tenorio, T.R., Botero, J.P., Hill, J.O. (2014). Effect of aerobic exercise on hunger feelings and satiety regulating hormones in obese teenage girls. *Pediatric Exercise Science, 26*(4), 463-469.

Rodrigues, A.N., Bissoli, N.S., Pires, J.G.P., & Abreu, G.R. (2004). A populational study on cariorespiratory and metabolic parameters in schoolchildren of Vitoria, Brazil: Preliminary results. *Journal of Hypertension, 22*, S51-S51.

Rodrigues, A.N., Perez, A.J., Carletti, L., Bissoli, N.S., & Abreu, G.R. (2006). Maximum oxygen uptake in adolescents as measured by cardiopulmonary exercise testing: a classification proposal. *Jornal de Pediatria, 82*(6), 426-430.

Rodrigues, A.N., Perez, A.J., Carletti, L., Bissolli, N.S., & Abreu, G.R. (2007). The association between cardiorespiratory fitness and cardiovascular risk in adolescents. *Jornal de Pediatria, 83*(5), 429-435.

Simmons, R.K., Griffin, S.J., Steele, R., Wareham, N.J., & Ekelund, U. (2008). Increasing overall physical activity and aerobic fitness is associated with improvements in metabolic risk: cohort analysis of the ProActive trial. *Diab tologia, 51*(5), 787-794.

Strong, W.B., Malina, R.M., Blimkie, C.J., Daniels, S.R., Dishman, R.K., Gutin, B. Hergenroeder, A.C., Must, A., Nixon, P.A., Pivarnik, J.M., Rowland, T., Trost, S., Trudeau, F. (2005). Evidence based physical activity for school-age youth. *Journal of Pediatrics, 146*(6), 732-737.

Swain, D.P., & Franklin, B.A. (2002). VO(2) reserve and the minimal intensity for improving cardiorespiratory fitness. *Medicine and Science in Sports and Exercise, 34*(1), 152-157.

Swain, D.P., & Leutholtz, B.C. (1997). Heart rate reserve is equivalent to %VO2 reserve, not to %VO2max. *Medicine and Science in Sports and Exercise, 29*(3), 410-414.

Swain, D.P., Leutholtz, B.C., King, M.E., Haas, L.A., & Branch, J.D. (1998). Relationship between % heart rate reserve and % VO2 reserve in treadmill exercise. *Medicine and Science in Sports and Exercise, 30*(2), 318-321.

World Health Organization, WHO. (2010). *Global recommendations on physical activity for health*. WHO Press: Geneva, Switzerland.

Autor's note

Kamilla Bolonha Gomes, Anselmo José Perez, Luciana Carletti are affiliated with the Federal University of Espírito Santo, Exercise Physiology Laboratory.

Adilson Marques is affiliated with the University of Lisboa, Interdisciplinary Centre for Human Performance Study.

Corresponding author

Kamilla Bolonha Gomes
Rua Vicente de Oliveira, 25, Vitória, ES, Brazil.
Email: kamilla.bolonha@outlook.com

4

Aging male symptoms: the relationship between physical activity and quality of life

Melissa de Carvalho Souza
Adriana Coutinho de Azevedo Guimarães
Universidade do Estado de Santa Catarina, UDESC, Florianópolis, SC, Brasil

Abstract—Objective To examine the relationship between physical activity (PA) and the aging male symptoms of middle-aged men in the quality of life (QOL). Methodology: Cross-sectional study with a probabilistic samples of 416 men (40-59 years old), all residents in two cities in southern of Brazil. A questionnaire was used. The studied population was divided into two groups: with and without symptoms. The analyses were carried out in a descriptive and inferential approaches. Results: Aging male symptoms were related to QOL. Men who perceive their overall QOL as good presented a13% lower probability of (95%CI = 0.77-0.98) being insufficiently active. For those with symptoms, QOL scores were higher in social and environmental domain in PA between 30-60 min/day, and the physical domain for more than 60min/day. Conclusion: Our findings show the importance of PA to achieve significant benefits in QOL and health of men in middle age with aging male symptoms.

Keywords: motor activity, quality of life, men, male ageing, health

Introduction

Middle age can be understood as a process of transition between adulthood and old age, including the age group from 40 to 59 years (Andrews, 2000). At this stage, physiological, morphological, and physical changes occur which appear distinctly in men and women (Antunes & Silva, 2013). For several years the characteristics of this stage in women (known as menopause) have been well documented, either being their effects on health as well as on the quality of life (Krajewska-Ferishah *et al.*, 2010; Waidyasekera, Wijewardema, Lindmark & Naessen, 2009). However, only in the years 2000 literature has been directing their studies more profoundly towards the modifications of the male population (Rohden, 2012). Such processes in men begin from about 40 years of age, along with symptoms, which are classified into; psychological symptoms including anxiety, depression, depressed mood, irritability and nervousness, sexual dysfunction with decreased ability/frequency of sexual activity, reduction in the number of morning erections, and decreased libido, and somatic symptoms with declining sense of well-being, decreased muscle strength, muscle and joint pain, insomnia and physical exhaustion. These symptoms may appear in mild, moderate or severe intensity (Heinemann, 2005).

According to some authors the prevalence of these symptoms affects the quality of life of men, even at lower intensities, considering the physical, psychological, social, and environmental domains (Salazar, Paravic & Barriga, 2012; Staerman & Léon, 2012). Regarding the aging process, quality of life is determined by the ability to maintain autonomy, decision-making, independence and ability to perform daily tasks (Freitas, Queiroz & Sousa, 2010), its decline may contribute to the risk of chronic degenerative diseases in different populations, mostly in men over the age of 40 years (Martits & Costa, 2004). Thus, it is important to maintain adequate levels of quality of life in this population (Perchon, Pintarelli, Bezerra, Thiel & Dambros, 2011).

Thus, clinical measures, such as hormone replacement, have been addressed to improve the quality of life of men experiencing aging symptoms, as well as for the lower prevalence of this symptomatology (Rohden, 2012). Other studies highlight the importance of the practice of physical activity as another measure to ease the symptoms, given its relevance to the physical, psychological and sexual aspects (Corrêa, Rombaldi & Silva, 2011; Corrêa, Silva & Rombaldi, 2014).

Recently, the practice of at least 150 minutes/week, according to the recommendations of the World Health Organization [WHO] (2011), was associated with a lower prevalence of symptoms, and the intensity in which they occur (Corrêa *et al.*, 2014). However, the influence of physical activity is still unknown, considering intensity and duration on quality of life in their domains, specifically, in men who are in the process of the aging symptoms. In addition, these symptoms have already reached a prevalence of over 40% in Brazilian middle-aged men up to the sixth decade of life (Abdo & Afif-Abdo, 2007). Unfortunately, only approximately 30% of men receive clinical diagnosis (Sociedade Brasileira de Urologia, SBU, 2012). Thus, it is important to investigate the influence of physical activity in these symptoms as well the health and quality of life of men, in order to contribute to the health promotion of this particular population. Thus, the present study aimed to verify the relationship between physical activity and quality of life according to the aging symptoms in middle-aged men.

Methodology

Study characterization

The exploratory analytical observational study with a cross-sectional delineation, consisted of middle aged men, within the age group of 40 to 59 years (Andrews, 2000), all residents in the greater Florianópolis region, located in the South of Brazil. The Ethics Committee on Human Research (CEPSH) of the Santa Catarina State University approved the study, Protocol number 535,729.

Population and sample

The cities were selected from the Greater Florianópolis area with more than 200 thousand inhabitants who presented similar economic characteristics, according to the last census by the *Brazilian Institute of Geography and Statistics* [IBGE] (2010). Corresponding to the cities of Florianopolis and São José, with a male population of 51,740 and 20,939, respectively, within the age group 40 to 59 years; thus, the study population was comprised of 72.679 men.

The population was stratified in conglomerates of socio-economic status according to the IBGE (2010), having as base the minimum wage (MW) of R$724, 00 valid in 2014. The individuals were classified as class A (above 20 MW); class B (10 to 20 MW); class C (4 to 10 MW); class D (2 to 4 MW) and class E (up to 2 MW).

In order to define the sample size, 20% was adopted on prevalence of male aging symptoms for men with age equal to or superior to 40 years (Heinemann, Zimmermann, Vermeulen, Thiel & Hummel, 1999), a four percentage point tolerable error, a 95% confidence level, and a 1.5 design effect (Luiz & Magnanini, 2000). Possible losses and refusals were increased to 10%, considering 631 men in the final sample. In accordance with the calculation in proportion to each socioeconomic class, the outcome showed 31 men belonging to class A, 193 to class B, 205 to class C, and 202 to class D following IBGE, neighborhoods considered to be class E were not characterized by the census for being sectors with low household density.

Research subjects presenting some clinically diagnosed sickness, such as cancer, cardiovascular diseases, diabetes, hypertension, and paraplegias, as well as institutionalized subjects (nursing homes, prisons, hospitals, and barracks), and those who presented inability to understand the questionnaire (mental illnesses).

In total 1,150 households were contacted, and in 338 households did not have men aged 40 to 59. During the data collection process, there were occasions of 396 refusals. Thus, the final sample by conglomerate random was of 416 men within the age of 49±6 years, 24 from class A, 89 from class B, 234 from class C, and 69 from Class D.

While the sample obtained was not sufficient to meet the accuracy specifications previously established in this study, this represented more than a half (66%) of 631 subjects provided in the final sample. The 416 men in the study would be sufficient considering a five percentage point tolerable error. Furthermore, a randomization process was observed in the sample selection.

Research Tools

For data collection in this study, a questionnaire was used divided into seven parts.

Sample Characteristics

Information related to age, marital status, schooling, occupation, presence of clinically diagnosed disease, use of medicines for both disease and sexual performance, and tobacco consumption.

Anthropometric Measurements

Body weight and stature (self referred) for body mass index - BMI (weight/stature^2). For the BMI classification (weight status), the World Health Organization [WHO] (2004) protocol with the cut off points below:

Underweight (BMI<18.5); regular weight (BMI within 18.5-24.9); overweight (BMI within 25.0-29.9), and obesity (BMI≥30.0). Underweight and regular weight categories were set into regular weight; and overweight and obesity categories were set into overweight, due to the low frequency of subjects within the underweight and obesity categories.

Socioeconomic Status

IBGE (2010) classifications were used to categorize individuals into socioeconomic status. Such classifications into socio-economic strata A, B, C, D, and E, was carried out by means of the average monthly family income, in particular, class A (above 20 MW), class B (10 to 20 MW), class C (4 to 10 MW), class D (2 to 4 MW), and class E (up to 2 MW).

For data analysis, the strata were set in high class (A and B), middle class (C), and lower class (D and E).

Physical Activity

The International Physical Activity Questionnaire (IPAQ - Short version) was adopted for assessment of physical activity. In Brazil, that questionnaire was validated by the Center of Studies of the Physical Fitness Research Laboratory in São Caetano do Sul – CELAFISCS, which is the IPAQ coordinator center in Brazil (Pardini, *et al.*, 1997). The Brazilian validity and reproducibility had significantly high Spearman correlation (rho= 0.69-0.71: $p<0.001$) (Matsudo *et al.*, 2001). In the current physical activity evaluation through IPAQ, the number of times in which an individual carried out at least 10 minutes of continuous walking, moderate intensity physical activity, and vigorous intensity physical activity was observed in the last week, in various involvements, in particular, labor, home, leisure, sports, and recreation. Physical activity was classified into walking, moderate, moderate+vigorous, vigorous, and total physical activity in minutes/day.

Thus, the individuals were classified as: insufficiently active – those who practiced at least 10 minutes of continuous physical activities per week, however, insufficient for classification as active. The sum of the duration and frequency of the different activities (moderate vigorous walking) is performed to establish the following criteria: active - has complied with the following recommendations: a) vigorous physical activity ≥ 3 days/week and ≥ 20 minutes/session; b) moderate ≥ 5 days/week and ≥ 30 minutes /session; c) any combined activity: ≥ 5 days/week and ≥ 150 min/week; very active - has fulfilled the indications: a) vigorous ≥ 5 days/week and ≥ 30 min/session; b) vigorous ≥ 3 days/week and ≥ 20 min/session moderate ≥ 5 days/week and ≥ 30 min/session. The individuals were set into sufficiently active (active+very active) and insufficiently active.

IPAQ - short version was used, since it is suitable for monitoring the level of physical activity, producing comparable results to the long version (Craig *et al.,* 2003).

Health Perception

Health perception was evaluated following the question model contained in BRFSS - Behavioural Risk Factors Surveillance System Questionnaire [CDC] (1999). It is composed of an issue that evaluates the individual's health perception. The answers are in a "Likert scale", in which 1 represents excellent; 2 very good; 3 good; 4 regular; 5 bad. For data analysis, due to the low presence of individuals in the categories excellent, good, and regular, answers 1 to 3 were set as very good and the answers 4 and 5 as bad.

Aging Male Symptoms

Aging Male Symptoms Scale (AMS) was used in a Portuguese version (Heinemann *et al.*, 2003). The reliability values of this version were significantly higher in the Pearson correlation considering the total score (r =0.74) and the score of psychological and sexual symptoms (r = 0.67). For the score of somatic symptoms the correlation coefficient was considered lower (r = 0.45) (Daig *et al.*, 2003). The scale is composed by 17 questions divided into three symptom blocks: psychological (five issues), somatic (7 questions), and sexual symptoms (five issues). The sum of the issues, which results variation from one to five points was considered as the general symptom score (Heinemann *et al.*, 1999). The general score for somatic, psychological, and sexual symptoms were categorized, being classified as having psychological symptoms the subjects who obtain scores ≥ 12 points; with somatic symptoms, the subjects who have scores ≥ 13 points; and with sexual symptoms those subjects who have scores ≥ 8 points. The general symptom score was dichotomized so that those who submit score ≥ 27 points were classified as having aging symptoms, while those with values below that score were classified without symptoms. The general score of male aging symptoms was also categorized so that those who submit score between 27 and 36 points were considered as having "smooth/mild symptoms"; those with a score between 37 to 49 points, considered as having "moderate" symptoms; and those with a score equal to or greater than 50, as having "severe symptoms" (Heinemann *et al.*, 1999). For the purposes of analysis the participants were divided into two groups: subjects with symptoms and without symptoms.

Quality of Life

Evaluated through World Health Organization Quality of Life (WHOQOL) short questionnaire, which is adapted to Portuguese of Brazil (Fleck *et al.*, 1999). This is a questionnaire is composed of 26 issues (of the original 100). There are 24 questions concerning the physical domain (physical pain, energy, mobility, daily living activities, medical treatment, work), psychological (positive feelings, concentration, self-esteem, self-image, negative feelings, spirituality), social (personal relationships, social support, sexual activity) and environment (physical security, housing, financial, healthcare, information, leisure, physical environment and transport) and two more general questions about quality of life. The result provides scores for each domain ranging from 0 to 100 points, the closer to 100, the better the quality of life score. The issue related to the overall quality of life was categorized according to the answers: very bad; bad; neither good nor bad; good; and very good, according to studies previously published (Conceição *et al.,* 2012; Pereira, Teixeira & Lopes, 2013). In this study, due to the low response in very bad; neither bad nor good, very good categories, they are grouped into: bad and good. The instrument showed adequate internal consistency, the amount of Cronbach's coefficient for the domains was 0.77. For discriminant validity, the control subjects showed higher scores in each of the four domains (physical = 16.6 ± 2.1, 15.6 ± 2.1 = psychological, social = 15.5 ± 2.6; environmental = 14.0 ± 2.1). Regarding the criterion validity they all showed a significant correlation (p <0.001) (Fleck *et al.,* 2000).

Data Collection

A team of seven individuals of both genders, holding at least complete high school education, carried out data collection. This team received 40 hours of training for application of the instrument from the main researcher of the study. In this training each question of the instrument was explained as well how to approach the subject and apply the questionnaire. After the procedure, questionnaires were forwarded for data collection. Interviewers conducted the interviews individually.

The zip code draw was held proportionally considering the four socioeconomic strata (A, B, C, and D) of the neighborhoods of Florianópolis and São José. The zip codes of each district were registered in a spreadsheet in the Excel program version

2010. The same program is currently used mostly for the draw of the zip codes of each district of the socioeconomic strata.

Thus, the streets corresponding to the zip codes were visited and the first home of the street was selected to be included in the study. The interval between the houses was in accordance with the quantity of households found in every street in which men aged 40 to 59 years could be found. The domicile was considered excluded from the study after the third failure to contact, and was also excluded when the individual refused to participate in the study. This process was replicated in all socioeconomic strata

The study questionnaire was applied in the format of an interview. In the block of sexual symptoms of the male aging symptoms scale, the participant had the option to answer individually if feeling uncomfortable or simply continue the interview.

Statistical Analysis

Statistical analysis was carried out using the Statistical Package for Social Sciences (SPSS) version 20.0, and Bioestat version 5.3. Descriptive statistics were used by means of the mean calculation, standard deviation, and percentage. The normality of the data was checked using the Kolmogorov-Smirnov test. The associations of personal characteristics among men with and without symptoms were carried out through the Chi-square test. The comparison of quality of life domains (physical, psychological, social, and environmental) among men with and without symptoms has been carried out through the Mann-Whitney U test. The comparison of the domains of quality of life and the characteristics of the sample was done by means of the Mann-Whitney U, and Kruskal-Wallis tests. The comparison between the three groups of physical activity (Group A <30 min/day; Group B 30-60 min/day; Group C >60 min/day) with the averages of the domains of quality of life was performed by Kruskall-Wallis test followed by the post hoc Student-Newman-Keuls. Multinomial Logistic Regression Analysis was performed to estimate raw and adjusted odds ratios between the levels of PA (dependent variables) and aging male symptoms and overall quality of life outcomes (independent variables). A simple and multiple models have been tested (adjusted for all variables). In the whole analysis, the significance adopted was the level of 5%.

Results

Table 1 presents the characteristics of participants among men with and without aging male symptoms. The significant variable differences were presented in the use of medicines for diagnosed diseases, health perception and physical activity level ($p = 0.032$; p; $p = 0.001$ 0.026 <), respectively. Men without symptoms presented lower use of drugs for diseases (92.5%), better health perception (92.5%) and sufficient levels of physical activity (66.9%).

Table 1. Characteristics of the sample according to the men symptomatology (%). Florianópolis and São José 2014. (n = 416)

	With Symptoms	IC95%	Without Symptoms	IC95%	p Value
Age					0.395
40-49 years	59.3	39-51	40.7	42-57	
50-59 years	63.3	49-61	36.7	43-58	
Schooling					0.265
Elementary School	14.8	10-19	9.4	05-14	
Secondary School	30.9	25-37	32.5	25-40	
Higher Education	33.4	48-60	22.4	50-66	
Socioeconomic Status					0.287
High	36.5	31-42	39.4	32-47	
Medium	33.3	28-39	37.5	30-45	
Low	30.2	25-36	23.1	17-30	
Profession					
Self-employed	58.8	52-65	61.6	54-69	0.646
Retired	4.6	02-07	2.6	0-05	
Civil Servant	36.2	30-42	35.8	28-43	
Marital Status					
Living together	80.7	76-86	83.8	78-90	0.434
Living apart	19.3	14-24	16.2	10-22	
Sickness Presence					
Yes	20.7	16-26	14.4	09-20	0.104
No	79.3	74-84	85.6	80-91	
Sickness Medicine					0.032
Yes	14.5	10-19	7.5	03-12	
No	85.5	81-90	92.5	88-97	
Sexual Medicine					0.258
Yes	2.3	0-04	0.6*	-01-02	
No	97.7	96-100	99.4	98-100	

continued...

Table 1. Continued.

	With Symptoms	IC95%	Without Symptoms	IC95%	p Value
Weight Status					0.636
Regular weight	27.8	22-33	30.0	23-37	
Overweight	72.2	67-78	70.0	63-77	
Health Perception					<0.001
Very good	77.0	72-82	92.5	88-97	
Bad	23.0	18-28	7.5	03-12	
Tobacco Smoking					
Yes	12.5	08-17	16.2	10-22	0.283
No	87.5	83-92	83.8	78-90	
PA Level#					0.026
Insufficiently active	44.1	38-50	33.1	26-40	
Sufficiently active	55.9	50-62	66.9	60-74	

Teste do Qui-squared. $\bar{x}$(sd): mean (standard deviation).
*Fisher Exact. #Physical Activity.

Even though significant difference could not be observed in other variables, the subjects without aging male symptoms, were mostly 40-49 years old (40.7%), high school graduates (32.5%), belonging to a high socioeconomic class (39.4%), self-employed (61.6%), living with a companion (83.8%) not presenting disease (85.6%), not using medicine for sexual performance (99.4%), within regular weight (30%), and non-smokers (83.8%).

The results of the comparison of the mean of the quality of life score between men with and without aging male symptoms are presented in Table 2. Significant results were observed in all the variables ($p < 0.001$), demonstrating that men without symptoms showed higher average scores in all areas of quality of life (63±8; 69±8; 77±12; 71±11).

In a comparison between the mean of the quality of life domains and the sample characteristics, the age group showed significant difference with only the physical domain, and individuals from 50 to 59 showed higher mean scores (61±8; p=0.004). The men with higher education and belonging to the high socioeconomic classes, require higher means in the psychological and environmental domain (67±9; p=0.010 e 69±12; p<0.001), concurrently. As for the PA level, sufficiently active men presented higher mean scores in the physical and psychological domains (61±8; p=0.003 e 67±9; p=0.048) (date not presented in the table).

Table 2. Comparison of quality of life between men with and without aging symptoms (mean and standard deviation). Florianópolis and São José 2014. (n=416)

	Median	Interquartile range	Total	With Symptoms $\bar{x}$(sd)	Without Symptoms $\bar{x}$(sd)	p Value
Physical Domain	61	14.29	60(9)	58(9)	63(8)	<0.001
Psychological Domain	67	8.33	65(9)	63(10)	69(8)	<0.001
Social Domain	75	8.33	71(15)	67(16)	77(12)	<0.001
Environmental Domain	68	17.86	66(13)	63(13)	71(11)	<0.001

Descriptive statistic. U deMann-Whitney Test

A comparison of the mean scores of quality of life domains with the intensities of physical activity in men with male aging symptoms is represented in Table 3. Quality of life scores were observed higher in social (72±14) and environmental (66±11) areas in the practice of physical activity at moderate intensity for the men of group B, in comparison to the other groups. In the moderate+vigorous physical activity, the mean scores of the physical domain were higher for group C (59±8), and the environmental field for the men of group B (66±12). Whereas at total physical activity practice, the scores on the physical domain of quality of life were higher for the group C (59±7), and the social and environmental fields for the men of group B (70±13; 66±12).

Table 4 presented the associations of physical activity level with aging male symptoms and overall quality of life. In the simple model the physical activity level was associated with both variables. When the model had been adjusted, only the overall quality of life remained associated. Men who perceive their overall quality of life as good presented a 13% lower probability (95%CI = 0.77-0.98), of being insufficiently active.

Table 3. Comparison of the averages of scores of quality of life domains with the intensity of physical activity of men with aging symptoms (mean and standard deviation). Florianópolis and São José, SC. 2014. (n=256)

	PA MODERATE				PA MODERATE+VIGOROUS				PA TOTAL			
	Group A	Group B	Group C	p value	Group A	Group B	Group C	p Value	Group A	Group B	Group C	p Value
Physical Domain $\bar{x}$(sd)	57(9)	59(8)	58(8)	0.476	56(10)[c]	57(9)[c]	59(8)[a.b]	0.018	55(10)[c]	56(8)[c]	59(7)[a.b]	0.014
Psychological Domain $\bar{x}$(sd)	62(10)	66(7)	64(9)	0.105	62(11)	63(8)	65(9)	0.138	62(11)	61(10)	65(9)	0.074
Social Domain $\bar{x}$(sd)	66(16)[b]	72(14)[c.a]	65(15)[b]	0.013	65(17)	71(14)	69(15)	0.079	63(17)[b]	70(13)[a]	69(15)	0.034
Environmental Domain $\bar{x}$(sd)	62(13)[b]	66(11)[a]	65(14)	0.031	61(13)[b]	66(12)[a]	65(12)	0.018	59(13)[b]	66(12)[a.c]	63(13)[b]	0.002

PA. Physical Activity. Group A= <30min./day; Group B= 30-60min./day; Group C= >60min./day.
Teste Kruskall-Wallis. Post hoc Student-Newman-Keuls.

Table 4. Raw and adjusted odds ratio in insufficiently active subjects in relation to the active subjects according aging male symptoms and quality of life. Florianópolis and São José - SC. 2014. (n=416).

Variables	PA level Raw OR (CI95%)	* p	PA level Adjusted OR (CI95%)	**p
Aging male symptoms		**0.023**		**0.081**
With symptoms	1.11(1.01-1.22)		1.08(0.99-1.19)	
Without symptoms	Reference		Reference	
Overall quality of life		**0.007**		**0.021**
Good	0.85 (0.76-0.95)		0.87 (0.77-0.98)	
Bad	Reference		Reference	

Poisson Regression. * The reference is the insufficiently active.

Discussion

This study aimed to verify the relation of physical activity with quality of life according to the aging male symptoms in middle-aged men. Physical activity was related to the scores of quality of life of the men, considering that those sufficiently active had higher mean scores compared to insufficiently active, mainly in the physical and psychological fields.

It is observed male population low levels of physical activity are related to a three time greater chance in the impairment of the physical domain and a two time greater chance in the psychological domain (Dey, Gmel & Mohler-Kuo, 2014). In this way, the fact that most men in this study reach the minimum recommendation of physical activity for health benefits (WHO, 2011) can generate higher mean scores of quality of life.

In the adjusted analysis performed in this study, it was identified that men who perceived their overall quality of life as good, were significantly less likely to be insufficiently active compared to those perceived as bad. Thus, the adhesion to an active lifestyle has been observed to have the influence of a good overall quality of life, regardless of the presence of aging male symptoms.

In addition to the relation with physical activity level, this study also showed relations between quantity and intensity of physical activity with the quality of life of men with aging symptoms. For those men, the practice of physical activity at moderate, moderate+vigorous, and total intensity, superior to 30 min/day may be related to more favourable characteristics in the social and environmental domains. In the physical domain, these relations seem to be found among those that practiced >60 min/day of moderate+vigorous, and total physical activity.

It is necessary to highlight that the physical domain of quality of life encompasses aspects related to physical pain, energy, locomotion, daily life activities, medical treatment, and work (Fleck *et al.*, 1999). According to the study, these aspects may present a certain decline over the years, reflecting in a lower quality of life in this area (Campolina, Dini & Ciconelli, 2011). This fact justifies the important contribution of physical activity in this period, observed in this study between the men who practiced physical activity with a greater duration (>60 min/day). These men presented higher scores on the physical domain of quality of life when compared to those that practiced lower amounts of physical activity (30-60 min/day; <30 min/day).

International studies of intervention have shown the positive influence of the physical activity practice at moderate+vigorous intensity of at least 120 min/week at the physical level of men in distinct health conditions. Benefits for aspects related to the physical domain of quality of life were identified, such as the reduction of pain, fatigue, and improvement of cardiorespiratory fitness (Galvão *et al.*, 2014; Giubilei *et al.*, 2007).

However, studies on aging male symptoms are not found in the national and international literature evaluating the influence of physical activity on the quality of life of the men. Thus, comparable results are identified in women who face menopause, equivalent process to the male aging symptoms (Guimarães & Baptista, 2011a; Fox, Stathi, McKenna & Davis, 2007).

As regards the results obtained for the social field of quality of life of men with symptoms, studies portray the positive influence of physical activity whereas intensities and specific quantities (Matsudo, 2009; Santana & Maia, 2009). For women in the menopause period, an analysis carried out in the South of Brazil suggests the practice of at least 60 min/day of total physical activity for which a significant improvement can be observed in the social field of quality of life (Guimarães & Baptista, 2011b). Exceeding quantity practiced by men of this study with higher scores in this area (30-60 minutes/day).

The present study, shall see the possibility of influence of male sexual aspect into the social domain of quality of life, since that aspect is one of the factors composing the social domain, including personal relations and social support (Fleck *et al.*, 1999), and it is present in the general of male aging symptoms (Heinemann, 2005). In this way, in male populations above 40 years of age, cross-sectional studies, cohort and quasi-experimental have already considered the importance of physical activity performed at moderate+vigorous intensity for improvement of male sexual aspect, which reflects in higher scores on their quality of life (Kratizik *et al.*, 2009; Revnic, Nica & Revnic, 2007).

Concerning the quality of life in the environmental domain, similar results were found to those in the social domain, and individuals who practiced 30-60 min/day of physical activity presented higher scores. It is important to mention that the environmental field is composed of dimensions related to physical security, housing, financial resources, health services, information, leisure, physical environment, and transport (Fleck *et al.*, 1999). Thus, the results concerning the relationship between duration of physical activity and the environmental domain may have an outcome due to some characteristics of the sample. Characteristics which according to some studies influence in the perception of quality of life, and are related to greater physical activity practice, such as higher levels of schooling and socioeconomic class (Beenackers *et al.*, 2012; Finger, Tylleskär, Thomas & Mensink, 2012).

The literature reports that in some populations was necessary to consider other factors besides physical activity which could influence the quality of life and its different areas (Giannouli *et al.*, 2012; Nakamura *et al.*, 2014). This study found that mainly the of male aging symptoms, schooling, and income can contribute into relations between physical activity and quality of life in the male physical, social, and environmental domains.

It is important to highlight that, although some authors demonstrate the effectiveness of physical activity for the physical, psychological, and social aspects related to quality of life (Cloix *et al.*, 2014; Joseph, Royse, Benitez & Pekmezi, 2014), there is still a gap in studies investigating the intensity and amount of physical activity for the improvement of the quality of life domains. Especially in the population of middle age men that present male aging symptoms. The already existent evidence in this area is limited to verify the benefits of physical activity for the lower prevalence of symptoms, or the impact on the male quality of life, without however associating the three variables (Corrêa *et al.*, 2014; Salazar *et al.*, 2012). Thus, this study seems to be the first to check in an indirect way the existence of significant relationships between intensity and amount of physical activity, directed to quality of life in the male aging symptoms in middle age.

The results of the present study need to be interpreted with caution, because the sample could not be representative of male population of middle age of the cities of Florianopolis and São José, the final sample did not reach the required minimum according to the calculated sample size. Since the collection was performed in their homes, there was some difficult to contact them, considering that such age group is active in the labour market (40 to 59). When the contact was made after business hours, they often refused to participate in the study by complaint of tiredness after a working day, besides the lack of interest. Other limitations should also be assessed, such as the cross-sectional design that makes it impossible the findings of cause and effect (Lopes, Toledo, Câmara, Menzel & Santos, 2014).

Concerning the advantages of the study, it is noteworthy the use of a probabilistic sample design, allowing the men of the study to be selected randomly. Still, the use of standardized questionnaires as the scale of the aging male symptoms, being the most used instrument in national and international studies related to the symptoms (Corrêa *et al.*, 2014; Hirokawa, Taniguchi, Fuji, Takaki & Tsutsumi, 2012), as well as the IPAQ, the most used instrument for evaluation of physical activity in Brazil (Hallal, Dumith, Bastos, Reichert, Siqueira & Azevedo, 2007), and the WHOQOL, considered one of the main instruments for assessing quality of life (Pucci, Rech, Fermino & Reis, 2012).

Then, the fact of investigating a theme not portrayed in the literature may enable a greater knowledge of the male health related to quality of life of men who are in the process of aging male symptoms within middle age. As well as encourage the practice of physical activity as a measure aimed at improvements in aspects related to the quality of life of this population in the physical, psychological, social, and environmental domains.

Conclusion

It is possible to identify the relevance of the practice of physical activity with specific intensity and amount as a means to obtain significant benefits to the physical, social, and environmental domain of male quality of life in middle age presenting the male aging symptoms. Nevertheless, other studies related physical activity to the quality of life in the process of this symptomatology, with randomized longitudinal and/or experimental being necessary, in order to check other important contributions of physical activity for the health and quality of life of men in middle age.

References

Abdo, C.H.N. & Afif-Abdo, J. (2007). Estudo populacional do envelhecimento (EPE): primeiros resultados masculinos. *Revista Brasileira de Medicina, 74*(8), 379-83.

Andrews, M. (2000). The seductiveness of agelessness. *Ageing and Society, 19*(3), 301-18.

Antunes, P.C. & Silva, A.M. (2013). Elementos sobre a concepção de meia idade, no processo de envelhecimento humano. *Revista Kairós Gerontologia, 19*(5), 123-40.

Beenackers, M.A., Kamphuis, C.B.M., Giskes, K., Brug, J., Kunst, A.E., Burdof, A., & Lenthe, F.J.V. (2012). Socioeconomic inequalities in occupational, leisure-time, and transport related physical activity among European adults: A systematic review. *International Journal of Behavioral Nutrition and Physical Activity*, 9. doi: 10.1186/1479-5868-9-116.

Campolina, A.G., Dini, P.S., & Ciconelli, R.M. (2011). Impacto da doença crônica na qualidade de vida de idosos da comunidade em São Paulo (SP, Brasil). *Ciência e Saúde Coletiva*, 16(6), 2919-25. http://dx.doi.org/10.1590/S1413-81232011000600029.

Center for Disease Control and Prevention (1999). Behavioral risk factor suveillance system questionnaire. Altanta: CDC.

Cloix, L., Caille, A., Helmer, C., Bourdel-Marchasson, I., Fagot-Campagna, A., Fournier, C., Lecomte, P., Oppert, J.M., & Jacobi, D. (2014). Physical activity at home, at leisure, during transportation and at work in French adults with type 2 diabetes: The ENTRED physical activity study. *Diabetes and Metabolism, 41*(1), 37-44. doi: 10.1016/j.diabet.2014.07.003.

Conceição, M.R., Costa, M.S., Almeida, M.I., Souza, A.M.A., Cavalcante, M.B.P.T., & Alves, M.D.S. (2012). Qualidade de vida do enfermeiro no trabalho docente: estudo com o whoqol-bref. *Escola Anna Nery Revista de Enfermagem, 16*(2), 320-25.

Corrêa, L.Q., Rombaldi, A.J., & Silva, M.C. (2011). Atividade física e sintomas do envelhecimento masculino em uma população do sul do Brasil. *Revista Brasileira de Medicina do Esporte*, 17(4), 228-31. http://dx.doi.org/10.1590/S1517-86922011000400002.

Corrêa, L.Q., Silva, M.C., & Rombaldi, A.J. (2014). Associação entre nível de atividade física nos diferentes domínios e sintomas do envelhecimento masculino. *Revista Brasileira de Atividade Física e Saúde, 19*(2), 186-94. http://dx.doi.org/10.12820/rbafs.v.19n2p186.

Craig, C.L. (2003). International physical activity questionnaires: 12-country reliability and validity. *Medicine and Science in Sports and Exercise, 35*(8), 1381-95.

Daig, I., Heinemann, L.A.J., Kim, S., Leugwattanakjj, S., Badia, X., Myon, E., Moore, C., Saad, F., Potthoff, P., & Thai, D.M. (2003). The Aging Males' Symptoms (AMS) scale: review of its methodological characteristics. *Health and Quality of Life Outcomes*, 1, 77. doi:10.1186/1477-7525-1-77.

Dey, M., Gmel, G., & Mohler-Kuo, M. (2014). Health-risk behaviors and quality of life among young men. *Quality of Life Research, 23*(3), 1009-17. doi: 10.1007/s11136-013-0524-4.

Finger, J.D., Tylleskär, T., Lampert, T., & Mensink, G.B.M. (2012). Physical activity patterns and socioeconomic position: the German National Health Interview and Examination Survey 1998 (GNHIES98). *BMC Public Health*, 12, 1079-90. doi: 10.1186/1471-2458-12-1079.

Fleck, M.P.A., Leal, O.F., Louzada, S., Xavier, M., Chachamovich, E., Vieira, G., Santos, L., & Pinzon, V. (1999). Desenvolvimento da versão em português do instrumento de avaliação de qualidade de vida da OMS (WHOQOL-100). *Revista Brasileira de Psiquiatria, 21*(1), 19-28. http://dx.doi.org/10.1590/S1516-44461999000100006.

Fleck, M.P.A., Louzada, S., Xavier, M., Chachamovich, E., Vieira, G., Santos, L., & Pinzon, V. (2000). Aplicação da versão em português do instrumento abreviado de avaliação da qualidade de vida "WHOQOL-bref". *Revista de Saúde Pública, 34*(2), 178-83. http://dx.doi.org/10.1590/S0034-89102000000200012.

Fox, K.R., Stathi, A., McKenna, J., & Davis, M.G. (2007). Physical activity and mental well-being in older people participating in the Better Ageing Project. *European Journal of Applied Physiology*, 100(5), 591-602.

Freitas, M.C., Queiroz, T.A., & Sousa, J.A.V. (2010). O significado da velhice e da experiência de envelhecer para os idosos. *Revista da Escola de Enfermagem da USP, 44*(2), 407-12.

Galvão, D.A, Spry, N., Denham, J., Taaffe, D.R., Cormie, P., Joseph, D., Lamb, D.S., Chambers, S.K., & Newton, R.U. (2014). A Multicentre Year-long Randomised Controlled Trial of Exercise Training Targeting Physical Functioning in Men with Prostate Cancer Previously Treated with Androgen Suppression and Radiation from TROG 03.04 RADAR. *European Urology, 65*(5), 856-64. http://dx.doi.org/10.1590/S0080-62342010000200024.

Giannouli, P., Zervas, I., Armeni, E., Koundi, K., Spyropoulou, A., Alexandrou, A., Kazani, A., Areti, A., Creatsa, M., & Lambrinoudaki, I. (2012). Determinants of quality of life in Greek middle-age women: A population survey. *Maturitas, 71*(2), 152-61. doi: 10.1016/j.maturitas.2011.11.013.

Giubilei, G., Mondain, N., Minervini, A., Saieva, C., Lapini, A., Serni, S., Bartoletti, R., & Carini M. (2007). Physical Activity of Men With Chronic Prostatitis/Chronic Pelvic Pain Syndrome Not Satisfied With Conventional Treatments - Could it Represent a Valid Option? The Physical Activity and Male Pelvic Pain Trial: A Double-Blind, Randomized Study. *Journal of Urology, 177*(1), 159-65.

Guimarães, A.C.A., & Baptista, F. Atividade física habitual e qualidade de vida de mulheres na meia-idade. (2011a). *Revista Brasileira de Medicina do Esporte, 17*(5), 305-9. http://dx.doi.org/10.1590/S1517-86922011000500002.

Guimarães, A.C.A., & Baptista, F. (2011b). Influence of habitual physical activity on the symptoms of climacterium/menopause and the quality of life of middle-aged women. *International Journal of Women's Health*, 3, 319-28. doi: 10.2147/IJWH.S24822.

Hallal, P.C., Dumith, S.C., Bastos, J.P., Reichert, F.F., Siqueira, F.V., & Azevedo, M.R. (2007). Evolução da pesquisa epidemiológica em atividade física no Brasil: uma revisão sistemática. *Revista de Saúde Pública*, 41, 453-60. http://dx.doi.org/10.1590/S0034-89102007000300018.

Heinemann, L.A. (2005). Aging Males' Symptoms scale: a standardized instrument for the practice. *Journal of Endocrinological Investigation*, 28, 34-8.

Heinemann, L.A.J., Zimmermann, T., Vermeulen, A., Thiel, C., & Hummel W. (1999). A new Aging Male's Symptoms' (AMS) rating scale. *Aging Male*, 2, 105-14. doi: 10.3109/13685539909003173.

Heinemann, L.A.J., Saad, F., Zimmerman, T., Novak, A., Myon, E., Badia, X., Potthoff, P., T'Sjoen, G., Pöllänen, P., Goncharow, N.P., Kim, S., & Giroudet, C. (2003). The Aging Males' Symptoms (AMS) scale: update and compilation of international versions. *Health and Quality of Life Outcomes, 1*(1). doi: 10.1186/1477-7525-1-15.

Hirokawa, K., Taniguchi, T., Fujii, Y., Takaki, J., & Tsutsumi, A. (2012). Job demands as a potential modifier of the association between testosterone deficiency and andropause symptoms in Japanese middle-aged workers: a cross-sectional study. *Maturitas*, *73*(3), 225-29. doi: 10.1016/j.maturitas.2012.07.006.

Instituto Brasileiro de Geografia e Estatística (Brasil). (2010). Projeção da população do Brasil/censo 2010. Retrieved from: [http//www.ibge.gov.br].

Joseph, R.P., Royse, K.E., Benitez, T.J., & Pekmezi, D.W. (2014). Physical activity and quality of life among university students: exploring self-efficacy, self-esteem, and affect as potential mediators. *Quality of Life Research, 23*(2), 659-67. doi: 10.1007/s11136-013-0492-8.

Krajewska-Ferishah, K.; Krajewska-Kułak, E., Terlikowski, S., Wiktor, H., Van Damme-Ostapowicz, K., Chadzopulu, A., Adraniotis, J., & Shpakou, A. (2010). Analysis of quality of life of women in menopause period in Poland, Greece, Belarus and Belgium using MRS Scale. A multicenter study. *Advances in Medical Sciences*, *55*(2), 191-95. doi: 10.2478/v10039-010-0042-3.

Kratzik, C.W., Lackner, J.E., Märk, I., Rücklinger, E., Schmidbauer, J., Lunglmayr, G., & Schatzl G. (2009). How much physical activity is needed to maintain erectile function? Results of the androx vienna municipality study. *European Urology*, *55*(2), 509-16. doi: 10.1016/j.eururo.2008.02.020.

Lopes, A.C.S., Toledo, M.T.T., Câmara, A.M.C.S., Menzel, H.J.K., & Santos, L.C. (2014). Condições de saúde e aconselhamento sobre alimentação e atividade física na Atenção Primária à Saúde de Belo Horizonte-MG. *Epidemiologia e Serviços de Saúde*, *23*(3), 305-16. http://dx.doi.org/10.5123/S1679-49742014000300010.

Luiz, M. & Magnanini, M.M.F. (2000). A lógica da determinação do tamanho da amostra em investigações epidemiológicas. *Cadernos de Saúde Coletiva*, *8*(2), 9-28.

Matsudo, S.M.M. (2009). Envelhecimento, atividade física e saúde. *Boletim do Instituto de Saúde*, 47, 76-9.

Matsudo, S., Araújo, T., Matsudo, V., Andrade, D., Andrade, E., Oliveira, L.C., & Braggion, G. (2001). Questionário internacional de atividade física (IPAQ): estudo de validade e reprodutibilidade no Brasil. *Revista Brasileira de Atividade Física e Saúde*, *6*(2), 5-18.

Nakamura, P.M., Teixeira, I.P., Smirmaul, B.P., Sebastião, E., Papini, C.B., Gobbi, S., & Kokubun, E. (2014). Health related quality of life is differently associated with leisure-time physical activity intensities according to gender: a cross-sectional approach. *Health and Quality of Life Outcomes*, 12. doi: 10.1186/1477-7525-12-98.

Pardini, R., Matsudo, S., Matsudo, V., Araújo, T., Andrade, E., & Braggion, G. (1997). Validation of international physical activity questionnaire (IPAQ): pilot study in brazilian young adults. *Medicine and Science in Sports and Exercise*, *29*(6), S5-S9.

Perchon, L.F.G., Pintarelli, V.L., Bezerra, E., Thiel, M., & Dambros, M. (2011). Quality of life in elderly men with aging symptoms and lower urinary tract symptoms (LUTS). *Neurourology and Urodynamics*, 30, 515-519. doi: 10.1002/nau.21008.

Pereira, E.F., Teixeira, C.S., & Lopes, A.S. (2013). Qualidade de vida de professores de educação básica do município de Florianópolis, SC, Brasil. *Ciência e Saúde Coletiva*, *18*(7), 1963-70. http://dx.doi.org/10.1590/S1413-81232013000700011

Pucci, G.C.M.F., Rech, C.R., Fermino, R.C., & Reis, R.S. (2012). Associação entre atividade física e qualidade de vida em adultos. *Revista de Saúde Pública*, *46*(1), 166-79. http://dx.doi.org/10.1590/S0034-89102012000100021

Revnic, C.R., Nica, A.S., & Revnic, F. (2007). The impact of physical training on endocrine modulation, muscle physiology and sexual functions in elderly men. *Archives of Gerontology and Geriatrics*, *44*(11), 339-42.

Rohden, F. (2012). A "criação" da andropausa no Brasil: articulações entre ciência, mídia e mercado e redefinições de sexualidade e envelhecimento. *Psicología, Conocimiento y Sociedad*, *2*(2), 196-219.

Salazar, A., Paravic, T., & Barriga, O.A. (2012). Percepción de los hombres y sus parejas sobre la calidad de vida en el climaterio masculino. *Revista Chilena de Obstetrícia y Ginecología, 77*(1), 11-7. http://dx.doi.org/10.4067/S0717-75262012000100003.

Santana, M.S., & Maia, E.M.C. (2009). Atividade Física e Bem-Estar na Velhice. *Revista de Salud Pública, 11*(2), 225-36. http://dx.doi.org/10.1590/S0124-00642009000200007.

SBU. Sociedade Brasileira de Urologia (2012). DAEM (Andropausa). Available from: [http://www.sbu.org.br/publico/?doencas-urologicas&p=350].

Staerman, F., León, P. (2012). Andropause (androgen deficiency of the aging male): Diagnosis and management. *Minerva Medica*, *103*(5), 333-42.

Waidyasekera, H., Wijewardena, K., Lindmark, G., & Naessen, T. (2009). Menopausal symptoms and quality of life during the menopausal transition in Sri Lankan women. *Menopause*, *16*(1), 164-170. doi: 10.1097/gme.0b013e31817a8abd.

World Health Organization (2004). Global Strategy on Diet, Physical Activity and Health. Available from:
[http://www.who.int/dietphysicalactivity/strategy/eb11344/strategy_english_web.pdf]

World Health Organization (US). (2010). Global Recommendations on Physical Activity for Health. Available from:
[http://www.who.int/dietphysicalactivity/physical-activity-recommendations-18-64years.pdf]

WHO. World Health Organization. Geneva: World Health Organization. [cited 2012 Sep 19]. MONICA Project. Smoking Questionnaire. Disponível em: Available from: http://www.ktl.fi/publications/monica/manual/index.htm. Aceddo em: 17 de junho 2014.

Author's note

Melissa de Carvalho Souza is Master of The Graduate Program in Human Movement from the Universidade do Estado de Santa Catarina (UDESC).

Adriana Coutinho de Azevedo Guimarães is PhD Professor of the Department of Physical Education at the Center for Health Sciences and Sports from the Universidade do Estado de Santa Catarina (UDESC).

Corresponding author

Melissa de Carvalho Souza
Laboratório de Pesquisa em Lazer e Atividade Físca (LAPLAF); Centro de Ciências da Saúde e do Esporte (CEFID); Universidade do Estado de Santa Catarina (UDESC).
Rua Pascoal Simone, 358, Coqueiros. Florianópolis, SC, Brazil.
Email: mecarvalho.s@gmail.com

5

Sociodemographic differences in walking for leisure and for commuting in Brazilian workers

Rodrigo de Rosso Krug
Giovâni Firpo Del Duca
Kelly Samara da Silva
Cecília Bertuol
Markus Vinicius Nahas
Universidade Federal de Santa Catarina, Florianópolis, SC, Brasil

Elusa Santina Antunes de Oliveira
Mauro Virgilio Gomes de Barros
Universidade de Pernambuco, Recife, PE, Brasil

Abstract—Walking is a great health promotion strategy due to its beneficial effects. Objetive: To identify the prevalence of walking for leisure and for commuting to work and its association with sociodemographic factors among 47,477 Brazilian workers. Walking and sociodemographic factors were obtained from a self-reported questionnaire. Poisson regression was used. Among men, walking for leisure was more frequent in those who were older, live with a partner, had a higher level of education and income, and worked in the Southeastern region of Brazil. When commuting, it was more prevalent among single men, who had a lower level of education and income and worked in the Southern region of this country. Among women, walking for leisure was more common in those who lived with a partner, had no children, and worked in the Southern region. There was an association between the outcome and age, education and family income. Regarding commuting, it was more prevalent among older individuals, without a partner, with a lower level of education and income, and working in the Southern region. Walking was associated with sociodemographic characteristics, with differences between sexes.

Keywords: leisure activities, occupational health, social class, cross-sectional studies

Introduction

The negative consequences of physical inactivity to health is considered of the most important risk behaviors for morbidity and mortality (Hallal *et al.*, 2007; World Health Organization, 2009; Lee *et al.*, 2012). The current physical activity recommendations have encouraged its practice during leisure time, domestic activities, transportation and work (WHO, 2009). In this context, walking is highly emphasized as a health promotion strategy, increasing the level of physical activity, due to its high rate of adherence, low cost, feasibility for the majority of the population, convenience, and beneficial health effects (Hallal *et al.*, 2005; Janssen *et al.*, 2010; Kruger, Ham, Berrigan & Ballard-Barbash, 2008; Lee & Buchner, 2008; Turi, Codogno, Fernandes & Monteiro, 2015; WHO, 2009).

Especially for leisure time, national and international studies indicate that walking is the main physical activity in adult populations (Lee, Sesso, Oguma, & Paffenbarger , 2004; Hallal *et al.*, 2005) with prevalence ranging from 8.8% to 35% (Gomes *et al.*, 2011; Parra *et al.*, 2011). This activity can provide better health perception, prevent disease, promote psychological well-being (Lee *et al.*, 2004; Gomes *et al.*, 2011), reduce expenses on medication (Codogno *et al.*, 2015; Turi *et al.*, 2015) and reduce mortality risk (Barros & Nahas, 2001; Lee *et al.*, 2004; Autenrieth *et al.*, 2011).

Concerning commuting to work among adults, walking is an alternative mode of transportation that is economically viable in both high-income countries, with effective public transport, and in low- and middle-income countries, where populations face more difficulties with public and private transport. The national prevalence of walking for commuting is 53% (Instituto Brasileiro de Opinião e Estatística, 2011). There is evidence that people who commute to work by walking have many health benefits (WHO, 2009; Lee *et al.*, 2004), a better health perception (Tassitano, Feitosa & Tenório, 2013), lower risk of chronic diseases, especially obesity (Gordon-Larsen *et al.*, 2009) and lower health expenses (Codogno *et al.*, 2015).

Understanding the differences in sociodemographic factors associated with walking during leisure time and commuting to work is very important for the development of public policies that helping to increase this behavior in society (Thomaz, Costa, Silva & Hallal, 2010), aiming to a more active and healthy lifestyle. In addition, it should be highlighted that women and men have different attitudes towards active behavior, especially walking (Hallal *et al.*, 2005; Kruger *et al.*, 2008), and that there are few studies addressing simultaneously walking during leisure time and commuting to work (Humpel, Owen, Iverson, Leslie, & Bauman, 2004; Teixeira, Nakamura & Kokubun, 2014; Turi *et al.*, 2015). Therefore, the objective of the study was to identify the prevalence of walking for leisure and for commuting to work and their association with socio demographic factors among Brazilian workers.

Method

This study is part of the survey entitled "Lifestyle and leisure activities of Brazilian industry workers". Data were collected between 2006 and 2008 and the survey included workers from 24 states of Brazil. Only the states of Rio de Janeiro, Sergipe and Piaui did not participate in the investigation, because they had not completed data collection in time.

Sample size calculation was performed independently for each state, according to the following parameters: prevalence of leisure-time physical inactivity of 45%, acceptable error of three percentage points, 95% confidence interval, an addition of 50% in the sample size to account for design effect and of 20% to account for possible losses and refusals. The planned sample size was 52,774 workers.

Sampling procedures included two stages. In the first stage, companies were randomly selected, according to the distribution of employees in large (≥ 500), medium (100-499) and small (<100) companies. In the second stage, the selection of workers was random and proportional to the size of the company. The industries that refuse to participate in the study were replaced by others that were similar in size and in the type of activity and that were located within the same geographical region.

The information used to develop the sampling plan and perform the random selection of companies and participating workers was provided by SESI's Regional Departments themselves. The number of companies selected in each stage can be consulted in the General Research Report (Nahas, Barros, Oliveira & Aguiar, 2009).

The instrument used was a questionnaire validated by Barros (1999). The workers answered the questions in groups of three to 15 individuals, under the supervision of evaluators, who were previously trained by videoconference. This instrument was previously tested for logic, content, clarity and reproducibility (Barros, 1999). A total of two senior researchers participated in the validation of logic and content. A pilot study was performed to assess clarity and to identify and resolve possible problems of interpretation. Analyses of reproducibility showed moderate to high levels of agreement in the physical activity section, with an interclass correlation coefficient varying from 0.60 to 0.84.

Study outcomes were walking for leisure and for commuting to work, which were self-reported by the workers as their main physical activity in each respective domain through the following questions: "Do you regularly perform some kind of physical activity in your leisure time, such as physical exercise (gymnastics, walking, running), sports, dance, or martial arts?"; and "How do you get to work from your home on most days of the week?" The answer options were walking, cycling, riding the bus, and taking a car/motorcycle. Those who selected the first option were categorized as practitioners walk.

The exposures investigated were sex (male and female), age (≤ 29, 30-39, 40-49 and ≥ 50 years), current marital status (with or without a partner), number of children (none, 1-2, ≥ 3), schooling (incomplete elementary education, complete elementary school, complete high school and complete undergraduation), gross family income in US dollars at the time of the study (≤ $280, $281-700, $701-1400, ≥ $1,401) and country region of the company (North, Northeast, Midwest, Southeast and South).

Data analysis was performed using Stata software, version 13.0 (Stata Corporation, College Station, USA). The results were expressed as absolute, relative frequencies and prevalence ratios with confidence intervals of 95% (95% CI), using Poisson regression with robust variance. Crude and adjusted analyses stratified by sex were carried out, using the following hierarchical model of analysis: Level 1 - age and region of the company; Level 2 - marital status and number of children; Level 3 - education and family income. The backward selection strategy was adopted and the variables in the same level were adjusted for each other and for the variables in subsequent levels. Variables with p value ≤ 0.20 were maintained in the model in order to control for confounding. Results with p value ≤ 0.05 were considered statistically significant.

Results

Among the 52,774 eligible workers, 47,477 participated in the study (89.90% response rate), mostly men (69.85%). Overall, the socio-demographic characteristics of the sample were similar for both sexes: most of the workers were ≤ 29 years old (45.31% men and 47.94% women), had one or two children (45.21% of men and 44.75% women), had completed high school (49.47% of men and 54.64% women) and had a gross family income equivalent to 281-700 US dollars at the time of the study (42.11% of men and 39.75% of women). By contrast, concerning marital status, most men (60.83%) reported having partners, while 54.18% of women reported being single. All variables showed statistical differences when sexes were compared. Further details on the workers' characteristics are shown in Table 1.

The prevalence of walking was 13.59% (95% CI: 13.27, 13.92) for leisure and 11.44% (95% CI: 11.16; 11.73) for commuting to work. 11.65% (95% CI: 11.30, 12.02) of men and 18.16% (95% CI: 17.51, 18.83) of women practiced walking during leisure time. Walking for commuting to work was reported by 10.18% (95% CI: 9.85, 10.51) of men and 14.38% (95% CI: 13.81, 15.00) of women. There was a significant difference between males and females for the two outcomes investigated ($p<0.001$).

Table 2 displays the results of the crude and adjusted analyses concerning walking for leisure and for commuting to work among males. There was an increasing trend of walking during leisure time among males with increasing age. However, age was not associated with walking for commuting to work. Workers with partners were 13% more likely to walk in leisure time and 14% less likely to walk for commuting to work. In addition, it was found that increasing education level and gross family income were associated with higher prevalence of walking in leisure time. Walking for commuting to work was significantly higher among socioeconomically disadvantaged workers. While workers from the Southeast region had the highest prevalence of walking for leisure (OR = 1.53), workers from the South had the highest prevalence of commuting to work (PR = 1.95).

Table 3 shows the crude and adjusted analyses of walking for leisure and for commuting to work among females. Increasing age was associated with walking for leisure and for commuting to work. Female workers with partners were 13% more likely to walk during leisure time and 9% less likely to walk for commuting to work compared to single female workers. The number of children was associated with lower prevalence of walking in leisure time ($p = 0.05$). i.e. working women with three or more children were 16% less likely to walk for leisure. However, the number of children was not significantly associated with walking for commuting to work. There was a positive trend between education level and the prevalence of walking for leisure, while the reverse occurred in the relation between education level and walking for commuting to work, i.e. less educated women were more likely to walk to commute to work. In relation to family income, women with lower income had higher prevalence of walking for both leisure and commuting. When compared with the North region, working in the South of Brazil was associated with higher prevalence of walking in both leisure time (OR = 1.32) and commuting to work (PR = 2.80).

Table 1. Characteristics of industry workers Brazilian according to sex. Brazil, 2008.

Variable	Male (n=33161)			Female (n=14316)		
	n	%	95% CI	n	%	95% CI
Age (years)						
≤29	14965	45.31	44.78; 45.85	6836	47.94	47.12; 48.76
30-39	10085	30.54	30.04; 31.04	4554	31.94	31.18; 32.71
40-49	5678	17.19	16.79; 17.60	2265	15.88	15.29; 16.49
≥50	2298	6.96	6.69; 7.24	604	4.24	3.92; 4.58
Marital status						
With partner	20117	60.83	60.31; 61.36	6547	45.82	45.00; 46.64
Without partner	12952	39.17	38.64; 39.69	7742	54.18	53.36; 55.00
Number of children						
None	11576	35.77	35.25; 36.30	6059	43.68	42.86; 44.51
1-2	14630	45.21	44.69; 45.75	6207	44.75	43.92; 45.58
3 or more	6154	19.02	18.59; 19.45	1605	11.57	11.05; 12.11
Education level						
Incomplete elementary school	7274	21.98	21.54; 22.43	1695	11.87	11.35; 12.41
Complete elementary school	5666	17.12	16.72; 17.53	1759	12.32	11.79; 12.87
Complete high school	16372	49.47	48.93; 50.01	7801	54.64	53.83; 55.46
Complete undergraduation	3782	11.43	11.09; 11.78	3021	21.16	20.50; 21.84
Family income						
≤280	10810	32.94	32.43; 33.45	4259	30.07	29.32; 30.83
281-700	13821	42.11	41.58; 42.65	5630	39.75	38.95; 40.56
700-1400	5337	16.26	15.87; 16.67	2879	20.33	19.67; 21.00
≥1401	2850	8.68	8.38; 8.99	1395	9.85	9.37; 10.35
Region of the company						
North	8722	26.30	25.83; 26.78	2918	20.38	19.73; 21.05
Northeast	10308	31.08	30.59; 31.59	4227	29.53	28.78; 30.28
Midwest	5815	17.54	17.13; 17.95	2335	16.31	15.71; 16.92
Southeast	4050	12.21	11.87; 12.57	1954	13.65	13.10; 14.22
South	4266	12.86	12.51; 13.23	2882	20.13	19.48; 20.80

Note: The variable number of children had the highest amount of missing information for both sexes (1246 missings in total, of which 801 were men and 445 were women). 95% CI: confidence intervals of 95%. p value <0,001 to comparison male and female.

Table 2. Descriptive and adjusted analysis of habitual practice walking for leisure and commuting to work among Brazilian male industry workers. Brazil, 2008.

	Walking for leisure				Walking for commuting to work			
	Descriptive analysis		Adjusted analysis		Descriptive analysis		Adjusted analysis	
Variable	**%**	**95% CI**	**PR (95% CI)**	**P value**	**%**	**95% CI**	**PR (95% CI)**	**P value**
Age (years)				**<0.001****				**0.689****
≤29	6.39	6.00; 6.81	1.00		10.60	10.11; 11.10	1.00	
30-39	11.10	10.48; 11.76	1.75 (1.60; 1.90)		9.38	8.83; 9.97	0.86 (0.82; 0.96)	
40-49	20.30	19.24; 21.41	3.18 (2.93; 3.46)		10.02	9.27; 10.84	0.94 (0.87; 1.04)	
≥50	26.57	24.75; 28.49	4.17 (3.80; 4.59)		11.30	10.06; 12.67	1.07 (0.94; 1.22)	
Marital status				<0.001*				<0.001*
With partner	13.70	13.21; 14.20	1.13 (1.05; 1.22)		9.70	9.30; 10.12	0.86 (0.80; 0.92)	
Without partner	8.44	7.99; 8.96	1.00		10.87	10.35; 11.42	1.00	
Number of children				0.794**				0.615**
None	8.22	7.71; 8.76	1.00		10.60	10.05; 11.17	1.00	
1-2	12.86	12.31; 13.43	1.06 (0.97; 1.16)		9.54	9.07; 10.03	0.95 (0.87; 1.04)	
3 or more	15.64	14.72; 16.60	1.00 (0.89; 1.12)		9.95	9.23; 10.73	0.98 (0.87; 1.09)	
Education level				<0.001**				<0.001**
Incomplete elementary school	9.68	9.00; 10.41	1.00		12.98	12.23; 13.78	1.00	
Complete elementary school	10.22	9.43; 11.07	1.29 (1.16; 1.44)		10.81	10.03; 11.65	0.80 (0.72; 0.88)	
Complete high school	11.22	10.73; 11.73	1.44 (1.31; 1.59)		9.81	9.37; 10.28	0.75 (0.69; 0.82)	
Complete undergraduation	19.73	18.43; 21.10	1.90 (1.68; 2.15)		5.22	4.56; 5.98	0.48 (0.40; 0.57)	
Family income				<0.001**				<0.001**
≤ 280	7.69	7.19; 8.23	1.00		11.99	11.39; 12.62	1.00	
281-700	11.50	10.96; 12.07	1.20 (1.10; 1.31)		10.69	10.18; 11.21	0.90 (0.83; 0.97)	
700-1400	15.46	14.48; 16.50	1.27 (1.14; 1.40)		8.30	7.59; 9.07	0.72 (0.64; 0.81)	
≥ 1401	20.26	18.75; 21.86	1.32 (1.17; 1.50)		4.34	3.64; 5.15	0.42 (0.35; 0.51)	
Region of the company				<0.001*				<0.001*
North	9.40	8.78; 10.06	1.00		8.16	7.60; 8.76	1.00	
Northeast	11.79	11.17; 12.44	1.12 (1.03; 1.22)		10.66	10.08; 11.28	1.31 (1.19; 1.43)	
Midwest	12.65	11.80; 13.55	1.31 (1.19; 1.44)		7.04	6.41; 7.73	0.86 (0.76; 0.97)	
Southeast	14.85	13.73; 16.04	1.53 (1.38; 1.69)		11.74	10.78; 12.77	1.44 (1.28; 1.62)	
South	11.53	10.52; 12.64	1.24 (1.10; 1.38)		15.93	14.86; 17.07	1.95 (1.76; 2.17)	

Note: PR: Prevalence ratio; 95% CI = 95% Confidence Interval; *= Heterogeneity test; **= Linear trend.

Table 3. Descriptive and adjusted analysis of habitual practice walking for leisure and commuting to work among Brazilian female industry workers. Brazil, 2008.

	Walking for leisure				Walking for commuting to work			
	Descriptive analysis		Adjusted analysis		Descriptive analysis		Adjusted analysis	
Variable	**%**	**95% CI**	**PR (95% CI)**	**P value**	**%**	**95% CI**	**PR (95% CI)**	**P value**
Age (years)				<0.001**				0.004**
≤29	15.16	14.28; 16.08	1.00		13.97	13.16; 14.81	1.00	
30-39	19.01	17.84; 20.23	1.28 (1.18; 1.40)		13.55	12.58; 14.57	0.97 (0.89; 1.07)	
40-49	23.21	21.44; 25.08	1.60 (1.45; 1.77)		15.99	14.54; 17.57	1.12 (1.00; 1.25)	
≥50	25.44	22.01; 29.20	1.81 (1.55; 2.11)		19.43	16.44; 22.81	1.34 (1.12; 1.59)	
Marital status				<0.001*				0.029*
With partner	19.97	18.97; 21.01	1.13 (1.05; 1.22)		14.21	13.38; 15.08	0.91 (0.84; 0.99)	
Without partner	16.64	15.79; 17.52	1.00		14.52	13.75; 15.32	1.00	
Number of children				0.053**				0.444**
None	16.66	15.69; 17.67	1.00		13.34	12.51; 14.22	1.00	
1-2	19.10	18.11; 20.14	0.96 (0.88; 1.06)		14.01	13.17; 14.90	0.92 (0.84; 1.02)	
3 or more	18.70	16.79; 20.77	0.84 (0.72; 0.97)		17.89	16.08; 19.85	0.97 (0.84; 1.13)	

continued...

Table 3. Continued.

	Walking for leisure				Walking for commuting to work			
	Descriptive analysis		Adjusted analysis		Descriptive analysis		Adjusted analysis	
Variable	%	95% CI	PR (95% CI)	P value	%	95% CI	PR (95% CI)	P value
Education level				<0.001**				<0.001**
Incomplete elementary school	17.41	15.56; 19.42	1.00		24.96	22.94; 27.08	1.00	
Complete elementary school	18.96	17.08; 20.99	1.20 (1.03; 1.40)		21.13	19.28; 23.11	0.85 (0.75; 0.96)	
Complete high school	17.30	16.44; 18.19	1.23 (1.08; 1.40)		13.87	13.12; 14.66	0.66 (0.59; 0.74)	
Complete undergraduation	20.33	18.87; 21.88	1.49 (1.28; 1.74)		5.80	5.02; 6.69	0.35 (0.29; 0.43)	
Family income				0.002**				<0.001**
≤ 280	17.75	16.57; 18.99	1.00		19.99	18.81; 21.22	1.00	
281-700	17.98	16.95; 19.05	0.92 (0.84; 1.01)		15.11	14.19; 16.07	0.82 (0.75; 0.90)	
700-1400	18.98	17.52; 20.53	0.89 (0.79; 0.99)		8.59	7.62; 9.68	0.52 (0.45; 0.61)	
≥ 1401	18.38	16.34; 20.62	0.81 (0.69; 0.94)		5.46	4.38; 6.79	0.38 (0.30; 0.48)	
Region of the company				<0.001*				<0.001*
North	17.25	15.87; 18.72	1.00		7.26	6.37; 8.26	1.00	
Northeast	15.20	14.13; 16.34	1.00 (0.74; 1.03)		17.33	16.21; 18.50	2.34 (2.02; 2.70)	
Midwest	19.14	17.54; 20.84	1.11 (0.99; 1.25)		10.36	9.18; 11.66	1.42 (1.19; 1.69)	
Southeast	19.64	17.85; 21.56	1.13 (1.00; 1.28)		14.45	12.96; 16.09	1.97 (1.67; 2.33)	
South	22.45	20.78; 24.22	1.32 (1.18; 1.48)		20.47	19.03; 21.99	2.80 (2.40; 3.25)	

Note: PR: Prevalence ratio; 95% CI = 95% Confidence Interval; *= Heterogeneity test; **= Linear trend.

Discussion

This study identified the prevalence and factors associated with walking during leisure time and commuting to work among Brazilian male and female workers. Walking prevalence, as the main physical activity in leisure time and in commuting to work, was considered low. In Brazil, there are few studies that have specifically assessed physical activity in adult workers simultaneously in both domains (Humpel *et al.*, 2004; Teixeira, Nakamura & Kokubun, 2014). This result can be partly explained by various environmental factors such as the rapid growth of cities, which could result in diminished opportunities for performing physical activity during leisure time, as well as greater difficulties for active commuting (Robroek *et al.*, 2011). In addition, issues such as working hours, high technological facilities (Robroek, Berg, Plat & Burdorf, 2011) and adverse weather conditions (Adamoli, Silva & Azevedo,2011) tend to decrease regular physical activity in general (Robroek *et al.*, 2011), including walking.

The prevalence of walking for leisure was slightly higher than walking for commuting to work in the study population, a result that is in agreement with other studies which show that, in Brazil, the prevalence of walking for leisure is usually higher than that for commuting to work (Gomes *et al.*, 2011; Parra *et al.*, 2011).

It is speculated that this finding can be explained by the worldwide increase in urban violence and insecurity (Handy, 2005). Some studies (Florindo, Salvador, Reis, & Guimarães, 2011; Gomes *et al.*, 2011; Parra *et al.*, 2011) showed that walking for leisure and commuting to work are influenced by the environment in different ways. Safety is one such way and it seems to have a greater influence on commuting to work.

Regarding sex, we observed that the prevalence of walking in both domains was higher among women than men. One possible explanation for this may be related to the fact that men practice more moderate and vigorous activities (Azevedo *et al.*, 2007; Thomaz *et al.*, 2010) and women, more walking and domestic activities (Thomaz *et al.*, 2010). In addition, men usually engage in collective activities such as football, while women opt for individual activities such as walking or gymnastics (Del Duca, Nahas, Hallal, & Peres, 2014).

In this study, it was shown that walking for leisure was more prevalent in older workers from both sexes. Similar results were found in other Brazilian studies (Del Duca *et al.*, 2014; Pitanga, Beck, Pitanga, Freitas, & Almeida, 2014). One explanation for this is that young and middle-aged adults engage in other more vigorous activities in their leisure time, while older adults engage in milder or moderate activities, such as walking (Hallal *et al.*, 2005). However, concerning walking for commuting to work, older age was positively associated with the outcome in women only. This result may be related to the fact that older women are more concerned about health issues, quality of life and aesthetics when compared to younger people, making them more involved with the practice of physical activities regardless of domain, intensity and duration (Azevedo *et al.*, 2007).

Concerning marital status, workers of both sexes who lived without a partner were more likely to walk for commuting to work. Similar results were found in another study involving adult residents of a Brazilian city (Dumith, Domingues & Gigante, 2009). On the other hand, walking for leisure was more common among men and women who had a partner. According to authors (Del Duca *et al.*, 2014) that observed similar findings, this relationship may be explained in part by the possibility of a joint practice, making physical activity more pleasant and enjoyable for those who live together.

In this study, having no children was associated with higher prevalence of walking for leisure in women only. Other studies (Barros & Nahas, 2001; Florindo *et al.*, 2009) have shown that, regardless of sex, the number of children influences physical activities during leisure time. It is possible that this discrepancy can be explained by existing family compositions. Typically, women are primarily responsible for taking care of their children during leisure time, which can reduce the time spent in walking in this domain (Florindo *et al.*, 2009).

In this study, walking for commuting to work was significantly higher among workers with lower levels of education and income, in both sexes. While in leisure time, walking was higher in individuals of higher educational levels for both sexes, men with higher income and women with lower income. It is possible that women with higher income choose other activities instead of walking, however there is no way to test this hypothesis with our data.

Kruger *et al.* (2008) also found that walking in leisure time was more frequent among educated people and higher family income, while walking for commuting to work was more frequent in individuals of lower socioeconomic status. In Brazilian studies (Barros & Nahas, 2001; Tassitano, Feitosa & Tenório, 2013; Pitanga *et al.*, 2014), the same trend of physical activity in leisure time, including walking (Barros & Nahas, 2001), or commuting is observed (Tassitano, Feitosa & Tenório, 2013; Pitanga *et al.*, 2014). It seems that the higher the educational level of Brazilian adults, the more physical activity is practiced for leisure and the less for commuting and for domestic purposes (Engbers, Poppel, Paw, & Mechelen, 2005). Possibly, this reality is most striking in middle and low income countries compared to high income countries, where the educational disparity is not so evident in the population. Among men, walking for leisure was more frequent in the Southeast, while walking for commuting was more frequent in the South. Among women, walking for both purposes was more frequent in those living in the South. Thus, walking was more common among workers of the richest regions of Brazil (South and Southeast). In the literature, wealthy regions with higher education levels tend to have more physically active people in leisure (Janssen *et al.*, 2010) but less in commuting (Kruger *et al.*, 2008; Tassitano, Feitosa & Tenório, 2013). Importantly, companies located in richer regions tend to have more financial resources, and consequently, better infrastructure and facilities (Matson-Koffman, Brownstein, Neiner & Greaney, 2005; Mutrie *et al.*, 2002) to perform physical activity in leisure time. It is believed that programs that encourage physical activity, as well as the availability of spaces suitable to the practice of these activities, are favorable aspects, and that companies could invest in this environment, by providing lectures on the benefits of regular physical activity, building sports courts, walking tracks, gyms and etc (Saelens & Handy, 2008).

On the other hand, the higher frequency of walking for commuting to work in less developed regions of Brazil can be explained by the absence of public transport in some localities and also by lower levels of violence compared to more developed regions and populated regions of the country. Studies (Dumith, Domingues & Gigante, 2009; WHO, 2009) show that there are many reasons that may hinder physical activity, among which are the increase in crime and high levels of traffic congestion.

This study had some limitations, such as the cross-sectional design, which restricts inferences about causal relationships between variables associated with walking for leisure and for commuting to work. The replacement of some companies, that refused to participate, by others of the same size and the replacement of selected workers, who were not at work at the time of collection or refused to participate, by the next name on the list of workers may have negative implications for the sampling procedure (non-respondent bias). One should also consider seasonal bias since data collection in each state occurred in different periods. The positive points of the study include the size and probability sample selection procedure, since this study was conducted with a large sample, sufficient for statistical analysis and representative of industry workers from 23 Brazilian states and the Federal District. Another important point was the high response rate.

Conclusion

Walking prevalence, as the main physical activity in leisure time and in commuting to work, was considered low. Sociodemographic factors associated with walking differ between the sexes, with different patterns for each domain. These differences may result in affirmative action for a physically active lifestyle, in which initiatives that support physical activity in different domains take into account some socio-demographic aspects of workers. Conducting cohort studies is important to better understand the "directionality" of these associations.

References

Adamoli, A.N.; Silva, M.C.; Azevedo, M.R (2011). Prática da caminhada no lazer na população adulta de Pelotas, RS. *Revista Brasileira de Atividade Física e Saúde, 16*(2), 113-119.

Autenrieth, C.S., Baumert, J., Baumeister, S.E., Fischer, B., Peters, A., Döring, A., & Thorand, B. (2011). Association between domains of physical activity and all-cause, cardiovascular and cancer mortality. *European Journal of Epidemiology, 26*(2), 91-99.

Azevedo, M.R., Araújo, C.L.P., Reichert, F.F., Siqueira, F.V., Silva, M.C., & Hallal, P.C. (2007). Gender differences in leisure-time physical activity. *International Journal of Public Health, 52*(1), 8-15.

Barros, M.V.G., & Nahas, M.V. (2001). Comportamentos de risco, auto-avaliação do nível de saúde e percepção de estresse entre trabalhadores da indústria. *Revista de Saúde Pública, 35*(6), 554-563.

Barros, M.V.G. (1999). *Atividades físicas no lazer e outros comportamentos relacionados à saúde dos trabalhadores da indústria no estado de Santa Catarina, Brasil.* Dissertação de mestrado, Programa de Pós-Graduação em Educação Física, Universidade Federal de Santa Catarina, Florianópolis, Santa Catarina, Brasil.

Codogno, J.S.; Turi, B.C.; Kemper, H.C.G.; Fernandes, R.A.; Christofaro, D.G.D.; Monteiro, L.H (2015). Physical inactivity of adults and 1-year health care expenditures in Brazil. *International Journal of Public Health, 60*(3), 309-316.

Del Duca, G.F., Nahas, M.V., Hallal, P.C., & Peres, K.G. (2014). Atividades físicas no lazer entre adultos de Florianópolis, Santa Catarina, Brasil: estudo populacional sobre as características das práticas e de seus praticantes. *Ciência & Saúde Coletiva, 19*(11), 4595-4604.

Dumith, S.C., Domingues, M.R., & Gigante, D.P. (2009). Epidemiologia das atividades físicas praticadas no tempo de lazer por adultos do Sul do Brasil. *Revista Brasileira de Epidemiologia, 12*(4), 646-658.

Engbers, L.H., Poppel, M.N,van., Paw, M.J.C.A., & Mechelen, W.van. (2005). Worksite health promotion programs with environmental changes: a systematic review. *American Journal of Preventive Medicine, 29*(1), 61-70.

Florindo, A.A., Guimarães, V.V., Cesar, C.L.G., Barros, M.B.A., Alves, M.C.G.P., & Goldbaum, M. (2009). Epidemiology of leisure, transportation, occupational, and household physical activity: prevalence and associated factors. *Journal of Physical Activity & Health, 6*(5), 625-632.

Florindo, A.A., Salvador, E.P., Reis, R.S., & Guimarães, V.V. (2011). Percepção do ambiente e prática de atividade física em adultos residentes em região de baixo nível socioeconômico. *Revista de Saúde Pública, 45*(2), 302-310.

Gomes, G.A.O., Reis, R.S., Parra, D.C., Ribeiro, I., Hino, A.A.F., Hallal, P.C., Malta, D.C., & Brownson, R.C. (2011). Walking for leisure among adults from three Brazilian cities and its association with perceived environment attributes and personal factors. *International Journal of Behavioral Nutrition and Physical Activity, 8*(1), 111-118.

Gordon-Larsen, P., Boone-Heinonen, J., Sidney, S., Sternfeld, B., Jacobs, D. R., & Lewis, C.E. (2009). Active commuting and cardiovascular disease risk: the CARDIA study. *Archives of Internal Medicine, 169*(13), 1216-1223.

Hallal, P.C., Azevedo, M.R., Reichert, F.F., Siqueira, F.V., Araújo, C.L., & Victora, C.G. (2005). Who, when, and how much? Epidemiology of walking in a middle-income country. *American Journal of Preventive Medicine, 28*(2), 156-161.

Hallal, P.C., Dumith, S.C., Bastos, J.P., Reichert, F.F., Siqueira, F.V., Azevedo, M.R. (2007). Evolução da pesquisa epidemiológica em atividade física no Brasil: uma revisão sistemática. *Revista de Saúde Pública, 41*(3): 453-460.

Handy, S. (2005). Critical assessment of the literature on the relationships among transportation, land use, and physical activity [Working paper Resource paper for TRB Special Report 282: 87]. *Transportation Research Board and Institute of Medicine Committee on Physical Activity, Health, Transportation, and Land Use*. Washington, USA.

Humpel, N., Owen, N., Iverson, D., Leslie, E., & Bauman, A. (2004). Perceived environment attributes, residential location, and walking for particular purposes. *American Journal of Preventive Medicine, 26*(2), 119-125.

Instituto Brasileiro de Opinião e Estatística – IBGE (2011). *Retratos da sociedade Brasileira: locomoção urbana*. Brasília: Confederação Nacional da Indústria (CNI).

Janssen, E., Sugiyama, T., Winkler, E., de Vries, H., te Poel, F., & Owen, N. (2010). Psychosocial correlates of leisure-time walking among Australian adults of lower and higher socio-economic status. *Health Education Research, 25*(2), 316-324.

Kruger, J., Ham, S.A., Berrigan, D., & Ballard-Barbash, R. (2008). Prevalence of transportation and leisure walking among US adults. *American Journal of Preventive Medicine, 47*(3), 329-334.

Lee, I.M., & Buchner, D.M. (2008). The importance of walking to public health. *Medicine and Science in Sports and Exercise, 40*(7 Suppl), S512-S518.

Lee, I.M., Sesso, H.D., Oguma, Y., & Paffenbarger, R.S. (2004). The "weekend warrior" and risk of mortality. *American Journal of Epidemiology, 160*(7), 636-641.

Lee, I.M., Shiroma, E.J., Lobelo, F., Puska, P., Blair, S.N., Katzmarzyk, P.T. (2012). Effect of physical inactivity on major non-communicable diseases worldwide: an analysis of burden of disease and life expectancy. *The Lancet, 380*(9838), 219-229.

Matson-Koffman, D.M., Brownstein, J.N., Neiner, J.A., & Greaney, M.L. (2005). A site-specific literature review of policy and environmental interventions that promote physical activity and nutrition for cardiovascular health: what works? *American Journal of Health Promotion, 19*(3), 167-193.

Mutrie, N., Carney, C., Blamey, A., Crawford, F., Aitchison, T., & Whitelaw, A. (2002). "Walk in to Work Out": a randomised controlled trial of a self help intervention to promote active commuting. *Journal of Epidemiology and Community Health, 56*(6), 407-412.

Nahas, M. V.; Barros, M. V. G.; Oliveira, E. S. A.; Aguiar, F. S. (2009). Estilo de vida e hábitos de lazer dos trabalhadores das indústrias brasileiras: relatório geral. Brasília: Serviço Social da Indústria/ Departamento Nacional, 2009, 163.

Parra, D.C., Hoehner, C.M., Hallal, P.C., Ribeiro, I.C., Reis, R., Brownson, R.C., Pratt, M., & Simoes, E.J. (2011). Perceived environmental correlates of physical activity for leisure and transportation in Curitiba, Brazil. *American Journal of Preventive Medicine, 52*(3), 234-238.

Pitanga, F.G., Beck, C.C., Pitanga, C.P.S., Freitas, M.M., & Almeida, L.A.B. (2014). Prevalência e fatores sociodemográficos e ambientais associados à atividade física no tempo livre e no deslocamento em adultos. *Motricidade, 10*(1), 3-13.

Robroek, S.J., Berg, T.I. van den, Plat, J.F., & Burdorf, A. (2011). The role of obesity and lifestyle behaviours in a productive workforce. *Occupational and Environmental Medicine, 68*(2), 134-139.

Saelens, B.E., & Handy, S.L. (2008). Built environment correlates of walking: a review. *Medicine and Science in Sports and Exercise, 40*(7 Suppl), S550-S566.

Tassitano, R.M., Feitosa, W.M.N., & Tenório, M.C.M. (2013). Fatores associados ao deslocamento ativo e indicadores de saúde em trabalhadores da indústria. *Revista Brasileira de Atividade Física & Saúde, 18*(4), 483-484.

Teixeira, I.P., Nakamura, P.M., & Kokubun, E. (2014). Prática de caminhada no lazer e no deslocamento e associação com fatores socioeconômicos e ambiente percebido em adultos. *Revista Brasileira de Cineantropometria & Desempenho Humano, 16*(3), 345-358.

Thomaz, P.M.D., Costa, T.H.M., Silva, E.F., & Hallal, P.C. (2010). Fatores associados à atividade física em adultos, Brasília, DF. *Revista de Saúde Pública, 44*(5), 894-900.

Turi, B.C.; Codogno, J.S.; Fernandes, R.A.; Monteiro, H.L (2015). Caminhada e gastos com saúde em adultos usuários do sistema public de saúde brasileiro: estudo transversal retrospective. *Ciência e Saúde Coletiva*, *20*(11), 3561-1568.

World Health Organization - WHO (2009). *Global health risks: mortality and burden of disease attributable to selected major risks.* Geneva: World Health Organization.

Autor's note

Rodrigo de Rosso Krug, Giovâni Firpo Del Duca, Kelly Samara da Silva, Cecília Bertuol and Markus Vinicius Nahas are affiliated whith the Federal University of Santa Catarina Sports Center, research Centre in Physical Activity and Health.

Mauro Virgilio Gomes de Barros and Elusa Santina Antunes de Oliveira are affiliated with the University of Pernambuco, Research Group in lifestyle and health.

Acknowledgments

The authors of this study acknowledge the financial and logistical support provided by the Social Service for Industry (SESI), which allowed the survey to be conducted successfully; the industry workers for participation, patience and commitment to research and the Coordination for the Improvement of Higher Education Personnel (CAPES) for master's and doctoral scholarships awarded to two authors of this paper.

Corresponding author

Rodrigo de Rosso Krug
Federal University of Santa Catarina Sports Center - Research Centre in Physical Activity and Health - Campus Universitário Reitor João David Ferreira Lima, Centro de Desportos. Florianopolis, SC, Brazil.
Email: rodrigo_krug@hotmail.com

6

Quantitative evaluation of trunk muscle strength in wheelchair basketball players

Sileno da Silva Santos
Angélica Castilho Alonso
Júlia Maria D'Andréa Greve
Universidade de São Paulo, São Paulo, SP, Brasil

Abstract—Trunk muscle strength affects trunk controlling playing an important role in performance and to define the classes of wheelchair basketball players. Trunk control capacity differs among players and quantitative assessments of trunk muscle strength have not been investigated. The aim of this study was to identify and correlate quantitative measures of trunk muscle strength with the wheelchair basketball players' classification. Forty-two male wheelchair basketball players with spinal cord injury, amputation, post-poliomyelitis sequelae, and cerebral palsy had their trunk extension and flexion strength evaluated with isokinetic dynamometer. The classes 1.0, 2.0, 3.0, and 4.0 were considered for statistical analysis. Comparison of trunk muscle strength differed significantly between classes: 1.0 and 3.0; 1.0 and 4.0; 2.0 and 3.0; and 2.0 and 4.0. High correlation was found between the trunk muscle strength and players' classes. The findings of the present study showed a strong correlation of trunk muscle strength and wheelchair basketball classes being able to distinguish players in their classes. However, this quantitative method of evaluation of the trunk muscle strength cannot be solely used to make a decision on the full trunk control.

Keywords: classification, functional performance, wheelchair sports

Introduction

The wheelchair basketball (WCB) is a paralympic sport which is very popular among people with disabilities (Malone, Gervais & Steadward, 2002; Yildirima, Comertb & Ozengina, 2010). Athletes with different physical disabilities such as spinal cord injuries (SCI), amputations, post-poliomyelitis sequelae, and cerebral palsy are eligible to join teams (Gil-Agudo, Ama-Espinosab, & Crespo-Ruizb, 2010). Depending on the particular disability, each player has a unique physical capacity affecting players' trunk control and the performance of WCB movements (Genthon & Rougier, 2006). To ensure that players with different physical capacity make part in the same team for competition, there is a player's classification following the rules of the International Wheelchair Basketball Federation (International Wheelchair Basketball Federation [IWBF], 2014). The official player classification manual, classifies athletes into eight classes ranging from 1.0 to 4.5 based on their physical capacity of trunk control, lower limb function, upper limb function and hand function. In particular, the trunk movement and stability form the basis for player classification (IWBF, 2014).

The classification process of a new player starts in the beginning of a competition. In a practice section, prior to the competition, a panel of classifiers observe the athlete's trunk movements capacity according to the volume of action (IWBF, 2014; Goosey-Trofey, 2010) which is standardized for each class. After this initial observation, the classifiers indicate a temporary class among one of the eight classes of WCB. During the games, classifiers continuously observe the performance of the player and, by the end of competition, the classifiers confirm or modify his initial classification (IWBF, 2014). According to this, the classification of wheelchair basketball player is an observation-based classification.

The International Paralympic Committee has encouraged studies based on scientific principles of athletes' classification in paralympic sport (Tweedy & Vanlandewijck, 2011). Some studies have been conducted relating WCB players' performance with physiological responses and their classes (Brasile 1986, 1990; Malone *et al*, 2002; Doyle *et al*, 2004; Molik, Laskin, Kosmol, Skucas, & Bida, 2010) The results of these studies have stated that the athletes' game performance was related to their class. Despite the indication that trunk muscle strength plays an important role for players' capacity of trunk movements and consequently for classification (IWBF 2014), quantitative studies assessing this variable have not been conducted. A quantitative evaluation of this variable would bring objective data of this important aspect of players' classification supporting the observed-based classification. According to this, the aim of this study was to identify and correlate quantitative measures of trunk muscle strength with wheelchair basketball players' classification.

Materials and Methods

Study Participants

Forty-two male wheelchair basketball players of mean age 28.3±7.4 years (16-46) participated in this study during a competitive season. All participants had previously received an official regional, national or international classification as following: class 1.0 (n = 11), 2.0 (n = 11), 3.0 (n = 9), and 4.0 (n = 11). Players of class 1.0 and class 4.5 are those with lower and higher physical capacity, respectively. Free and informed consent form was signed by all participants before evaluations of their trunk muscle strength. The Ethics Committee of the University of Sao Paulo College of Medicine approved this study (n# 063/10). All tests were performed at the Movement Study Laboratory, Institute of Orthopedics and Traumatology of Hospital das Clinicas-SP.

Table 1. Characteristics of participants.

Class	n	Age (Years)	Body Mass (kg)	High (cm)	BMI (kg/cm²)
1	11	28.0 ± 8.6	61.9 ± 16.5	166.5 ± 14.0	22.5±7.1
2	11	26.5 ± 6.5	61.2 ± 14.0	157.9 ± 13.8	24.7±5.4
3	9	27.0 ± 9.3	68.7 ± 12.4	157.9 ± 13.8	24.9±9.4
4	11	27.9 ± 8.6	74.6 ± 17.2	172.1 ± 11.3	25.5±4.5
Group	42	28.3 ± 7.4	66.5 ± 15.7	165.0 ± 15.8	24.7±6.0

Data are expressed as mean and Standard deviation (±).
n= number of subjects; Kg= kilogram; cm=centimeters; Kg/cm² =Kilogram/square centimeter.

Table 2. Distribution of subjects according to disabilities and wheelchair basketball classes.

	Disabilities						
Class	sci	amp	polio	sb	cd	art	CP
1	9			1		1	
2	5	1	4	1		1	
3	2	1	3	1			1
4	1	8	1		1		
Total	17	10	8	3	1	2	1

Sci=spine cord injury; amp=amputation; polio=poliomyelitis sequelae; sb= spine bifida; cd=congenital deformity, art=arthrogryposis; cp=cerebral palsy.

Testing Protocol

Trunk muscle strength evaluation: isokinetic dynamometry

For this study, we used the Biodex System-3 isokinetic equipment (model: Biodex Multi Joint System, Biodex System Inc.; software version 4.5) to measure trunk muscle strength in isometric mode (Fleck & Kraemer, 1999). The athletes had undergone prior spinal joint warm-up and familiarization with the equipment. They were positioned in accordance with the manufacturer's standards, in a semi-standing position (Biodex, 2013). The initial position of the trunk was at 90° in relation to the femur, and the knees were flexed at 45° in relation to the lower legs. Stabilizing bands secured using Velcro were positioned around the trunk, waist, legs and feet. The axis of the dynamometer was aligned with the iliac crest with the range of motion limited to -15° of extension and 15° of flexion. During the test, the athletes were instructed applying force into a fixed bar in front of their chest for flexion and, against a back hold support for trunk extension. They exerted maximum trunk flexion and extension strength alternately for five seconds each, in a total of ten repetitions, with intervals of 15 seconds of rest between the repetitions. In order to define the angular amplitude and number of repetition, it was conducted a pilot test with athletes who had higher level of impairments. The mean of highest peak torque (PT) and the radio between the peak torque in flexion and extension were the variables selected to be analyzed. These isokinetic variables describe the muscle's strength capabilities (Biodex, 2013).

Statistical analysis

All data were analyzed with SPSS software for Windows (v.18) and Minitab (v.16) and are expressed as means within the athletes' distributed into WCB classes. The Shapiro-Wilk test confirmed that the data presented a non-normal distribution, and comparisons between the classes were made using the Kruskal-Wallis test with Bonferroni correction. The Spearman correlation coefficient was used to correlate the trunk muscle strength with the wheelchair basketball classes. A p-value <0.05 was accepted as significant (Fisher & Van-Belle, 1993).

Results

Trunk muscle strength

Trunk muscle strength progressively increased with the athletes' classes. Players of class 1.0 and 4.0 showed the lowest and the highest values, respectively. Comparing the athletes of different classes, there were significant differences between the mean peak torque during trunk flexion and extension between the following classes: 1.0 and 3.0; 1.0 and 4.0; 2.0 and 3.0; and 2.0 and 4.0. The ratio between the trunk flexion and extension was also significantly different in the comparisons between classes 1.0 and 3.0; 1.0 and 4.0; and 2.0 and 4.0 (Table 3).

Correlation of trunk muscle strength and WCB classes

There was a strong correlation between wheelchair basketball classes and all isokinetic variables measured during extension and flexion of the trunk: (Peak torque extension; Peak torque in flexion; and, Ratio between flexion/extension (Table 4).

Table 3. Comparison of isokinetic variables of trunk muscle strength according to the WCB classes.

Variable	Class 1	Class 2	Class 3	Class 4	
PT extension					1 vs. 3 p = 0.004*
(N/m)	65.0	108.0	218.5	341.3	1 vs. 4 p < 0.001*
					2 vs. 4 p = 0.003*
PT flexion					1 vs. 3 p = 0.006*
(N/m)	43.5	69.9	144.7	129.5	1 vs. 4 p < 0.002*
Flex/Ext ratio					1 vs. 4 p = 0.002*
(%)	107.3	77.9	51.0	42.8	2 vs. 4 P = 0.007*

Kruskal-Wallis test with post-hoc Bonferroni correction;
* $p \leq 0.05$; PT, peak torque; Legend: N/m=Newton per meter; Flex/Ext=Flexion/Extension; %=percentage.

Table 4. Correlation of isokinetic variables stratified by WCB classes.

Class	PT extension r(p-value)	PT flexion r(p-value)	Flex/Ext ratio r(p-value)
1.0	0.509(0.110)	0.196(0.282)	-0,836(<0.001)*
2.0	0.864(<0.001)*	-.109(0.375)	-0.482(0.067)
3.0	0.117(0.383)	0.733(0.012)	-0.433(0.122)
4.0	0.082(0.405)	0.645(<0.05)*	-0.491(0.063)
Total	0.806(<0.001)*	0.691(<0.001)*	-0.631(<0.001)*

r=Spearman's correlation coefficient; PT=peak torque; *p*-value=level of significance $p<0.05$.

Discussion

This study aimed to identify and correlate quantitative measures of trunk muscle strength with the wheelchair basketball players' classification. The mean peak torque during players' flexion and extension of the trunk has shown that the lowest values were found among players of classes 1.0 and 2.0. Athletes with cervical and upper- and mid-thoracic spinal cord injuries, who have partial control over the trunk, are the classic examples of athletes in classes 1.0 and 2.0. The lower peak torque of the trunk extensor musculature, i.e., the musculature working against gravity, may provide the conditions for developing postural abnormalities and respiratory disorders (Schilero, Spungen, Bauman, Radulovic, and Lesser, 2009). This contributed to lower levels of players' physical capacity seen in class 1.0 and 2.0. The highest trunk muscle strength was found in athletes of classes 3.0 and 4.0, which were composed of athletes with higher physical capacity. Athletes in classes 3.0 and 4.0 were those with amputations or impairments after polio and they had less loss of their physical capacity due to the preservation of upper body musculoskeletal structures (lower limb amputees). These important factors contribute towards the higher peak torque values seen in classes 3.0 and 4.0. The results of flexion/extension ratio (Brown, 2008) have shown that the athletes in classes 1.0 and 2.0 had higher flexion/extension ratios than did the athletes in classes 3.0 and 4.0. These results always need to be discussed with care. It means that flexor trunk muscle strength predominated over extensor trunk muscle strength in classes 1.0 and 2.0, but not in the other classes. All isokinetic results are concordant with studies that have analyzed physical and physiological performance of WCB players and their classes (Brasile 1986, 1990; Malone *et al.*, 2002; Doyle *et al.*, 2004; Vanlandewijck *et al.*, 2004; Molik *et al.*, 2010).

Due the indication that disabilities impact the capacity of trunk control (IWBF, 2014), it is easier to identify players of class 1.0 and 4.0. In this case, an observation-based classification is enough to identify players of these classes. On the other hand, it is not easy to identify players of classes 1.0 and 2.0; 2.0 and 3.0; and 3.0 and 4.0. These are "neighboring classes" and the impact of disability on the trunk capacity control present a greater variability.

This situation can be verified comparing the trunk muscle strength with WCB classes. The results have shown differences in players of classes 1.0 and 4.0; 1.0 and 3.0; and, 2.0 and 4.0 showing that an observation-based classification might bring doubts for classifiers in the "neighboring classes". The strong correlation found in this study support the indication that trunk muscle strength must be considered as important aspect of players' classification (IWBF 2014; Gil-Agudo *et al.*, 2010).

The players' classification is well established in WCB, but scientific evidence is still pursued once it is an observed-based classification (Tweedy & Vanlandewijck, 2011). Despite the indication that quantitative evaluation of disability cannot be taking account into wheelchair basketball players' classification (Brasile, 1990), a combined system of observed-based and quantitative evaluation of players' capacity can contribute to a justified and fair classification of athletes (Vanlandewijck, Spaepen, Lysens, 1995). It is necessary to have in mind that a quantitative evaluation of the trunk muscle strength cannot be solely used to make a decision of full trunk control. It is necessary to consider other factors such as disabilities, wheelchair and, players' strategies to maintain their balance in the seated position, and function of the upper and lower limbs (IWBF 2014).

Conclusion

No studies have investigated quantitatively the trunk muscle strength of WCB players. This study suggests that a quantitative assessment of trunk muscle strength might contribute towards providing objective data about players' trunk control, thereby supporting the current classification of WCB players. The findings of the present study showed a strong correlation of trunk muscle strength and wheelchair basketball classes being able to distinguish players in their classes. However, this quantitative method of evaluation of the trunk muscle strength cannot be solely used to make a decision on the full trunk control.

References

Biodex. (2013). Biodex Multi-Joint System Pro. *Setup/Operation Manual.* Retrivied from: http://www.biodex.com/sites/default/files/835000man_06159.pdf.

Brasile, F.M. (1986). Wheelchair basketball skills proficiencies versus disability classification. *Adapted Physical Activity Quarterly,* 3, 6-13.

Brasile, F.M. (1990). Performance Evaluation of Wheelchair Athletes: More Than a Disability Classification Level Issue. *Adapted Physical Activity Quarterly,* 7, 289-297.

Brown L.E. (2008). *Isokinetics in Human Performance.* Champagne IL/USA: Human Kinetics.

Doyle T.L.A., Davis R.W., Humphries B., Dugan E.L., Horn B.G., Shim J.K., & Newton R.U. (2004). Further Evidence to Change the Medical Classification System of The National Wheelchair Basketball Association. *Adapted Physical Activity Quarterly,* 21, 63-70

Fisher L.D. & Van-Belle G. 1993. *Biostatistics.* New York/EUA: John Wiley & Sons.

Fleck S.J., & Kraemer W.J. (1999). *Fundamentos do treinamento de forca muscular.* Porto Alegre, 2ª Edição: Artmed Bookman.

Genthon N., & Rougier P. (2006). Does the Capacity to Appropriately Stabilize Trunk Movements Facilitate the Control of Upright Standing? *Motor Control,* 10, 232-243.

Gil-Agudo A., Ama-Espinosab A.D., & Crespo-Ruizb B. (2010). Wheelchair Basketball Quantification. *Physical Medicine Rehabilitation Clinic North America,* 21, 141–156.

Goosey-Trofey V. (2010). *Wheelchair Sport.* Loughborough, UK: Human Kinetics.

International Wheelchair Basketball Federation IWBF. (2014). Oficial player classification manual. *International Wheelchair Basketball Federation,* Retrivied from: http://www.iwbf.org/images/a_classification/ClassificationManual2014-2018EnglishFinal.pdf.

Malone L.A., Gervais P.L., & Steadward R.D. (2002). Shooting mechanics related to player and free throw success in wheelchair basketball. *Journal of Rehabilitation Research & Development,* 39(6), 701-710.

Molik B., Laskin J.J., Kosmol A., Skucas K., & Bida U. (2010). Relationship Between Functional Classification Levels and anaerobic performance of wheelchair basketball athletes. *Research Quarterly for Exercise and Sport, 81*(1), 69-73.

Schilero G.J., Spungen A.M., Bauman W.A., Radulovic M., & Lesser M. (2009). Pulmonary function and spinal cord injury. *Respiratory physiology and neurobiology, 166*(3), 129-141.

Tweedy S.M., & Vanlandewijck Y.C. (2011). International Paralympic Committee position stand—background and scientific principles of classification in Paralympic sport. *British Journal of Sports Medicine,* 45, 259-69. doi:10.1136/bjsm.2009.065060

Vanlandewijck ,Y.C., Spaepen, A.J., Lysens, R.J. (1995). Relationship between the level of physical impairment and sports performance in elite wheelchair basketball players. *Adapted Physical Activity Quarterly*, 12, 139-150.

Vanlandewijck, Y.C. *et al.* (2004). The relationship between functional potential and field performance in elite female wheelchair basketball players. *Journal of Sports Science*, 22, 668–675.

Yildirima, N.U., Comertb, E., & Ozengina, N. (2010). Shoulder pain: A comparison of wheelchair basketball players with trunk control and without trunk control. *Journal of Back Musculoskelet Rehabilitation*, 23, 55–61.

Authors' note

Sileno da Silva Santos, Angélica Castilho Alonso, Júlia Maria D'Andréa Greve are affiliated with the University of Sao Paulo College of Medicine. Movement Study Laboratory, Institute of Orthopedics and Traumatology of Hospital das Clinicas-SP.

Corresponding author

Sileno da Silva Santos
Av. João Peixoto Viegas, 195 Apto. 164, São Paulo, SP, Brazil.
Email: sileno@usp.br

7

Previous participation in FIFA World-Cup: the key to success?

Ronaldo Kobal
Núcleo de alto rendimento esportivo de São Paulo, SP, Brasil

Renato Barroso
Universidade Estadual de Campinas, Campinas, SP, Brasil

Cesar Cavinato Cal Abad
Kátia Kitamura
Núcleo de alto rendimento esportivo de São Paulo, SP, Brasil

Everton Crivoi do Carmo
Centro Universitário Senac, São Paulo, SP, Brasil

Lucas Pereira
Núcleo de alto rendimento esportivo de São Paulo, SP, Brasil

Fábio Yuzo Nakamura
Núcleo de alto rendimento esportivo de São Paulo, SP, Brasil
Universidade Estadual de Londrina, Londrina, PR, Brasil

Irineu Loturco
Núcleo de alto rendimento esportivo de São Paulo, SP, Brasil

Abstract—This qualitative-descriptive investigation examining the influence exerted by experienced soccer-players on the ranking obtained from the four best-ranked by their teams in the last four FIFA World Cups (WC). They were divided into experienced-players (at least one WC participation [+1WC]) or non-experienced players (no previous participation [1WC]). Thereafter, they were classified according to their contribution in each of the playoff matches in a given WC: STARTER (started all matches); START/SUBST (started at least one match); SUBST/BENCH (did not start any matches, but replaced a player in at least one match); and BENCH (did not participate in matches). The sample was composed of 33.7% experienced and 66.3% non-experienced players. The number of players +1WC in finalist teams was significantly higher than in the non-finalist teams ($p<0.05$). In addition, when compared with the non-finalist teams, the finalists presented significantly higher number of players STARTER with +1WC ($p<0.05$). Possibly, the selection of experienced players to participate in WC may be an effective strategy to achieve better competitive performance.

Keywords: competitive performance, tactical, soccer, experienced players, strategy

Introduction

Soccer is the most popular sport in the world, played in almost every country, both as a leisure activity and competitively. The most important soccer tournament worldwide is the FIFA World Cup (WC), in which the best players from 32 national teams represent their countries every four years. The first tournament was held in Montevideo, Uruguay in 1930. Since then, eight different national teams have won the FIFA WC: Brazil (5 times), Italy and Germany (4 times), Argentina and Uruguay (twice) and England, France and Spain (once).

Performance in soccer is highly complex. Depending on the interaction of multiple factors, such as technical aspects, tactical strategies, nutritional and psychological factors, fitness abilities (power, speed, anaerobic and aerobic demands) and individual soccer skills (Ali, 2011; Arnason, Sigurdsson, Gudmundsson, Holme, Engebretsen & Bahr, 2004; Barnes, Archer, Hogg, Bush, & Bradley, 2014; Castagna, Impellizzeri, Chamari, Carlomagno &

Rampinini, 2006; Kobal *et al.*, 2014; Stolen, Chamari, Castagna, & Wisloff, 2005; Wisloff, Castagna, Helgerud, Jones, & Hoff, 2004). Although these physiological/technical aspects have been extensively investigated by sport scientists, there is a lack of data regarding other parameters which could be related to successful team performance trajectories during important tournaments.

There are some methodological difficulties in investigating teams participating in the FIFA WC due to the restricted access to information and the short-period of preparation and competition. Therefore, using observational and qualitative data available on specialized soccer websites (i.e. www.fifa.com) might contribute to the development of new studies investigating the particular/crucial characteristics presented by successful national teams during the WC. Certainly, the match outcome is the primary (and most important) criterion for evaluating specific performances in team sports. Thus, establishing the data capable of defining the "closeness of the game" (i.e., winning and losing margin) may provide substantial information about the success obtained during the competitions (Liu, Gomez, Lago-Penas & Sampaio, 2015). These additional data would allow head coaches and technical staff to identify team skills/qualities more associated with the winning teams.

Some studies have already shown that athletes with competitive experience perform specific motor tasks more efficiently than novice athletes (Gabbett, Jenkins & Abernethy, 2011; Garcia-Gonzalez, Moreno, Moreno, Iglesias, & del Villar, 2012; Gil, Moreno, Moreno, Garcia-Gonzalez, Claver & Del Villar, 2013; Lex, Essig, Knoblauch, & Schack, 2015; Vanttinen, Blomqvist, Luhtanen, & Hakkinen, 2010; Vaz, Leite, Joao, Goncalves, & Sampaio, 2012). For instance, Gabbett *et al.* (2011) demonstrated that rugby players selected to play in the first National Rugby League were older, more experienced, faster, had superior power and aerobic capacities, and skill qualities than non-selected players. Moreover, Lex *et al.* (2015) showed that more experienced soccer players, in contrast to less experienced soccer players, possess a functionally organized cognitive representation of team-specific tactics in soccer and reacted faster in tactical decisions. That is experienced players have a perceptual advantage in tactical decision-making in soccer.

These studies reported that experienced athletes possess more extensive, organized, structured and complete understanding of the game in comparison to novice players. This information allows coaches to produce/create more efficient athletes for identifying relevant technical/tactical aspects of the game and, as a consequence, make more appropriate decisions to execute the specific soccer tasks (Del Villar, Garcia Gonzalez, Iglesias, Perla Moreno, & Cervello, 2007; Garcia-Gonzalez *et al.*, 2012), thereby affecting their match performance. Based on these previous statements, it is highly likely that top-level soccer players with previous experience in world tournaments may present better performance in the WC and thus impact on the competitive performance presented by their teams. If confirmed, this hypothesis would allow soccer managers and head coaches to plan more efficient/successful long-term strategies for their national teams in order to attain better results during the WC.

In addition to the role of the athletes' experience in the competition results, understanding the influence of the experienced starters (i.e., players starting the match who have previously participated in the WC) and experienced non-starters (i.e., bench-players with previous experience of WC participation) on the rate of success reached by their national teams during the WC could assist the technical staff to select the better/more suited players to compose their squads for competing in this tournament. Moreover, this information could help the head coaches to choose the best formation to start the games even during the course of the WC. Therefore, the primary purpose of this study was to investigate, in the 4 most highly ranked teams from the last 4 FIFA WCs (i.e., 2002, 2006, 2010 and 2014), the influence exerted by the total number of experienced players in the final classification reached by their teams during the FIFA WCs. Secondly, the role played by experienced starters (experienced soccer players who started the games) in determining the success rate of their teams was examined.

Methods

Sample

Three hundred and sixty-eight top level soccer players from the four best-ranked teams of the last four FIFA World Cups (23 players from each team) were analysed in this qualitative and descriptive investigation. The teams which represent the population of this study are described in Table 1.

Table 1. Ranking of the last four FIFA World Cups.

	Champion	**2nd place**	**3rd place**	**4th place**
2002	Brazil	Germany	Turkey	Republic of Korea
2006	Italy	France	Germany	Portugal
2010	Spain	Netherlands	Germany	Uruguay
2014	Germany	Argentina	Netherlands	Brazil

Procedures

The data used in this study were obtained through the official FIFA website (www.fifa.com/worldcup). All selected players were classified according to their participation in previous WCs, into experienced (at least one WC participation, [+1WC]) or non-experienced (no previous participation, [1WC]) in the FIFA World Cup. Next, each player was classified according to their contribution in each playoff match (round of 16; quarter-finals; semi-finals, and final or third place) in a given WC. Contribution categories were: STARTER (started all playoff matches); START/SUBST (started at least one playoff match); SUBST/BENCH (did not start any playoff matches, but replaced a player in at least one playoff match); and BENCH (did not participate in the playoff matches). The group's matches were excluded because most of the previous classified teams used the START/SUBST, SUBST/BENCH, and/or BENCH players as starters in the last match of this stage.

Statistical Analyses

To test for differences between experienced (+1WC) and non-experienced (1WC) players by ranking (champion, second, third, and fourth places) the Kruskal-Wallis test was used. Since this statistical analysis does not reveal the direction the differences, finalists (champion and second place) and non-finalists (third and fourth places) were grouped. Sequentially, the Chi-square (x^2) test was applied to check for differences between +1WC and 1WC by subgroup (finalists and non-finalists). Subsequently, the Kruskal-Wallis test was used to search for differences between +1WC and 1WC (players by ranking in each specific contribution as STARTER, START/SUBST, SUBST/BENCH, and/or BENCH). Afterward, the Chi-square test was used to compare +1WC and 1WC (contributions of players in finalists and non-finalists). Finally, a Spearman rank-order correlation was used to analyze the relationships between ranking places (champion, second, third, and fourth place) and the respective number of players classified STARTER with +1WC. Data of the soccer players age are presented as mean ± standard deviation (SD). An independent t-test was used to test the difference between ages of the two groups (+1WC) and (1WC). The level of significance was set at $p \leq 0.05$ in all analysis.

Results

Of the 368 soccer players, 66.3% had never participated in a previous WC (1WC, n=244) and 33.7% had participated in at least one WC (+1WC, n=124). +1WC players were significantly older than 1WC players (29.8 ± 3.2yrs; 26.4 ± 3.5yrs, $p<0.05$). On average the champion teams had 60.9 ± 9.4% of 1WC and 39.1± 9.4% of +1WC players. The second place teams contained 57.6 ± 12.5% of 1WC and 42.4 ± 12.5% of +1WC, the third place teams had 72.8 ± 18.9% of 1WC and 27.2 ± 18.9% of +1WC and the fourth place teams 73.9 ± 12.8% of 1WC and 26.1 ± 12.8% of +1WC (Figure 1A). In addition, the finalist teams demonstrated significantly higher percentage of +1WC than non-finalist teams (Figure 1B) ($x^2 = 8.222$; $p \leq 0.05$). Figure 2 (A, B, C, and D) presents the STARTER, START/SUBST, SUBST/BENCH, and BENCH players classified as 1WC and +1WC among the final ranking. No significant differences were found between players +1WC by contribution in finalists and non-finalists, except by STARTERs ($x^2 = 9.655$; $p \leq 0.05$) (Figure 2E). Figure 3 presents the eleven starting players in the most important matches of the WCs (final and 3rd place) according to their classification in 1WC and +1WC. Figure 4 presents the numbers of started players with +1WC distributed by each stage of the playoff matches. Significant and large correlations between ranking places and STARTERs with +1WC were found ($r = 0.70$; $p \leq 0.05$). From the all STARTER players (n=117), 58 were +1WC and of these, 50 (86.2%) had started at least one match in a previous WC.

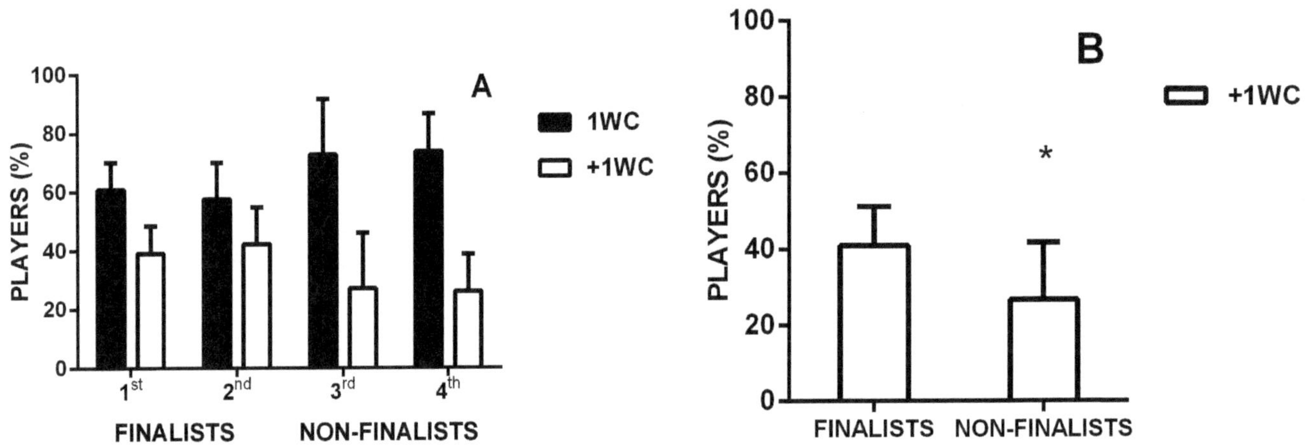

Figure 1. Panel A - Classification of all players in experienced (+1WC) and non-experienced (1WC) (mean and SD) among first, second, third, and fourth places of the last four WCs. Panel B –Experienced players (+1WC) between finalists (first and second place) and non-finalists (third and fourth place). * $p \leq 0.05$ lower than finalists.

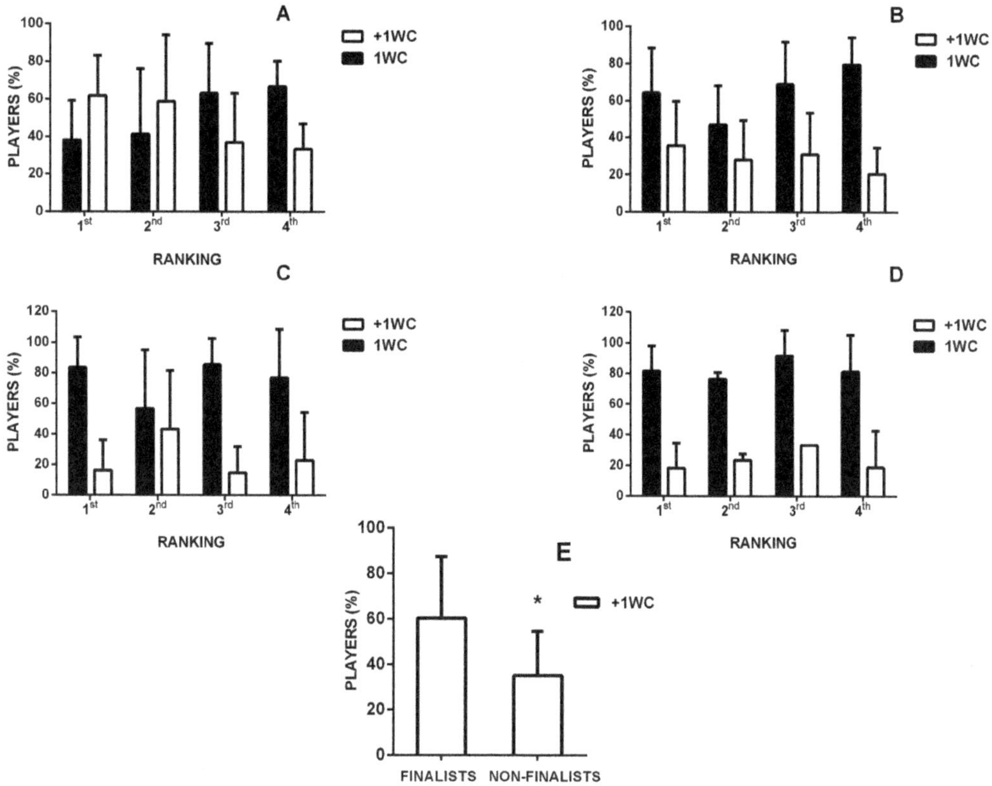

Figure 2. Distribution of players experienced (+1WC) and non-experienced (1WC) (mean and SD): Panel -A- STARTER, Panel -B- START/SUBST, Panel -C- SUBST/BENCH, Panel –D- BENCH, among first, second, third, and fourth places of the last four WCs. Panel –E- STARTER experienced players (+1WC) between finalists (first and second place) and non-finalists (third and fourth place). * $p \leq 0.05$ lower than finalists.

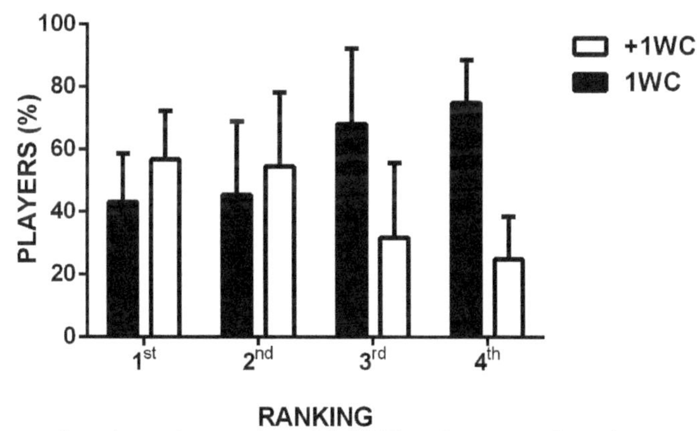

Figure 3. Classification of the eleven starting players in experienced (+1WC) and non-experienced (1WC) in final and 3rd place matches.

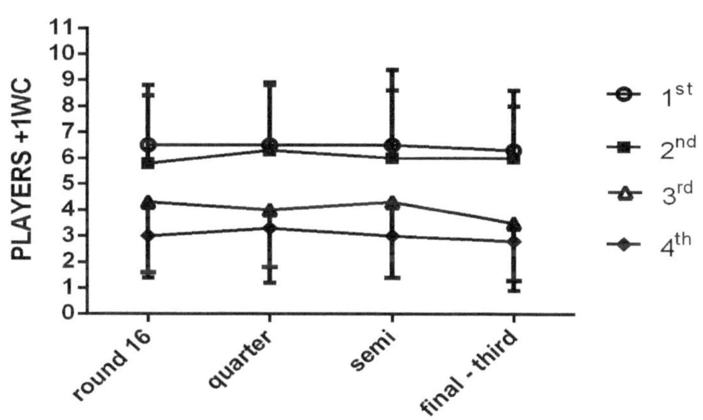

Figure 4. Number of players experienced (+1WC) (mean and SD) in each playoff match by ranking.

Discussion

The purpose of this study was to verify the influence exerted by experienced soccer players on the final ranking obtained by their teams in the last four FIFA World Cups. In addition, we verify the respective contributions of these experienced soccer players according to their participation in the playoff matches (i.e., STARTER, START/SUBST, SUBST/BENCH, and BENCH). The main findings reported herein were: 1) overall, among all soccer players in the 4 analyzed WCs, the number of 1WC players was greater than the number of +1WC players; 2) the percentage of +1WC players was significantly higher in the finalists (compared to non-finalists); 3) importantly, the finalists demonstrated significantly higher number of STARTER players with +1WC when compared to the non-finalists; 4) there was a large correlation ($r = 0.70$) (Hopkins, 2002) between ranking places and the numbers of STARTER players with +1WC 5) ≈ 55% of the twenty-two started players in the finalist teams were +1WC.

At least for the four FIFA WCs examined in this study, our findings demonstrated that the experience of players played a crucial role in the final classification reached by a national team in the WC. This can be confirmed by analyzing the higher number of +1WC among the finalist teams (≈ 40% of +1WC) when compared to the third and fourth place teams (≈ 26% of +1WC) (Figure 1B). For reasons to be further explored it seems that these players have a great influence on the match outcomes; especially in the semi-finals, when teams with higher numbers of +1WC played against teams with lower numbers of +1WC (Figure 4). Indeed, Sedeaud, Marc, Schipman, Tafflet, Hager & Toussaint (2012) demonstrated similar relevance of previous participation in the Rugby World Cup from 1987 to 2007. For these Rugby WCs, the winning teams contained a significantly higher number of experienced players (i.e., players who participate in WC before) than all the other teams. Additionally, the percentage of experienced players increased from the quarter-finalists (33.4%) to the winning teams (39.6%). According to the authors, it is likely that the "time playing together" exerted a substantial influence on the results achieved by a given team during a specific tournament (i.e., the longer the time, the better the team performance).

Another advantage for the experienced players was investigated by Thelwell, Weston, Lane, and Greenlees (2006), who demonstrated that more experienced soccer players, presented a more positive general mood profile than less experienced players. Particularly during away matches, that represent an uncomfortable and stressful situation, the less experienced players reported significantly more tension than the more experienced ones. When playing in the FIFA WC playoffs, players are probably submitted to similar or worse situations. Thus, it is conceivable that experienced athletes would also present less tension than non-experienced athletes, which may positively influence the team performance.

In this sense, we found that ≈20% of the players did not participate (BENCH) in any playoff matches. Accordingly, 16.3% of the players participated as SUBST/BENCH in (at least one) playoff matches (Figure 2C and 2D). Consequently, of the 23 players selected by each specific national team, about eight players had little or no participation in the playoffs. Importantly, the majority of these players were debuting in the WC in all ranked places. This highlights the importance of the athletes' experience during the crucial phases of the WC.

The selection of soccer players with previous participation in the WC seems to be crucial to achieve higher levels of competitive performance. However, it appears that the number of experienced players do not differ between first and second place teams. Curiously, there is a particularity in the FIFA WC finalist teams: a higher number of +1WC players participating as STARTER in the finalist teams (Figure 2 E). It is important to emphasize that, among all STARTER players with +1WC, 86.2% had started at least one match in a previous WC. It seems reasonable to suggest that not only "being in a WC" is important for the athletes to become more experienced, but rather, it is important to have participated as a starter in at least one match in a previous WC. Of note, a comparison between the champions and the runner-up reveals only a small difference in the number of players STARTER with + 1WC playing in these teams (first place ≈ 62% *vs* second place ≈ 59%). This similarity between the number of STARTER players +1WC playing in the finalist teams was also observed in the closely matched final games, as demonstrated by the need for extra-time in the last three FIFA WCs (2006, 2010 and 2014).

Indeed, it is likely that selecting more experienced players as starters in a team throughout the training process and competition could be an advantage in the technical and/or tactical factor, especially in short-tournaments. For instance, Vaz *et al.* (2012) compared physical exertion and game performance indicators of experienced (more than five years in regular national or international competitions) and novice (one or less years of rugby playing experience) players in Rugby Union, when playing small-sided games. In spite of the absence of differences in the physical exertion, the results from the game performance indicators (i.e., passes, tries and tackles made) demonstrated significant differences between the two groups, with a clear advantage in favor of the more experienced players. Probably, in team sports, the "athlete's experience" plays a central role in determining the level of performance in specific technical/tactical game actions.

Two studies have investigated the game actions able to discriminate the performance obtained by national teams during the last four FIFA WCs (2002, 2006, 2010 and 2014). Castellano, Casamichana and Lago (2012) found that shot and shot on target were two variables that significantly differentiated winning, drawing and losing teams in 2002, 2006 and 2010. Furthermore, ball possession was also able to discriminate the team performances in the 2010 and 2006 WCs. Analyzing the data from the 2014 FIFA WC, Liu *et al.* (2015) observed that an increase in the number/amount of some specific game actions (i.e., number of shots, shot on target, ball possession and short pass) resulted, respectively, in 13, 48, 11 and 12% higher probabilities of winning the matches. Based on these results, it is highly suggested that coaches use "collective training strategies" in their teams, capable of developing in their athletes the capacity to keep ball possession and, as a consequence, increase the number of crucial game actions (i.e., assistances and shots on target). This is surely a characteristic of teams formed by highly experienced players who have been playing together (under the same formation) for a long time.

In summary, this study may assist the technical staff to choose the best players for participating in FIFA WCs. Using the information presented here, the national head coaches can discriminate their national players into specific sub-groups (STARTER, START/SUBST, SUBST/BENCH and BENCH) and, consequently, adopt the best strategy to form their teams. Since the more experienced players have a central role in determining the rate of success of the national teams during the FIFA WCs, it is highly suggested that the coaches increase the participation of these athletes during the competitions. Secondly, the inclusion of novice players in the national teams and their participation in at least one match during the FIFA WCs seems to have a great influence on the experience accumulated by this player, which consequently influences the results, obtained in future WCs.

Conclusion

To conclude, our findings suggest that experienced soccer players who participate in playoffs can significantly contribute to influencing the performance obtained by their national teams during FIFA WCs. It could be highlighted when observing the large level of correlation between the number of experienced STARTER and the ranking places reached by their respective teams. Increasing the experience level of the novice soccer players by including these athletes during partial times of the matches might also be an important strategy to form winning teams.

References

Ali, A. (2011). Measuring soccer skill performance: a review. *Scandinavian Journal of Medicine and Science in Sports, 21*(2), 170-183. doi:10.1111/j.1600-0838.2010.01256.x.

Arnason, A., Sigurdsson, S.B., Gudmundsson, A., Holme, I., Engebretsen, L., & Bahr, R. (2004). Physical fitness, injuries, and team performance in soccer. *Medicine Science in Sports Exercise, 36*(2), 278-285. doi:10.1249/01.MSS.0000113478.92945.CA.

Barnes, C., Archer, D.T., Hogg, B., Bush, M., & Bradley, P.S. (2014). The Evolution of Physical and Technical Performance Parameters in the English Premier League. *International Journal of Sports Medicine.* doi:10.1055/s-0034-1375695.

Castagna, C., Impellizzeri, F.M., Chamari, K., Carlomagno, D., & Rampinini, E. (2006). Aerobic fitness and yo-yo continuous and intermittent tests performances in soccer players: a correlation study. *Journal of Strength Conditioning Research, 20*(2), 320-325. doi:10.1519/R-18065.1.

Castellano, J., Casamichana, D., & Lago, C. (2012). The Use of Match Statistics that Discriminate Between Successful and Unsuccessful Soccer Teams. *Journal of Human Kinetics, 31*, 139-147. doi:10.2478/v10078-012-0015-7.

Del Villar, F., Garcia Gonzalez, L., Iglesias, D., Perla Moreno, M., & Cervello, E.M. (2007). Expert-novice differences in cognitive and execution skills during tennis competition. *Perceptual and Motor Skills, 104*(2), 355-365. doi:10.2466/pms.104.2.355-365.

Gabbett, T.J., Jenkins, D.G., & Abernethy, B. (2011). Relative importance of physiological, anthropometric, and skill qualities to team selection in professional rugby league. *Journal of Sports Science, 29*(13), 1453-1461. doi:10.1080/02640414.2011.603348.

Garcia-Gonzalez, L., Moreno, A., Moreno, M.P., Iglesias, D., & del Villar, F. (2012). Tactical knowledge in tennis: a comparison of two groups with different levels of expertise. *Perceptual and Motor Skills, 115*(2), 567-580. doi:10.2466/30.10.25.PMS.115.5.567-580.

Gil, A., Moreno, M.P., Moreno, A., Garcia-Gonzalez, L., Claver, F., & Del Villar, F. (2013). Analysis of the relationship between the amount of training and cognitive expertise. A study of young volleyball players. Journal of Strength Conditioning Research, 27(3), 698-702. doi:10.1519/JSC.0b013e31825d99c9.

Hopkins, W.G. (2002). A scale of magnitudes for effect statistics. Avaliable at: *http://www.sportsci.org/resource/stats/effectmag.html.*

Kobal, R., Loturco, I., Gil, S., Cavinato Cal Abad, C., Cuniyochi, R., Barroso, R., & Tricoli, V. (2014). Comparison of physical performance among brazilian elite soccer players of different age-categories. The *Journal of Sports Medicine and Physical Fitness.*

Lex, H., Essig, K., Knoblauch, A., & Schack, T. (2015). Cognitive representations and cognitive processing of team-specific tactics in soccer. *PLoS One, 10*(2), e0118219. doi:10.1371/journal.pone.0118219.

Liu, H., Gomez, M.A., Lago-Penas, C., & Sampaio, J. (2015). Match statistics related to winning in the group stage of 2014 Brazil FIFA World Cup. *Journal of Sports Science*, 1-9. doi:10.1080/02640414.2015.1022578.

Sedeaud, A., Marc, A., Schipman, J., Tafflet, M., Hager, J.P., & Toussaint, J.F. (2012). How they won Rugby World Cup through height, mass and collective experience. *British Journal of Sports Medicine, 46*(8), 580-584. doi:10.1136/bjsports-2011-090506.

Stolen, T., Chamari, K., Castagna, C., & Wisloff, U. (2005). Physiology of soccer: an update. *Sports Medicine, 35*(6), 501-536.

Thelwell, R.C., Weston, N.J., Lane, A.M., & Greenlees, I.A. (2006). Relation of game location and experience on mood states. *Perceptual and Motor Skills, 102*(1), 157-162. doi:10.2466/pms.102.1.157-162.

Vanttinen, T., Blomqvist, M., Luhtanen, P., & Hakkinen, K. (2010). Effects of age and soccer expertise on general tests of perceptual and motor performance among adolescent soccer players. *Perceptual and Motor Skills, 110*(3 Pt 1), 675-692. doi:10.2466/PMS.110.3.675-692.

Vaz, L., Leite, N., Joao, P.V., Goncalves, B., & Sampaio, J. (2012). Differences between experienced and novice Rugby Union players during small-sided games. *Perceptual and Motor Skills, 115*(2), 594-604. doi:10.2466/30.10.25.PMS.115.5.594-604.

Wisloff, U., Castagna, C., Helgerud, J., Jones, R., & Hoff, J. (2004). Strong correlation of maximal squat strength with sprint performance and vertical jump height in elite soccer players. *British Journal of Sports Medicine, 38*(3), 285-288.

Authors' note

Ronaldo Kobal, Cesar Cavinato Cal Abad, Kátia Kitamura, Lucas Pereira and Irineu Loturco are affiliated with the NAR - Nucleus of High Performance in Sport, São Paulo, SP, Brazil.

Renato Barroso is affiliated with the Faculty of Physical Education, State University of Campinas, SP, Brazil.

Everton Crivoi do Carmo is affiliated with the Department of Physical Education, University Center – Senac, SP, Brazil.

Fábio Yuzo Nakamura is affiliated with the Department of Physical Education, State University of Londrina, PR, Brazil and NAR - Nucleus of High Performance in Sport, São Paulo, SP, Brazil.

Corresponding author

Ronaldo Kobal
Nucleus of High Performance in Sport, São Paulo
Av. Padre José Maria, 555 São Paulo, SP, Brazil.
Email: ronaldo.kobal@narsp.com.br

8

Effects of 22 weeks of training on functional markers and match performance of young soccer players

Rodrigo Leal de Queiroz Thomaz de Aquino
Universidade do Porto, Porto, Portugal

Luiz Guilherme Cruz Gonçalves
Lucas de Paula Oliveira
Hugo Tourinho Filho
Enrico Fuini Puggina
Universidade de São Paulo, Ribeirão Preto, SP, Brasil

Abstract—The aim of this study was to verify the effects of 22 weeks of training on functional markers and match performance through the use of earned points in competition. Twenty male soccer players were submitted to the same group of tests in four moments of the periodization: before the preparatory stage (T0); after the preparatory stage (T1); after the competitive stage I (T2); after the competitive stage II (T3). The functional markers were measured using the vertical and horizontal jump, T-40; Shuttle Run Test and RAST. The match performance was obtained by earned points in competition. An increase were found for all the variables analyzed for functional markers when T0 was compared with T3. In relation to the match performance, the team obtained 83.33% success in competitive stages. It is possible to conclude that training plan was efficient to improve technical-tactical skills and physical fitness of the studied athletes.

Keywords: periodization, motor skills, match performance, soccer

Introduction

The increasing professionalization and commercialization of sport followed by the growing investments has leading the athletes in searching of success to attract new investments (Gomes, 2009; Tourinho, 2001). However, high performance in sport implies in technological and scientific knowledge to prepare athletes according to their needs. Studies aiming to extend this knowledge to the annual training plan, called periodization, may contribute to the sports science based on practice, which may substitute the empiricism based on practice (Lopez, Marques, Tillaar, & Gonzalez-Badillo, 2011).

Training periodization consists in establishing and guiding the athlete physical preparation process, in an attempt to achieve the best specific fitness in a target competition (Barbanti, 2010). Along with this, the physical fitness is understood as a biological adaptation process due to the training stimulus, manifested after a long-term preparation to the competition (Matvéiev & Ruas, 1986). According to Borin, Gomes, & Leite (2008), periodization is the process to unify the physical, technical, tactical and psychological variables that characterizes the athlete training to compete.

Currently, the periodization in soccer presents some difficulties. In the most part of the cases, the training is planed to immediate results, being directed to the team performance in just a part of the official matches. However, the player must acquire and maintain the physical fitness during annual cycles of training and competitions. Thus, the main objective of periodization in soccer is to reach the maximum level of performance aiming to succeed during the competitive season (Zakharov, 1992). Thus, one of the most common critics about the training programs for soccer players is that the competitive calendar does not allow to peak performance and to recover after the competitions (Sargentim, 2010).

Regarding to that, it was demonstrated that the team sports calendar, especially in soccer, are designed with an excess of matches in the competitions with very short periods to perform the pre season. Based on this statement, it was proposed the selective loads model of periodization, that consists in an annual cycle of 52 weeks, divided in two stages with 26 weeks each, characterizing a double periodization (Bompa, 2002; Gomes, 2009). The training load remains almost the same during the competition season, focusing on velocity performance. Thus, the proposition suggests that in the first training drive, the stimulations must be directed to the functional aspects of the body, alternating the emphasis to the neuromuscular training followed by velocity training.

In the model proposed by Gomes (2009) specific resistance, power manifestations (maximal power, fast power and endurance power), flexibility/coordination, technique and tactics and velocity are considered physical attributes of the athlete. The effectiveness of the model on functional markers were early investigated in basketball players (Moreira, 2006; Moreira, Okano, Souza, Oliveira, & Gomes, 2005; Moreira, Oliveira, Ronque, Okano, & Souza, 2008), soccer (Souza, 2006), and futsal (Thiengo *et al.*, 2013).

However, considering the training and competitive season of the players, as well the studies in providing scientific and practice knowledge in physical education and sport field, this study aimed to adapt the selective loads periodization model considering the execution and evaluation of the strategy verifying its efficacy. Thus, the original model proposed by Gomes (2009) consists in stimulate predominantly the technical and tactical capacities in all stages of the season. Considering that it is very important for the performance in the field. In other words, the functional and metabolic capacities of the players must be connected to the technical execution and tactical application of the game elements (Garganta, 2001). Based on that, the objective of this study was to investigate the effects of 22 weeks of training on functional markers and performance in the game in young soccer players.

Methods

Participants

Twenty male soccer players belonging to the under 17 category were selected to participate in the study. They have regularly trained and participated in the first division of professional league of the São Paulo state representing a club that they belong– Brazil.

For characterization of the participants, body composition (body mass, body fat, height), O2MAX and the peak height velocity were evaluated according to previous studies (Léger & Lambert, 1982; Mirwald, Jones, Bailey, & Beunen, 2002; Machado, Oikawa & Barbanti, 2013). Data are summarized in Table 1.

Table 1. Sample characteristics expressed in mean ± sd of age, height, body mass, body fat, peak height velocity and O2MAX.

	Mean ± SD
Age (years)	15.1 ± 0.3
Height (cm)	171.5 ± 6.1
Body Mass (kg)	60.4 ± 5.5
Body Fat (%)	11.5 ± 2.8
Peak height velocity (years)	1.42 ± 0.5
O_{2MAX} ($ml.kg^{-1}.min^{-1}$)	48.68 ± 4.67

The participants were submitted to a periodization training program developed to improve the physical, technical and tactical components of soccer. The inclusion criteria were the participation in all of the sample collection and one uninterrupted year of soccer training.

The present study was approved by the ethics Commitee of the Ribeirão Preto Medical School of the University of São Paulo (n°. 710.998). The participants and their legal responsible signed an informed consent and instructed about the procedures of the study.

Overview of experimental design

In this study, the periodization was consisted of 22 weeks, with 4 training sessions per week (Mondays, Tuesdays, Wednesdays and Thursdays), totalizing 96 training sessions of 100-120 minutes of duration, divided in three stages: preparatory stage (six weeks), competitive stage I (eight weeks) and competitive stage II (eight weeks). Ten official matches were performed during the target competition, divided into four in the competitive stage I and six in the competitive stage II. During the preparatory stage, two friendly matches were performed.

The subjects were evaluated in four moments: at beginning of the training season (TO), the end of the training season (T1), end of the competitive stage I (T2) and end of the competitive stage II (T3). The tests and retests to measure the functional markers were performed on the same time (approximately 05:30 PM) in the training field, always in the beginning of the week (Monday and Tuesday). The sequence of testing was standardized for the every moments of collection, starting with a standardized warm-up.

1° day of evaluation: afternoon –T-40 test (cyclic and acyclic velocity of displacement) and Running-based Anaerobic Sprint Test – RAST (anaerobic power).

2° day of evaluation: afternoon – vertical jump and horizontal jump from stand position (fast power) and Shuttle Run Test (aerobic power).

The soccer players performed a familiarization session with the tests one week before starting of the experimental protocol. The T-40 test, RAST, Shuttle Run Test were conducted on the grass field with soccer boots. The vertical and horizontal jump tests were performed inside the changing room with participants in barefoot.

Determination of Displacement Speed Cyclic-Acyclic

Aiming to evaluate the cyclic and acyclic velocity of displacement, T-40 test was applied to all participants (Moreira *et al.*, 2005). The participant was positioned behind the start-stop line and started the test after the command. After the command, the volunteer ran 10 m straight to the first cone; after touching the hand in the cone of the center, quickly changed the direction to the left, toward the next cone positioned 5 meters from the center cone; after touch the left cone, the player returned to the previous direction, but moving to the cone on the right positioned 5 meters from the center cone, running 10 meters; after touching the right cone, the subject returned and touched the center cone and move toward to the start/stop cone, totalizing 40 m with four sudden stops, followed by changes of direction.

The time expend to perform the test was measured using a professional manual chronometer from TIMEX® (Waterburry, USA). Three attempts were done with two to three minutes rest between the attempts, considering the mean of the two best attempts.

Determination of Anaerobic Power

To measure the aerobic power (fatigue index, minimum power, peak power and average power) of the players, the Running-based Anaerobic Sprint Test - RAST (Zacharogiannis, Paradisis, & Tziortzis, 2004) was used. The athlete ran six times 35 m with ten seconds of passive rest between the sprints. The starts of the races were performed in the stop stand position and the time elapsed in each sprint was measured a professional manual chronometer from TIMEX®, as well as the interval between the sprints.

Determination of Lower Limb Power

Horizontal and vertical jump tests were used to assess the fast power of the power of the lower limbs. The vertical jump test was performed using the Ergojump System® (Bosco *et al.*, 1995). The participants were instructed to perform the vertical jump using the countermovement technique. They were positioned in a stand position over the carpet with their feet parallel and hands on hips. It was not allowed to perform any movement with the arms when performing the jump, while the flexion and extension of the lower limbs were allowed (Smirniotou *et al.*, 2008).

Horizontal jump test was also performed from the stand position. The subject started the attempt with his feet parallel and slightly apart, with toes behind the start line. After the command, the volunteer performed an arm swing and a semi flexion of the knees followed by jump itself aiming to reach the longest distance as possible from the starting line. The best attempt of vertical and horizontal jumps among three were considered for the further analysis (Moreira, Souza, & Oliveira, 2003).

Determination of O2MAX and VMAX

In order to access aerobic power of the participants, the Shuttle Run Test was performed (Léger & Lambert, 1982). At the beep from an audio metronome, the participant started a 20 m running. After the first race, the athlete returned to the start line that should be reached exactly when the next beep was provided, running 40 m (scored as a stage). The test was started at 8,5 km/h, and the speed was increased in 1 km/h at the end of each stage.

The time expend to cover the 40 m was progressively reduced. The aim of this test was to complete as many times as possible the distance of 40 m (completing the largest number of stages), finishing the test when the subject was not able to complete the stage two times or interrupted the test voluntarily. The last stage was computed for the O2MAX determination (Krustrup *et al.*, 2006). The Kuipers, Verstappen, Keizer, Geurten, and Kranenburg (1985) equation was used to calculate the maximum intensity (VMAX) reached during the protocol as shown below:

$$VMAX = Ecom + (t/DE) * I$$

Where "Ecom" represents the speed (km/h) in the last stage, "t" is the time (hours) elapsed in the last incomplete stage, "DE" means time (hours) of a complete stage and "I" is the intensity increment (1km/h).

Training Program

The specific game endurance was stimulated during the technical-tactical activities (small sided games) characterized by the use of the same rules of the sport with reduced field and number of players, and formal games (same rules of the game with maximum metabolic intensity) (Moreira, 2006). However, to ensure the development of aerobic power during the preparatory phase, the load of reduced and formal games was increased. The distribution of training content during the preparatory stage is shown in Table 2.

Table 2. Distribution of the training content among different capacities and skills during the preparatory stage.

Training Content	Distribution % (weeks)					
	1	2	3	4	5	6
Aerobic Power	15	15	15	15	15	0
Flexibility/Coordination	15	15	15	15	15	15
Strength	20	20	20	20	20	25
Velocity	15	15	15	15	15	20
Technique-Tactics	35	35	35	35	35	40
Stages	Preparatory					

It is possible to observe that in the sixth week, the aerobic training load was interrupted due to the increase of technical-tactical training, considered intense to maintain the specific game endurance (Coelho *et al.*, 2008; Impellizzeri *et al.*, 2006). There was also an increase in strength and velocity training load.

The distribution of training loads during the competitive stage I and II are described in Table 3. It is observed in the competitive stage, the predominance of technical-tactical training and speed.

Table 3. Distribution of the training content among different capacities and skills during the competitive stage I and II.

Training Content	Distribution % (months)			
	1	2	3	4
Aerobic Power	0	0	0	0
Flexibility/Coordination	10	10	10	10
Strength	25	20	15	15
Velocity	20	25	25	25
Technique-Tactics	45	45	50	50
Stages	Competitive I		Competitive II	

Regarding the training load of the sessions, the training program was organized aiming to respect the progressive increase of stimulus principle of sports training (Moreira *et al.*, 2005).

Training load was measured by multiplying the total time expend to perform the training session by the perception of effort reported by the athletes at the end of training (Foster, 1998), given that it presents a strong correlation between heart rate and high applicability in athletes of collective sports as well as it is a simple, practical and inexpensive method (Impellizzeri, Rampinini, Coutts, Sassi, & Marcora, 2004; Putlur *et al.*, 2004). The dynamics of these variables (load and perceived exertion) along the timeline of this study is presented in Figure 1.

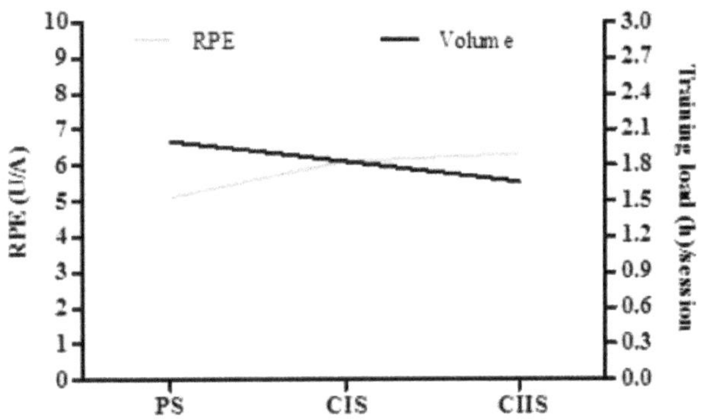

Figure 1. Training load (h) and ratings of perceived exertion (U/A) during the stages of periodization.

PS: Preparatory Stage; CIS: Competitive I Stage; CIIS: Competitive II Stage; RPE: Ratings of perceived exertion.

The training session to develop aerobic power during the preparatory stage in the 1st and 2nd weeks was consisted of five series of three minutes at 90% of VMAX with 90 seconds of active recovery. The 3rd, 4th and 5th weeks were consisted by three sets of five minutes at 95% of VMAX with 90 seconds of active rest. In the competitive stages, the aerobic training was replaced by increasing technical and tactical sessions, performed at high metabolic intensities. In the technical-tactical training sessions, the competition method was carried out aiming to increase the specificity of motor and cognitive-motor adaptations.

The coordinative exercises were used to improve the running technique in high speed, aiming to enable a specific economy of movement in soccer. Regarding flexibility, active stretching and ballistic exercises were performed. Maximum strength and power of lower limbs were stimulated with traction exercises followed by accelerations; jumps; pliometric exercises; active displacements (Tourinho, 2001). The cyclic-acyclic velocity of displacement was stimulated using maximum velocity sprints with and without changes of direction, and in an attempt to make the training sessions more specific, it was emphasized displacements belonging to the soccer game (front, back, side, diagonal) with 10 s of duration and a maximum of 30 m long (Sargentim, 2010).

Statistical analysis

The statistical analysis was performed using the Statistical Package for Social Sciences (SPSS) software for Windows®, version 17.0. The distribution of the data was assessed by Shapiro-Wilk test and external functional markers in the four moments of collection (T0, T1, T2, T3) was tested by repetitive measurements ANOVA and when necessary followed by Tukey-Kramer post test. Performance in the field was characterized using descriptive statistics. The level of significance was set at 5% ($p \leq 0.05$).

Results

Figure 2 illustrates the cyclic-acyclic velocity of displacement dynamics on the four moments of collection. It was found significant differences in the comparisons among T0 with T2 ($p < 0.001$), T0 with T3 ($p < 0.001$), T1 with T2 ($p < 0.001$), T1 with T3 ($p < 0.001$) and T2 with T3 ($p = 0.01$). These results indicate that the training stimulus was not capable to promote increases in the T-40 test in the preparatory stage while in the competitive stages I and II was observed a significant increase.

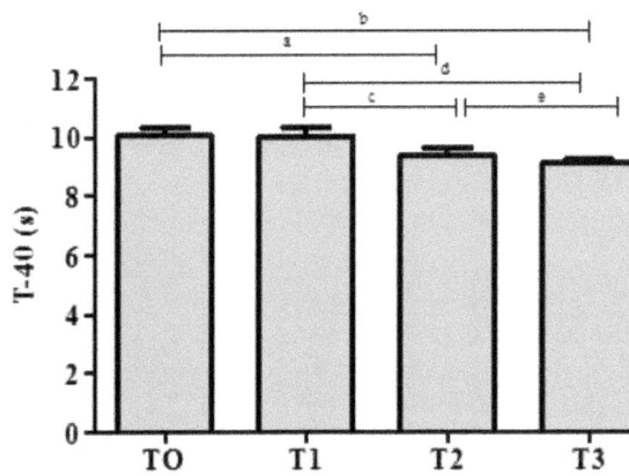

Figure 2. Cyclic-acyclic velocity displacement during the periodization.

a = T0 x T2 ($p < 0.001$); b = T0 x T3 ($p < 0.001$); c = T1 x T2 ($p < 0.001$); d = T1 x T3 ($p < 0.001$); e = T2 x T3 ($p = 0.01$).

Figure 3 shows the RAST test results (average power – A; peak power – B; minimum power – C; fatigue index – D). The average power was significantly increased when T0 was compared to T1, T2 and T3 ($p < 0.001$). However, no differences were found in the comparisons among T1 with T2, T1 with T3 and T2 with T3 ($p > 0.05$). Similar result was found for peak power.

Minimum power was improved when T0 was compared to – T1, T2, T3 (p < 0.001) and T1 with T2 ($p = 0.04$). In the comparisons among T1 to T3 and T2 with T3 no changes were found ($p > 0.05$). For the fatigue index, a difference was found only between T0 and T2 ($p = 0.005$) and T0 and T3 ($p = 0.008$).

In sum, in all variables obtained through the RAST, excepting the fatigue index, training sessions applied in the preparatory stage produced significant increases in the variables. Another important information is that the stimuli of competitive stage I and II were intense enough to maintain the performance levels acquired during the preparatory stage.

Regarding the performance in the horizontal jump (Figure 4 - A), there was significant difference in the comparison between T0 and T2 ($p = 0.006$), T0 and T3 ($p < 0.001$), T1 and T2

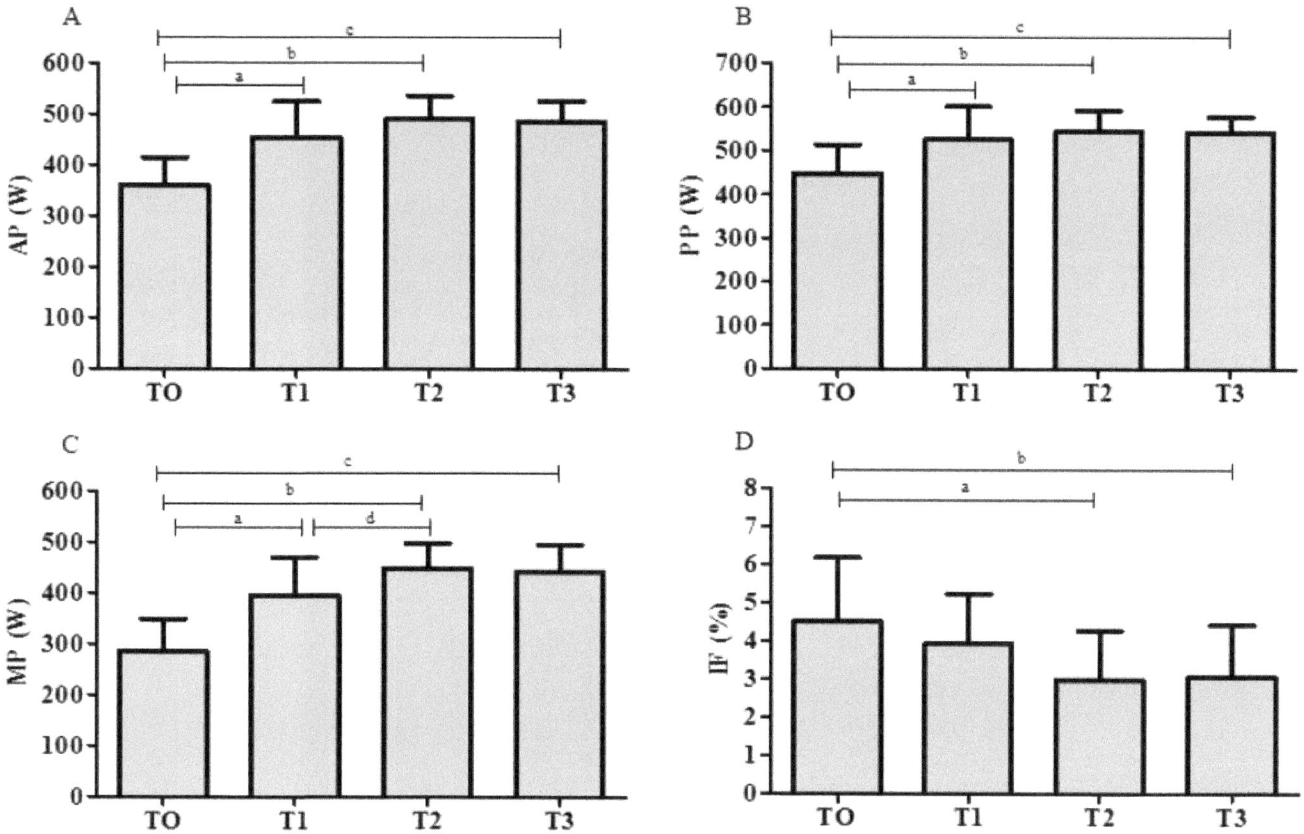

Figure 3. RAST test results.

Average Power (AP) – A, Peak Power (PP) - B, Minimium Power (MP) - C and Index of Fatigue (IF) - D during the periodization. A – a = T0 x T1 ($p < 0.001$); b = T0 x T2 ($p < 0.001$); c = T0 x T3 ($p < 0.001$). B – a = T0 x T1 ($p = 0.001$); b = T0 x T2 ($p < 0.001$); c = T0 x T3 ($p < 0.001$). C - a = T0 x T1 ($p < 0.001$); b = T0 x T2 ($p < 0.001$); c = T0 x T3 ($p < 0.001$); d = T1 x T2 ($p = 0.04$). D – a = T0 x T2 ($p = 0.005$); b = T0 x T3 ($p = 0.008$).

(p = 0:02), T1 and T3 ($p < 0.001$) and T2 with T3 ($p < 0.001$). When comparing T0 with T1 collections, there was not significant difference ($p > 0.05$). The performance in the vertical jump (Figure 4 - B) showed similarities to the horizontal jump, obtaining significant difference ($p \leq 0.05$), in all comparisons between the collections, except in the comparison between T0 with T1 ($p > 0.05$). Therefore, the stimuli offered during the preparatory phase were not able to significantly improve the performance in horizontal and vertical jump. However, during the competitive stage I and II, these variables were significantly increased.

Figure 5 illustrates the average values of O2MAX (A) and VMAX (B). Both variables revealed similar behavior for both indicators. There was a significant difference when T0 was

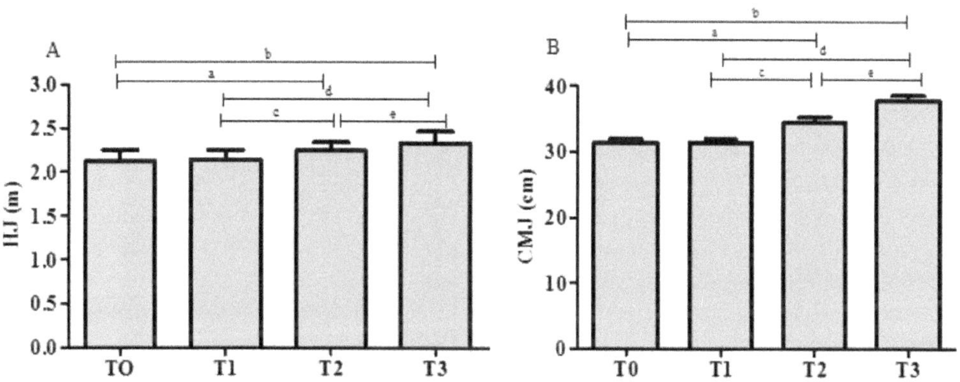

Figure 4. Performances in jumps.

Horizontal Jump (HJ) - A and Countermovement Jump (CMJ) – B tests during the periodization. A – a = T0 x T2 ($p = 0.006$); b = T0 x T3 ($p < 0.001$); c = T1 x T2 ($p = 0.02$); d = T1 x T3 ($p < 0.001$); e = T2 x T3 ($p < 0.001$). B – a = T0 x T2 ($p = 0.01$); b = T0 x T3 ($p < 0.001$); c = T1 x T2 ($p = 0.04$); d = T1 x T3 ($p < 0.001$); e = T2 x T3 ($p = 0.006$).

compared with the other collection times - T1, T2, T3 (p <0.001). Therefore, it is possible to report that preparatory stage was efficient to promote improvements in O2MAX and VMAX. In addition, the competitive stages I and II were able to maintain the performance levels acquired during the preparatory phase.

The match performance analysis during the competition is described in Table 4.

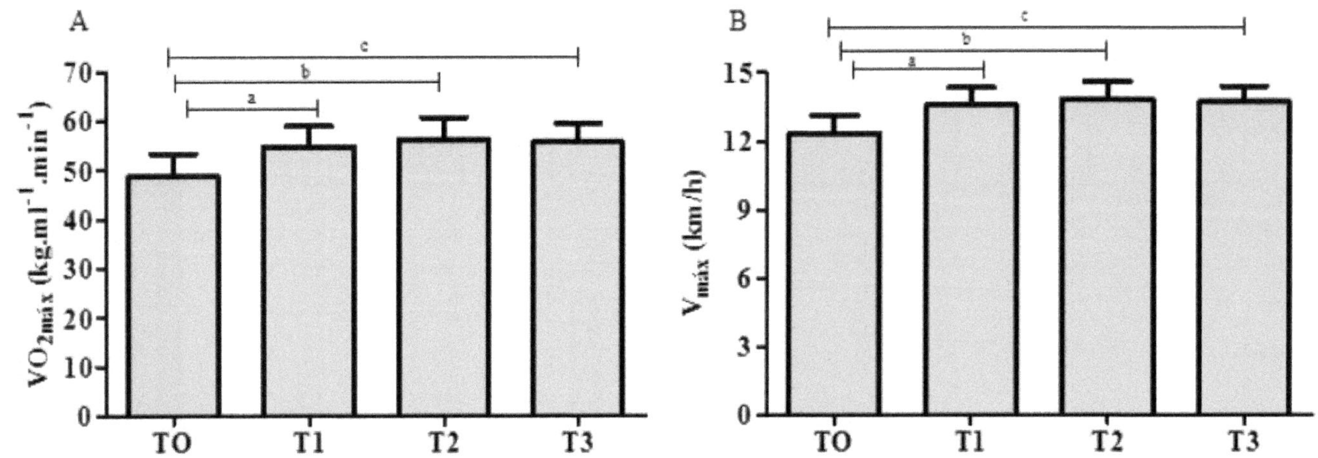

Figure 5. O2MAX and VMAX during the periodization.

A – a = T0 x T1 (p < 0.001); b = T0 x T2 (p < 0.001); c = T0 x T3 (p < 0.001). B – a = T0 x T1 (p = 0.001); b = T0 x T2 (p < 0.001); c = T0 x T3 (p < 0.001).

Table 4. Match performance in the competition during the stages of the periodization.

	Competitive I Stage	Competitive II Stage
N° of Oficial Games	4	6
Disputed Points	12	18
Earned Points	10	15
Use of points (%)	83,33	83,33
Placing	2°	2°

Discussion

The aim of the present study was to observe possible changes in the external markers resulting from an adaptation of the selective loads model and to examine the match performance of the young soccer players, in an attempt to optimize the development of motor and technical-tactical skills along the training program.

The results showed that the proposed periodization significantly affected performance in T-40 test, RAST, horizontal jump, vertical jump and Shuttle Run Test of young soccer players. Concomitantly, there was a satisfactory match performance during the competitive stages (83.33% games won), reaching the final stage and second position in the tournament. Accordingly, previous study analyzed the lower limbs power, acceleration and aerobic power during a macro cycle based on selective loads model in young soccer players of 18-20 years where it was found that eight weeks were not sufficient to promote any increase in this variable (Souza, 2006). However, for acceleration, the same author found significant change after eight weeks of training, which differs from the present study. One possible explanation lies on the structural characteristics of the test used. In our study, it was used the T-40 test, which has rapid and constant changes of direction (cyclic-acyclic), being close to the soccer demands. In contrast, the previous study the analysis of the acceleration was carried out by a linear run of 40 meters (cyclic) (Souza, 2006). This difference in the results was also found by Moreira (2002).

Moreira *et al.* (2005) have demonstrated the effects of a preparatory stage composed by a five week meso cycle based on the selective loads model on lower limbs power and velocity in professional female basketball players. Using the T-40, vertical jumps (squat and countermovement), horizontal jump and unilateral triple horizontal jump (left and right legs), it was observed a significant increase in both variables, differently from our data, showing that these variables did change just after the competitive stage I. It is possible to attribute this difference to the training content used in the preparatory stage in our study, with emphasis on specific endurance (technical-tactical training), aerobic power and strength endurance. Other possible explanation is the fitness of the participants.

Thus, in the present study a trend in increasing cyclic-acyclic speed associated with the lower limbs power was found, showing a similarity of the behavior of these variables along with periodization. In agreement with our study, previous studies found this association (Driss, Vandewalle, & Monod, 1998; Hennessy & Kilty, 2001; Young, McLean, & Ardagna, 1995).

The necessity imposed by soccer imposes a simultaneous training of the strength, endurance and velocity. Therefore, the improvement in one of these variables may affect the development of the other. Thus, the adaptive responses to training is specific to the stimulus offered and may cause an incompatibility between the adjustments, causing the "phenomenon of interference" (Hakkinen *et al.* 2003).

Although the training program of the present study have been proposed the simultaneous stimulus of the different capacities, it is possible to suggest that there was no negative interference of a capacity on the performance in the others. Accordingly, a previous study shows no effects simultaneous training on different capacities in futsal players (Tourinho, 2001).

Although there is need of aerobic in the beginning of the preparatory stage to support the development of other capacities during the periodization, in soccer there is also a need to improve strength (Nunez, Grigoletto, Castillo, Poblador, & Lanc ho, 2008). Therefore, due to the age of the participants (15.1 ± 0.3 years) and the short experience with strength training reported by the athletes, the periodization was used the maximum strength training during the preparatory stage (Gomes, 2009), and the endurance strength. Subsequently, in the competitive stages I and II, the training of power in the legs was conducted. Thus, due to structural characteristics of strength training used in this study, the significant changes in power of the lower limbs were found after 14 weeks of training.

Meylan and Malatesta (2009) verified the influence of a plyometric training program on power related actions of young soccer players (13.1 ± 0.6 years). After eight weeks of training, the authors found increases in cyclic velocity, cyclic-acyclic velocity and power of the lower limbs, demonstrating the efficacy of the plyometric training to develop strength/velocity, corroborating with this study.

In relation to O2MAX and VMAX values, it was found a significant increase after the preparatory stage, occurring the maintenance of the values in competitive stages I and II. It is considered in this study that this maintenance was due to the increase of the training load of technical and tactical skills, stimulated by reduced and formal games. This result corroborates with studies reported in the literature that demonstrate the effectiveness of training programs composed by small sided games on physiological variables, mainly related to aerobic power (Hoff, Wisloff, Engen, Kemi, & Helgerud, 2002; Impellizzeri *et al.*, 2006; Owen, Wong del, Paul, & Dellal, 2012).

Despite the predominance technical and tactical training over the other skills, which may have contributed to the match performance, it was feasible to significantly develop the external functional markers suggesting that the training organization was effective for the technical-tactical and physical improvement in the studied players.

In modern sport, mainly in collective sports, the training programs have been focused on motor skills, maybe under influence of sports physiology. However, it may not be useful to athlete excellent levels of functional markers whether they are not suitable to match situations. This reflection suggests a form of training that encompasses activities in the specific context of game, especially in sports training for young athletes (Pinho, Alves, Greco, & Schild, 2010).

In this study, the periodization was proposed to develop the technical and tactical skills during the stages of the training program, concerning the cognitive processes related to perception, anticipation, decision making capacity and the indexes of strength and velocity.

In addition, a limitation of the present study was the use of T-40 test aiming to measure the agility capacity, since there are other motor tests already recognized and validated to verify this capacity in soccer players, as the Zig Zag Test (Little, & Williams, 2005) eve though the test employed in our study has already been used in previous studies involving collective sports such as basketball, futsal and soccer (Moreira *et al.*, 2005; Thiengo *et al*, 2013; Váczi, Tollár, Meszler, Juhász, & Karsai, 2013).

We conclude that the periodization proposed in this study was effective in significantly raising the indices of the external markers, promoting a satisfactory performance when evaluated by scoring technical abilities along with competitive stages.

References

Barbanti, V.J. (2010). *Treinamento esportivo: as capacidades motoras dos esportistas* (1 ed.). Barueri: Manole.

Bompa, T.O. (2002). *Periodização: teoria e metodologia do treinamento* (4 ed.). São Paulo: Phorte.

Borin, J., Gomes, A., & Leite, G.d.S. (2008). Preparação desportiva: aspectos do controle da carga de treinamento nos jogos coletivos. *Revista da educação física/UEM, 18*(1), 97-105. Retrieved from: http://www.periodicos.uem.br/ojs/index.php/RevEducFis/article/view/3321

Bosco, C., Belli, A., Astrua, M., Tihanyi, J., Pozzo, R., Kellis, S., . . . Tranquilli, C. (1995). A dynamometer for evaluation of dynamic muscle work. *European Journal of Applied Physiology and Occupational Physiology, 70*(5), 379-386. doi: 10.1007/BF00618487

Coelho, D., Matos Rodrigues, de.V., Condessa, L.A., Mortimer, L.d.Á.C.F., Soares, D.D., & Silami-Garcia, E. (2008). Intensidade de sessões de treinamento e jogos oficiais de futebol. *Revista Brasileira de Educação Física e Esporte, 22*(3), 211-218. Retrieved from: http://www.revistasusp.sibi.usp.br/pdf/rbefe/v22n3/v22n3a05.pdf

Driss, T., Vandewalle, H., & Monod, H. (1998). Maximal power and force-velocity relationships during cycling and cranking exercises in volleyball players. Correlation with the vertical jump test. *Journal of Sports Medicine and Physical Fitness 38*(4), 286-293. Retrieved from: http://europepmc.org/abstract/MED/9973770

Foster, C. (1998). Monitoring training in athletes with reference to overtraining syndrome. *Medicine and science in sports and exercise, 30*(7), 1164-1168. doi: 10.1097/00005768-199807000-00023

Garganta, J. (2001). A análise da performance nos jogos desportivos. Revisão acerca da análise do jogo. *Revista Portuguesa de Ciências do Desporto, 1*(1), 57-64. Retrieved from: http://observatorio.esportes.mg.gov.br/wp-content/uploads/2012/07/2001-A-an%C3%A1lise-da-performance-nos-jogos-desportivos-Revis%C3%A3o-acerca-da-an%C3%A1lise-do-jogo-garganta.pdf

Gomes, A.C. (2009). *Treinamento Desportivo: Estrututuração e Periodização* (2ed.). Porto Alegre: Artmed.

Hakkinen, K., Alen, M., Kraemer, W.J., Gorostiaga, E., Izquierdo, M., Rusko, H., . . . Paavolainen, L. (2003). Neuromuscular adaptations during concurrent strength and endurance training versus strength training. *European Journal of Applied Physiology, 89*(1), 42-52. doi: 10.1007/s00421-002-0751-9

Hennessy, L., & Kilty, J. (2001). Relationship of the stretch-shortening cycle to sprint performance in trained female athletes. *Journal of Strength and Conditioning Research, 15*(3), 326-331. Retrieved from: http://journals.lww.com/nsca-jscr/pages/results.aspx?txtkeywords=Relationship+of+the+stretch-shortening+cycle+to+sprint+performance+in+trained+female+athletes.

Hoff, J., Wisloff, U., Engen, L.C., Kemi, O.J., & Helgerud, J. (2002). Soccer specific aerobic endurance training. *British Journal of Sports Medicine, 36*(3), 218-221. Retrieved from: http://bjsm.bmj.com/content/36/3/218

Impellizzeri, F.M., Marcora, S.M., Castagna, C., Reilly, T., Sassi, A., Iaia, F.M., & Rampinini, E. (2006). Physiological and performance effects of generic versus specific aerobic training in soccer players. *International Journal of Sports Medicine, 27*(6), 483-492. doi: 10.1055/s-2005-865839

Impellizzeri, F.M., Rampinini, E., Coutts, A.J., Sassi, A., & Marcora, S.M. (2004). Use of RPE-based training load in soccer. *Medicine and Science in Sports and Exercise, 36*(6), 1042-1047. Retrieved from: http://journals.lww.com/acsm-msse/pages/articleviewer.aspx?year=2004&issue=06000&article=00018&type=abstract

Krustrup, P., Mohr, M., Nybo, L., Jensen, J.M., Nielsen, J.J., & Bangsbo, J. (2006). The Yo-Yo IR2 test: physiological response, reliability, and application to elite soccer. *Medicine and Science in Sports and Exercise, 38*(9), 1666-1673. doi: 10.1249/01.mss.0000227538.20799.08

Kuipers, H., Verstappen, F.T., Keizer, H.A., Geurten, P., & Kranenburg, G. van, (1985). Variability of aerobic performance in the laboratory and its physiologic correlates. *International Journal of Sports Medicine, 6*(4), 197-201. doi: 10.1055/s-2008-1025839

Léger, L.A., & Lambert, J. (1982). A maximal multistage 20-m shuttle run test to predict VO2 max. *European Journal of Applied Physiology and Occupational Physiology, 49*(1), 1-12. Retrieved from: http://download.springer.com/static/pdf/932/art%253A10.1007%252FBF00428958.pdf?auth66=1420575507_108db3fef49de319e0e417a804a81a03&ext=.pdf

Little, T., Williams, A.G. (2005). Specificity of acceleration, maximum speed, and agility in professional soccer players. *Journal of Strength and Conditioning Research, 19*(1), 76-78.

Lopez-Segovia, M., Marques, M.C., Tillaar, R. van den, & Gonzalez-Badillo, J.J. (2011). Relationships between vertical jump and full squat power outputs with sprint times in u21 soccer players. *Journal of Human Kinetics, 30*, 135-144. doi: 10.2478/v10078-011-0081-2

Machado, D., Oikawa, S., & Barbanti, V. (2013). The multicomponent anthropometric model for assessing body composition in a male pediatric population: a simultaneous prediction of fat mass, bone mineral content, and lean soft tissue. *Journal of Obesity, 2013*, 428135. doi: 10.1155/2013/428135

Matvéiev, L., & Ruas, M. (1986). *Fundamentos do treino desportivo* (1 ed.) Lisboa: Livros Horizontes.

Meylan, C., & Malatesta, D. (2009). Effects of in-season plyometric training within soccer practice on explosive actions of young players. *Journal of Strength and Conditioning Research, 23*(9), 2605-2613. doi: 10.1519/JSC.0b013e3181b1f330

Mirwald, R.L., Baxter-Jones, A., Bailey, D.A., & Beunen, G.P. (2002). An assessment of maturity from anthropometric measurements. *Medicine and Science in Sports and Exercise, 34*(4), 689-694. doi: 10.1097/00005768-200204000-00020

Moreira, A. (2002). *Basquetebol: sistema de treinamento em bloco-organização e controle.* (Mestrado), Universidade Estadual de Campinas, Campinas. Retrieved from: http://boletimef.org/biblioteca/705/Basquetebol-sistema-de-treinamento-em-bloco-organizacao-e-controle

Moreira, A. (2006). *A eficácia ea heterocronia das respostas de adaptação de basquetebolistas submetidos a diferentes modelos de estruturação da carga de treinamento e competição.* . (Doutorado), Universidade Estadual de Campinas, Campinas. Retrieved from: http://www.nuteses.temp.ufu.br/tde_busca/arquivo.php?codArquivo=6501&acordo=

Moreira, A., Okano, A.H., Souza, M., Oliveira, P.R., & Gomes, A.C. (2005). Sistema de cargas seletivas no basquetebol durante um mesociclo de preparação: implicações sobre a velocidade e as diferentes manifestações de força. *Revista Brasileira de Ciência e Movimento, 13*(3), 7-16. Retrieved from: http://portalrevistas.ucb.br/index.php/RBCM/article/viewFile/639/650

Moreira, A., Oliveira, P.R., Ronque, E.R.V., Okano, A.H., & Souza, M. (2008). Análise de diferentes modelos de estruturação da carga de treinamento e competição no desempenho de basquetebolistas no Yo-yo intermittent endurance test. *Revista Brasileira de Ciências do Esporte, 29*(2). Retrieved from: http://www.rbceonline.org.br/revista/index.php/RBCE/article/view/124

Moreira, A., Souza, M., & Oliveira, P.R. (2003). A velocidade de deslocamento no basquetebol. *Revista Brasileira de Ciências do Esporte, 24*(2). Retrieved from: http://rbceonline.org.br/revista/index.php/RBCE/article/view/367

Nunez, V.M., Da Silva-Grigoletto, M.E., Castillo, E.F., Poblador, M.S., & Lancho, J.L. (2008). Effects of training exercises for the development of strength and endurance in soccer. *Journal of Strength and Conditioning Research, 22*(2), 518-524. doi: 10.1519/JSC.0b013e318163468f

Owen, A.L., Wong del, P., Paul, D., & Dellal, A. (2012). Effects of a periodized small-sided game training intervention on physical performance in elite professional soccer. *Journal of Strength and Conditioning Research, 26*(10), 2748-2754. doi: 10.1519/JSC.0b013e318242d2d1

Pinho, S.T., Alves, D.M., Greco, P.J., & Schild, J.F.G. (2010). Método situacional e sua influência no conhecimento tático processual de escolares. *Motriz, 16*(3), 580-590. Retrieved from: http://www.scielo.br/pdf/motriz/v16n3/a05v16n3.pdf

Putlur, P., Foster, C., Miskowski, J.A., Kane, M.K., Burton, S.E., Scheett, T.P., & McGuigan, M.R. (2004). Alteration of immune function in women collegiate soccer players and college students. *Journal of Sports Science and Medicine, 3*(4), 234-243. Retrieved from: http://www.ncbi.nlm.nih.gov/pmc/articles/PMC3938062/pdf/jssm-03-234.pdf

Sargentim, S. (2010). *Treinamento de força no futebol* (1 ed.) São Paulo: Phorte.

Smirniotou, A., Katsikas, C., Paradisis, G., Argeitaki, P., Zacharogiannis, E., & Tziortzis, S. (2008). Strength-power parameters as predictors of sprinting performance. *Journal of Sports Medicine and Physical Fitness 48*(4), 447-454. Retrieved from: http://europepmc.org/abstract/MED/18997647

Souza, E.N. (2006). *Alterações das capacidades físicas de jovens futebolistas durante o macrociclo de treinamento: estudo a partir da periodização de cargas seletivas.* (Mestrado), Universidade Metodista de Piracicaba, Piracicaba. Retrieved from: http://www.unimep.br/phpg/bibdig/pdfs/2006/GHKTCUYCMFWV.pdf

Thiengo, C.R., Talamoni, G.A., Silva, R.N.B.d., Morceli, H.d.S., Porfírio, J.C., Santos, J.W., & Drigo, A.J. (2013). Effect of the periodization model with selective loads on motor abilities during a preparatory mesocycle in futsal players. *Revista Brasileira de Ciências do Esporte, 35*(4), 1035-1050. Retrieved from: http://www.scielo.br/pdf/rbce/v35n4/15.pdf

Tourinho, H. Filho. (2001). *Periodização de regimes de treinamentos antagônicos: um estudo sobre o futsal.* (Doutorado), Universidade de São Paulo, São Paulo. Retrieved from: http://www.nuteses.temp.ufu.br/tde_busca/arquivo.php?codArquivo=5731&acordo=

Váczi, M., Tollár, J., Meszler, B., Juhász, I., Karsai, I. (2013). Short-term high intensity plyometric traning program improves strength, power and agility in male soccer players. *Journal of Human Kinetics, 36*, 17-21. Retrieved from: http://www.ncbi.nlm.nih.gov/pmc/articles/PMC3661889/pdf/jhk-36-17.pdf

Young, W., McLean, B., & Ardagna, J. (1995). Relationship between strength qualities and sprinting performance. *Journal of Sports Medicine and Physical Fitness 35*(1), 13-19. Retrieved from: http://europepmc.org/abstract/MED/7474987

Zacharogiannis, E., Paradisis, G., & Tziortzis, S. (2004). An evaluation of tests of anaerobic power and capacity. *Medicine and Science in Sports and Exercise, 36*(5), S116. doi: 10.1249/00005768-200405001-00549

Zakharov, A. (1992). *Ciência do treinamento desportivo* (1 ed.) Rio de Janeiro: Palestra Sport.

Autor's note

Rodrigo Leal de Queiroz Thomaz de Aquino is affiliated with University of Porto, Portugal. Luiz Guilherme Cruz Gonçalves, Lucas de Paula Oliveira, Hugo Tourinho Filho and Enrico Fuini Puggina are affiliated with University of São Paulo. Research group in Physical Performance and Sport Training.

Acknowledgments

CAPES (Coordenação de Aperfeiçoamento de Pessoal de Nível Superior) for the financial support.

Corresponding author

Enrico Fuini Puggina
Av. Bandeirantes, 3900, Monte Alegre, Ribeirão Preto, SP, Brazil.
Email: enrico@usp.br

9

Technical-tactical performance profile of the block and dig according to competition category in men's volleyball

Antonio García-de-Alcaraz
Faculty of Physical Activity and Sport Sciences, Polytechnic University of Madrid, Spain

Enrique Ortega
Faculty of Sport Sciences, University of Murcia, Spain

José M. Palao
University of Wisconsin-Parkside, United States

Abstract—The aim of this study was to analyse the technical-tactical performance profile of blocking and court defence actions for various age groups and categories of competition in men's volleyball. The sample comprised 16,454 blocks and 8,321 digs performed in 299 sets in several categories of competition (from U-14 to Olympic Games). A descriptive and correlational inter- and intra-group observational design was used. The variables studied were: category of competition, opponent's spike tempo, and block and dig performance. The results showed a significant increase in the percentage of blocks and digs derived from fast attacks and a significant improvement in performance of these actions to counteract slow attacks. Thus, improving in blocking and digging performance was observed at higher categories when the attack is performed slowly. This paper discusses various reasons for the evolution in defensive performance and the effects on the training process for various categories of competition in volleyball.

Keywords: team sports, performance, match analysis, volleyball

Introduction

In a volleyball play, the defending team tries to neutralise or restrain the opponent's offense through defensive actions such as blocking and court defence. The block is a team's first line of defence, and it aims to intercept, stop, or restrain the opponent's offensive actions (Selinger & Ackermann-Blount, 1985). The main objective of court defence is to control the ball that was attacked by the opponent to send it to the setter and, thus, counterattack (Stone, 2002). Block and court defence performance depend on how an opponent's spike (e.g. attack tempo, distance from the ball, previous displacements) is performed (Selinger & Ackermann-Blount, 1985) as well as on variables that determine the opponent′s offense (e.g. setter's zone, available hitters, attack area) (Afonso & Mesquita, 2011). The interaction of various game actions determines the performance of defensive actions such that performance may vary according to the age group and/or competition level. These changes are determined by players′ maturity (e.g. greater height, weight, reach) (Malina & Bouchard, 1991), progress in the training process (e.g. higher speed, better technical execution), and changes in game regulations (e.g. net height, libero), which may occur as players progress from one category to the next.

Block performance is associated with players′ anthropometric features (e.g. height, weight, etc.), and behavioural and psychological abilities (e.g. reaction time) (Stamm, Stamm, & Thomson, 2005). One reason for this association is the fact that the height reached over the net is crucial (Grgantov, Katic, & Jankovic, 2006; Stanganelli, Dourado, Oncken, Mancan, & Costa, 2008), as it enables an appropriate technical-tactical execution. On the other hand, court defence performance requires the development of physiological factors (e.g. strength, flexibility, etc.), technical-tactical factors (hand-eye coordination, etc.), and psychological factors (optimal activation for a quick reaction to the opponent's attack) (Stone, 2002). Most of these performance factors are limited when the opponent's spike is carried out quickly. These quick attacks force defenders to react and move in the shortest possible time. Thus, quick attacks have greater efficiency (Bergeles & Nikolaidou, 2011; Castro, Souza, & Mesquita, 2011; Costa *et al.*, 2011; Palao, Santos, & Ureña, 2007) on account of the conditions in which the block is performed (Afonso, Mesquita, Marcelino, & Silva, 2010) and limited defensive movements.

Despite the relationship between the spike and defensive actions, there is a lack of reference values in the scientific literature pertaining to technical-tactical performance of the block and court defences that take into consideration the opponent's spike tempo according to the various categories of competition. Reference values may be helpful in guiding training process and improving the performance of these actions. This study is the first step in establishing a technical-tactical performance profile of blocking and court defence. The aim was to assess technical-tactical performance profiles of blocking and court defence for various categories of competition in men's volleyball.

Method

Population and sample

The sample was made up of teams and players participating in matches and sets in Spain´s U-14, U-16, and U-19 men's championships (2008-2009 season), Spain´s first division (national senior category, 2008-2009 and 2009-2010 seasons), and the 2008 Olympic Games (international senior category). The analysed actions comprised 16,454 blocks and 8,321 digs. These actions were played by 99 teams in 299 sets. Fifty-nine sets were randomly selected from the Olympic Games, while sixty sets were randomly selected from the other categories. The sets were stratified in terms of "performance level" (one of three rankings) and "quality of opposition" (six different options according to rival's level of performance). Given the different structure of the fifth set (FIVB, 2008), it was not included in the sample.

All matches were video recorded after the organizing committee had given consent. In the case of the Olympics, matches were not filmed, but downloaded from open online channels such as NBC. The process did not affect players´ and teams´ spontaneous behaviour, as filming is a common, non-invasive procedure typically used by coaches. This study complied with the Bioethics Commission of the University of Murcia (Spain) and with the ethical principles stated by the Declaration of Helsinki.

Design

A descriptive, correlational, observational (nomothetic, intra sessional, and multidimensional) design were implemented through of a category system (Anguera, 2003). The study´s variables were: a) category of competition (U-14, U-16, U-19, national senior, and international senior); b) attack tempo (first, second, or third tempo); and c) the performance of the block and dig. A first, second, or third tempo block or dig was an action or attempted action responding to a first, second, or third tempo spike, respectively. Block and dig performance were measured in terms of the defending team's ability to counterattack under the best possible conditions. The performance of the block was measured in terms of the opponent's ability to continue the play when the ball is returned to their court or in terms of the defending team's ability to continue the play when the ball remains in their court (Table 1). Performance of the dig was measured in terms of the defending team's ability to continue the play (Table 2).

Table 1. Variables for block performance.

Value	Category	Description
0	Error	Block error. Point is lost after block contact
0	Error (fault)	Block error. Point is lost because blocker commits a fault (touching the net, penetration, etc.)
1	Negative block	Block continuity. The blocking team cannot set up a counterattack, but when the ball is in the opponent's court, the opposing team can counterattack
3	Positive block	Block continuity. The blocking team can set up a counterattack, and if the ball remains in the opponent's court, the opponent cannot counterattack
4	Point	Block point. The player who blocks sends it to the court on the other side of the net

Table 2. Variables for dig performance.

Value	Category	Description
0	Error	Dig error. Point is lost after dig contact
1	Negative dig	Dig continuity. The digging team continues the play but is not able to set up a counterattack, or the ball is sent to the opponent's court after digging
3	Positive dig	Dig continuity. The digging team continues the play and maintains the possibility of setting up a counterattack

Procedure and instruments

Competitions were recorded on video cameras placed at the end of the court and at a height higher than the net, except for the matches from the Olympic Games where filming took place from the sides and back of the court. It was ensured that the official court area (18 x 9 m) would be recorded, at a minimum, to allow clear viewing of all actions. Regular video cameras positioned on tripods and plugged in with extension cords were used. For the national senior category, matches were also downloaded from an official website.

Technical-tactical actions were observed by a single observer, who was licensed in sport science, was a volleyball coach with the highest coach certification in Spain, and had over ten years of experience in volleyball training and performance analysis. To assess the adequacy of data coding and variables, a training process which included analysing twelve national senior-category matches was undertaken before starting the research study. The videos were observed in the month after the end of each tournament. The consistency analysis (Cronbach's Alpha) was conducted with two observers who were volleyball coaches with over two years of experience in performance analysis, and in the use of the observational software used in this study, and who held the highest national coach certification. For the inter-observer reliability analysis, 25% of sets from the national senior category were randomly selected and observed. Analyses showed a reliability of 0.865 for blocking and 0.820 for court defence. For intra-reliability analysis, 20% of sets from each category of competition were randomly selected and observed. Analyses showed a reliability of 0.872 for blocking and 0.864 for court defence.

While observing, variables were recorded with the Data Volley software (Data Volley 2007, Data Project Sport Software, Bologna, Italy). Recorded actions were then synchronised with video images by means of Data Video (Data Video 2007, Data Project Sport Software, Bologna, Italy), so that the quality of the data could later be analysed. The data were collected and exported from Data Volley 2007 software using the observation tool´s internal spreadsheets. Each spreadsheet contained players´ and teams´ performance during sets. All spreadsheets were merged into a single matrix in which contextual variables (category, team level, type of match, set result, game system, initial line-up, substitutions, and role of players) were added. SPSS 15.0.0 (Statistical Package for the Social Sciences, IBM, Armonk, United States) was used for descriptive and inferential analyses. The sample size was analysed in order to check the stability of data (Hughes & Daniel, 2003). For all tested categories, stability occurred starting at the 17th set, in the case of the block, and starting at the 10th set, in the case of court defence.

Statistical analysis

A descriptive analysis for the various actions and types of actions in every category of competition was performed. Frequency (number of actions or type of actions), relative frequency (relative measure for frequency), mean actions (team´s mean value for the entire set), coefficient (mean value of performance of an action or type of action), efficacy (percentage of maximum performance of an action or type of action), efficiency (percentage of maximum value of an action when subtracting errors), and ratios (block point-to-error or positive-dig-to-negative-dig) were calculated. Coefficient, efficacy, efficiency and ratio were calculated using players' mean values per set. The following inferential tests were performed: a) Kolmogorov-Smirnov test to analyse normality of data; b) Kruskal-Wallis test ($p < 0.05$) to identify differences among categories; c) Wilcoxon test ($p < 0.05$) to analyse differences within each category; and d) Mann Whitney U procedure with post hoc Bonferroni ($p < 0.01$) to analyse specific differences between categories.

Results

Results showed that at the initial stages (U-14, U-16, and U-19), the percentage of blocks with ball contact was significantly lower than the percentage of blocks with no ball contact (Table 3). These differences were not significant at later stages. At higher categories, the percentage of ball contacts increased significantly. Beginning with the U-14 category, the percentage of attack situations in which there were no block actions decreased significantly. The percentage of block attempts decreased significantly starting in the U-19 category. Regarding the tempo utilised to block, a predominance of third tempo blocks was observed in initiation stages (U-14, U-16 and U-19), and a predominance of second tempo blocks was observed in the senior stage. In higher categories; however, first and second tempo blocks increased significantly, while third tempo blocks decreased significantly. Starting at the U-16 category, all changes were significant, except for first and third tempo blocks, which changed significantly starting at the U-19 category.

Table 3. Number of blocks, mean team blocks per set, percentage of blocks per player per set, and statistically significant differences among categories.

	U-14			U-16			U-19			National			International		
	n	Mean	%	n	Mean	%	n	Mean	%	n	Mean	%	n	Mean	%
Attempted blocks	1710	14.25	56.58^{A}	1887	15.73	54.31^{A}	1769	14.74	$50.91^{\uparrow A}$	1636	13.63	$49.38^{\uparrow *}$	1445	12.25	$46.15^{\uparrow * \downarrow}$
1st tempo	37	0.31	2.22	98	0.82	$5.26^{\uparrow}$	360	3.00	$20.72^{\uparrow *}$	397	3.31	$24.20^{\uparrow *}$	351	2.97	$23.94^{\uparrow *}$
2nd tempo	0	0.00	0.00^{a}	56	0.47	$2.80^{\uparrow a}$	125	1.04	$7.33^{\uparrow a}$	771	6.43	$47.57^{\uparrow * \downarrow a}$	834	7.07	$58.02^{\uparrow * \downarrow \backslash a}$
3rd tempo	1673	13.94	97.78^{ab}	1733	14.44	$91.94^{\uparrow ab}$	1284	10.70	$71.95^{\uparrow * ab}$	468	3.90	$28.24^{\uparrow * \downarrow b}$	260	2.20	$18.03^{\uparrow * \downarrow \backslash ab}$
Contacted blocks	642	5.35	20.70	1172	9.77	$33.04^{\uparrow}$	1347	11.23	$38.39^{\uparrow *}$	1541	12.84	$46.19^{\uparrow * \downarrow}$	1516	12.85	$47.82^{\uparrow * \downarrow}$
1st tempo	37	0.31	6.63	76	0.63	6.34	231	1.93	$17.82^{\uparrow *}$	315	2.63	$20.34^{\uparrow *}$	242	2.05	$16.28^{\uparrow *}$
2nd tempo	0	0.00	0.00^{a}	34	0.28	$2.40^{\uparrow a}$	88	0.73	$6.61^{\uparrow * a}$	755	6.29	$49.30^{\uparrow * \downarrow a}$	831	7.04	$54.96^{\uparrow * \downarrow \backslash a}$
3rd tempo	605	5.04	93.37^{ab}	1062	8.85	91.27^{ab}	1028	8.57	$75.57^{\uparrow * ab}$	471	3.93	$30.36^{\uparrow * \downarrow ab}$	443	3.75	$28.76^{\uparrow * \downarrow ab}$
No blocks	660	5.50	22.72^{B}	443	3.69	$12.65^{\uparrow AB}$	350	2.92	$10.19^{\uparrow * AB}$	149	1.24	$4.43^{\uparrow * \downarrow AB}$	187	1.58	$6.04^{\uparrow * \downarrow \backslash AB}$
Total	3012	25.10	100	3502	29.18	100	3466	28.88	100	3326	27.72	100	3148	26.68	100

Note. $^{\uparrow}p < .01$ when compared to U-14. $^{*}p < .01$ when compared to U-16. $^{\downarrow}p < .01$ when compared to U-19. $^{\backslash}p < .01$ when compared to national category. [A] Significant differences when compared to "Contacted blocks". [B] Significant differences when compared to "Attempted blocks". [a] Significant differences when compared to "1st tempo block". [b] Significant differences when compared to "2nd tempo block".

When analysing the performance of first tempo blocks (Table 4), a predominance of block points in the U-14 category and of block errors in the other categories were observed. Block errors increased significantly beginning in the U-19 category, while block errors due to faults decreased significantly starting at U-16. When analysing the performance of second tempo blocks (Table 4), a predominance of block errors in all categories was found, except for the U-14 category in which there were no such attacks. A statistically significant increase in positive blocks was detected when comparing senior categories (national and international) with U-19. As to the performance of third tempo blocks (Table 4), a predominance of block errors in all categories was observed. Regarding the national category, the evolution of performance of third tempo blocks showed a statistically significant decrease in errors due to faults and negative blocks. In contrast, a statistically significant increase in block points was found.

Table 4. Performance of contacted blocks with regard to spike tempo, and statistically significant differences between categories.

		U-14			U-16			U-19			National			International		
		n	Mean	%	n	Mean	%	n	Mean	%	n	Mean	%	n	Mean	%
1st tempo block	Error	4	0.03	11.67	21	0.18	25.98	73	0.61	30.07$^{\uparrow}$	113	0.94	37.02$^{\uparrow}$	105	0.89	42.88$^{\uparrow *}$
	Error (rule)	6	0.05	16.67	1	0.01	1.09$^{\uparrow a}$	10	0.08	3.82^{a}	8	0.07	2.08^{a}	4	0.03	2.18$^{\uparrow a}$
	Negative block	7	0.06	16.67	22	0.18	24.60^{b}	54	0.45	20.91^{b}	77	0.64	21.90^{ab}	34	0.29	15.00^{ab}
	Positive block	8	0.07	25.00	18	0.15	24.96^{b}	47	0.39	23.33^{b}	63	0.53	20.25^{ab}	61	0.52	25.00^{abc}
	Point	12	0.10	30.00	14	0.12	23.37^{b}	47	0.39	21.87^{b}	54	0.45	18.74^{ab}	38	0.32	14.94^{abd}
Total		37	0.31	100	76	0.63	100	231	1.93	100	315	2.63	100	242	2.05	100
2nd tempo block	Error	0	0.00	-	13	0.11	41.12	36	0.30	49.28	358	2.98	46.36	393	3.33	48.62
	Error (rule)	0	0.00	-	0	0.00	0.00^{a}	2	0.02	1.90^{a}	16	0.13	2.36^{a}	13	0.11	1.83^{a}
	Negative block	0	0.00	-	8	0.07	22.89^{b}	14	0.12	16.42^{ab}	118	0.98	16.92^{ab}	105	0.89	12.78^{ab}
	Positive block	0	0.00	-	6	0.05	19.69^{b}	15	0.13	11.33^{ab}	140	1.17	18.19$^{\downarrow ab}$	162	1.37	18.78$^{\downarrow abc}$
	Point	0	0.00	-	7	0.06	16.30^{b}	21	0.18	21.06^{ab}	123	1.03	16.17^{ab}	158	1.34	18.00^{abc}
Total		0	0.00	-	34	0.28	100	88	0.73	100	755	6.29	100	831	7.04	100
3rd tempo block	Error	225	1.88	38.01	359	2.99	33.90	359	2.99	36.70	157	1.31	33.87	140	1.19	32.10
	Error (rule)	35	0.29	6.26^{a}	71	0.59	7.29^{a}	55	0.46	5.87^{a}	12	0.10	2.81$^{\uparrow * \downarrow a}$	6	0.05	1.36$^{\uparrow * \downarrow a}$
	Negative block	119	0.99	17.89^{ab}	211	1.76	18.44^{ab}	229	1.91	20.27^{ab}	83	0.69	17.14^{ab}	68	0.58	15.14$^{* \downarrow ab}$
	Positive block	123	1.03	21.49^{ab}	243	2.03	22.47^{abc}	235	1.96	22.49^{ab}	92	0.77	18.30^{ab}	117	0.99	25.24^{bc}
	Point	103	0.86	16.35^{ab}	178	1.48	17.90^{abd}	150	1.25	14.68^{abcd}	127	1.06	27.88$^{\uparrow * \downarrow bcd}$	112	0.95	26.15$^{\downarrow bc}$
Total		605	5.04	100	1062	8.85	100	1028	8.57	100	471	3.93	100	443	3.75	100

Note. $^{\uparrow}p < .01$ when compared to U-14. $^{*}p < .01$ when compared to U-16. $^{\downarrow}p < .01$ when compared to U-19. $^{\backslash}p < .01$ when compared to national category. [a] Significant differences when compared to "error". [b] Significant differences when compared to "rule error". [c] Significant differences when compared to "negative block". [d] Significant differences when compared to "positive block".

As for statistical parameters of total blocks (Table 5), a statistically significant decrease in the block point-to-error ratio between U-14 and senior categories (national and international) and a statistically significant increase in this same variable between U-14 and U-19 were found. Also, a statistically significant increase in efficacy starting at the national senior category was found. When analysing statistical parameters of first and second tempo blocks, there was a significant increase in the block point-to-error ratio as of the national senior category. Furthermore, there was a significant increase in the percentage of errors in first tempo blocks between the U-16 and international senior categories. Regarding the third tempo block, an increase in the coefficient, efficacy, and efficiency beginning with the senior national category was observed, while a statistically significant decrease in percentage of error (between the initiation categories and the international senior category) and in the block point-to-error ratio (beginning with U-19) was also observed.

For court defence (Table 6), there was a significant predominance of digs with ball contact versus digs without ball contact throughout all categories. From the senior category upwards, a significant decrease in the percentage of digs with ball contact and a significant increase in the percentage of digs without ball contact were observed. For both types of dig, a predominance of third tempo actions at initial stages (U-14, U-16 and U-19) and of second tempo actions at senior stages (national and international) were found. A statistically significant increase in digs for first and second tempo attacks and a statistically significant decrease in digs for third tempo attacks were observed. These changes were significant beginning with U-16, except for first and third tempo digs with ball contact, which increased significantly from the U-19 category upwards.

Table 5. Block performance values and statistically significant differences between categories.

Type of block	Statistical data	U-14		U-16		U-19		National		International	
		Mean	SD	Mean	SD	Mean	SD	Mean	SD	Mean	SD
Total Blocks	Coefficient	1.51	0.85	1.59	0.58	1.50	0.48	1.54	0.43	1.57	0.52
	Efficacy (%)	17.28	17.90	18.14	14.42	15.98	11.70	20.02↓	11.39	19.72↓	11.61
	Error (%)	43.80	27.41	40.17	16.64	41.11	16.67	43.35	12.92	45.32	15.53
	Efficiency (%)	-26.52	38.53	-22.03	24.54	-25.13	22.93	-23.33	20.60	-25.60	23.21
	Point:error	1:2.35	1.78	1:2.34	1.79	1:2.45↑	2.01	1:2.18↑	1.90	1:2.15↑	1.82
1st tempo block	Coefficient	2.12	1.60	1.93	1.46	1.78	1.24	1.58	1.15	1.50	1.16
	Efficacy (%)	30.00	44.72	23.37	40.28	21.87	31.24	18.74	28.19	14.94	26.41
	Error (%)	28.33	42.92	27.07	39.55	33.89	35.29	39.10	35.41	45.06*	37.27
	Efficiency (%)	1.67	73.68	-3.70	65.67	-12.02	56.09	-20.36	53.55	-30.13	52.75
	Point:error	1:0.83	0.32	1:1.57	0.60	1:1.77	0.96	1:2.24↑	1.05	1:2.87↑	0.73
2nd tempo block	Coefficient	.	.	1.47	1.13	1.35	1.38	1.36	0.69	1.41	0.73
	Efficacy (%)	.	.	16.30	19.84	21.06	31.54	16.17	15.20	18.00	16.97
	Error (%)	.	.	41.12	38.41	51.19	42.10	48.72	20.94	50.45	20.09
	Efficiency (%)	.	.	-24.82	46.93	-30.13	66.62	-32.55	30.95	-32.45	32.95
	Point:error	.	.	1:1.86	0.66	1:1.81	0.68	1:3.04↓	1.70	1:2.57↓	1.64
3rd tempo block	Coefficient	1.48	0.87	1.58	0.58	1.46	0.59	1.84↑*↓	0.94	1.95↑*↓	1.03
	Efficacy (%)	16.35	17.83	17.90	14.83	14.68	13.14	27.88↑*↓	24.66	26.15↓	27.36
	Error (%)	44.27	28.34	41.19	17.80	42.57	20.71	36.68	26.05	33.46↑*↓	28.59
	Efficiency (%)	-27.92	39.59	-23.29	25.05	-27.89	27.91	-8.80↑*↓	44.13	-7.31↑*↓	47.64
	Point:error	1:2.52	1.80	1:2.42	1.82	1:2.76↑	1.69	1:1.33↑*↓	0.95	1:1.30↑*↓	1.08

Note. ↑$p < .01$ when compared to U-14. *$p < .01$ when compared to U-16. ↓$p < .01$ when compared to U-19. \$p < .01$ when compared to national category.

Table 6. Number of digs, mean team digs per set, percentage of digs per player per set, and statistically significant differences between categories.

	U-14			U-16			U-19			National			International		
	n	Mean	%	n	Mean	%	n	Mean	%	n	Mean	%	n	Mean	%
Non-contacted dig	344	2.87	18.42^{A}	389	3.24	20.68^{A}	362	3.02	22.01^{A}	500	4.17	$34.19^{\uparrow * \downarrow A}$	544	4.61	$38.73^{\uparrow * \downarrow A}$
1st tempo	19	0.16	5.72	54	0.45	$13.35^{\uparrow}$	94	0.78	$25.67^{\uparrow *}$	182	1.52	$37.74^{\uparrow * \downarrow}$	175	1.48	$31.39^{\uparrow *}$
2nd tempo	0	0.00	0.00^{a}	14w	0.12	$3.96^{\uparrow a}$	31	0.26	$6.91^{\uparrow a}$	221	1.84	$43.64^{\uparrow * \downarrow}$	306	2.59	$57.28^{\uparrow * \downarrow \backslash a}$
3rd tempo	325	2.71	94.28^{ab}	321	2.68	$82.69^{\uparrow ab}$	237	1.98	$67.42^{\uparrow * ab}$	97	0.81	$18.61^{\uparrow * \downarrow ab}$	63	0.53	$11.32^{\uparrow * \downarrow \backslash ab}$
Contacted digs	1592	13.27	81.58	1481	12.34	79.32	1256	10.47	77.99	998	8.32	$65.81^{\uparrow * \downarrow}$	855	7.25	$61.27^{\uparrow * \downarrow}$
1st tempo	114	0.95	6.80	115	0.96	7.68	258	2.15	$20.81^{\uparrow *}$	218	1.82	$22.21^{\uparrow *}$	172	1.46	$20.19^{\uparrow *}$
2nd tempo	0	0.00	0.00^{a}	38	0.32	$2.33^{\uparrow a}$	72	0.60	$6.28^{\uparrow a}$	444	3.70	$44.67^{\uparrow * \downarrow a}$	448	3.80	$51.44^{\uparrow * \downarrow \backslash a}$
3rd tempo	1478	12.32	93.20^{ab}	1328	11.07	89.99^{ab}	926	7.72	$72.90^{\uparrow * ab}$	336	2.80	$33.13^{\uparrow * \downarrow ab}$	235	1.99	$28.37^{\uparrow * \downarrow ab}$
Total	1936	16.13	100	1870	15.58	100	1618	13.48	100	1498	12.48	100	1399	11.86	100

Note. ↑$p < .01$ when compared to U-14. *$p < .01$ when compared to U-16. ↓$p < .01$ when compared to U-19. \$p < .01$ when compared to national category. [A] Significant differences when compared to "Contacted digs". [a] Significant differences when compared to "1st tempo dig". [b] Significant differences when compared to "2nd tempo dig".

When analysing first tempo digs (Table 7), predominance of positive digs in U-14, U-16, and U-19 and of dig errors in the senior national and international categories were observed. An increase in errors beginning at U-19 and a statistically significant decrease in negative and positive digs starting at the national senior category were found. Concerning second tempo digs (Table 7), there was a predominance of dig errors in all categories, except for U-14 as no data were recorded. There were no differences between categories for the evolution of performance of this action, yet a decrease in negative digs and an increase in positive digs were observed. Regarding the analysis of third tempo digs (Table 7), a predominance of positive digs in all categories was observed. There was a significant decrease in dig errors (between the U-14 and international senior categories) as well as in negative digs (starting with the U-19 category). On the other hand, an increase in positive digs beginning with the U-16 category was observed.

When analysing the statistical data of the total number of digs and first tempo digs (Table 8), there was a significant increase in the percentage of error and in the positive-dig-to-negative-dig ratio as well as a significant decrease in the coefficient, efficiency, and effectiveness. All these changes were significant starting at the national senior level, except for the first tempo defence ratio variable, which showed a significant increase in the beginning at the U-19 category. For the second tempo dig, a significant increase in the positive-dig-to-negative-dig ratio between the national category and U-16 was observed. For the third tempo defence, there were an increase in the coefficient, efficiency (starting at U-19), and efficiency (starting with the national category) and decrease in the percentage of errors (for the international senior category) and in the ratio (starting at the national category).

Table 7. Performance of contacted digs with regard to spike tempo, and statistically significant differences between categories.

		U-14			U-16			U-19			National			International		
		n	Mean	%	n	Mean	%	n	Mean	%	n	Mean	%	n	Mean	%
1st tempo dig	Error	22	0.18	17.63	29	0.24	21.64	79	0.66	$30.48^{\uparrow}$	118	0.98	$55.15^{\uparrow *\downarrow}$	89	0.75	$53.83^{\uparrow *\downarrow}$
	Negative dig	2 9	0.24	25.72	27	0.23	23.23	63	0.53	23.55	32	0.27	$13.72^{\downarrow a}$	15	0.13	$7.87^{\uparrow *\downarrow a}$
	Positive dig	63	0.53	56.64^{ab}	59	0.49	55.13^{ab}	116	0.97	45.98^{b}	68	0.57	$31.13^{\uparrow *\downarrow ab}$	68	0.58	$38.30^{\uparrow b}$
Total		114	0.95	100	115	0.96	100	258	2.15	100	218	1.82	100	172	1.46	100
2nd tempo dig	Error	0	0.00	-	14	0.12	40.08	37	0.31	54.97	227	1.89	52.66	222	1.88	48.47
	Negative dig	0	0.00	-	13	0.11	36.31	13	0.11	21.78	70	0.58	14.31^{a}	58	0.49	13.87^{a}
	Positive dig	0	0.00	-	11	0.09	23.61	22	0.18	23.25	147	1.23	33.03^{ab}	168	1.42	37.65^{b}
Total		0	0.00	-	38	0.32	100	72	0.60	100	444	3.70	100	448	3.80	100
3rd tempo dig	Error	405	3.38	30.11	351	2.93	25.77	238	1.98	27.26	89	0.74	28.39	52	0.44	$25.60^{\uparrow}$
	Negative dig	408	3.40	26.58	329	2.74	24.60	203	1.69	$20.29^{\uparrow a}$	47	0.39	$13.31^{\uparrow *\downarrow a}$	20	0.17	$7.81^{\uparrow *\downarrow a}$
	Positive dig	665	5.54	43.31^{ab}	648	5.40	$49.63^{\uparrow ab}$	485	4.04	$52.45^{\uparrow ab}$	200	1.67	$58.29^{\uparrow ab}$	163	1.38	$66.59^{\uparrow *\downarrow ab}$
Total		1478	12.32	100	1328	11.07	100	926	7.72	100	336	2.80	100	235	1.99	100

Note. $^{\uparrow}p < .01$ when compared to U-14. $^{*}p < .01$ when compared to U-16. $^{\downarrow}p < .01$ when compared to U-19. $^{\backslash}p < .01$ when compared to national category. [a] Significant differences when compared to "error". [b] Significant differences when compared to "negative dig".

Table 8. Dig performance values and statistically significant differences among categories

Types of court defence	Statistical data	U-14		U-16		U-19		National		International	
		Mean	SD	Mean	SD	Mean	SD	Mean	SD	Mean	SD
Total dig	Coefficient	1.59	0.51	1.72	0.48	1.69	0.52	$1.37^{\uparrow *\downarrow}$	0.55	1.50^{*}	0.62
	Efficacy (%)	44.33	17.80	48.90	17.82	49.31	19.18	$41.24^{*\downarrow}$	19.06	46.55	21.65
	Error (%)	29.31	18.52	26.33	15.35	29.93	17.22	$45.40^{\uparrow *\downarrow}$	19.86	$42.74^{\uparrow *\downarrow}$	20.88
	Efficiency (%)	15.07	33.73	22.57	30.52	19.29	33.84	$-4.11^{\uparrow *\downarrow}$	36.62	$3.78^{*\downarrow}$	40.56
	Positive:error ratio	1:0.59	0.76	1:0.55	0.84	1:0.57	1.03	$1{:}1.05^{\uparrow *\downarrow}$	1.23	$1{:}0.91^{\uparrow *\downarrow}$	1.22
1st tempo dig	Coefficient	1.96	1.06	1.89	1.16	1.61	1.03	$1.07^{\uparrow *\downarrow}$	1.08	$1.23^{\uparrow *}$	1.17
	Efficacy (%)	56.65	43.30	55.12	45.15	45.98	38.95	$31.11^{\uparrow *\downarrow}$	36.87	$38.29^{\uparrow}$	39.88
	Error (%)	17.62	31.68	21.65	37.30	$30.43^{\uparrow}$	35.22	$55.17^{\uparrow *\downarrow}$	40.94	$53.84^{\uparrow *\downarrow}$	41.86
	Efficiency (%)	39.01	65.48	33.50	73.40	15.49	66.35	$-24.01^{\uparrow *\downarrow}$	72.89	$-15.53^{\uparrow *\downarrow}$	78.42
	Positive:error ratio	1:0.35	0.45	1:0.49	0.61	$1{:}0.68^{\uparrow *}$	0.55	$1{:}1.74^{\uparrow *}$	1.01	$1{:}1.31^{\uparrow *}$	0.86
2nd tempo dig	Coefficient	.	.	1.07	1.02	0.92	0.95	1.13	0.79	1.27	0.89
	Efficacy (%)	.	.	23.62	37.65	23.23	31.96	33.03	27.86	37.65	31.30
	Error (%)	.	.	40.05	42.79	54.97	43.29	52.67	29.23	48.48	30.61
	Efficiency (%)	.	.	-16.43	68.69	-31.73	66.45	-19.64	52.98	-10.83	58.67
	Positive:error ratio	.	.	1:1.27	0.47	1:1.68	1.61	$1{:}1.54^{*}$	1.27	1:1.32	0.92
3rd tempo dig	Coefficient	1.57	0.53	1.74	0.47	$1.78^{\uparrow}$	0.61	$1.88^{\uparrow}$	0.98	$2.08^{\uparrow *\downarrow}$	1.03
	Efficacy (%)	43.35	18.67	49.65	18.19	$52.48^{\uparrow}$	22.46	$58.30^{\uparrow}$	35.26	$66.61^{\uparrow *\downarrow}$	36.02
	Error (%)	30.12	19.18	25.81	15.57	27.29	20.12	28.40	32.43	$25.57^{\uparrow}$	34.44
	Efficiency (%)	13.19	35.17	23.88	29.97	25.16	39.44	$29.94^{\uparrow}$	63.86	$40.97^{\uparrow *\downarrow}$	67.65
	Positive:error ratio	1:0.61	0.99	1:0.54	0.79	1:0.49	0.88	$1{:}0.45^{\uparrow *\downarrow}$	0.54	$1{:}0.32^{\uparrow *\downarrow}$	0.45

Note. $^{\uparrow}p < .01$ when compared to U-14. $^{*}p < .01$ when compared to U-16. $^{\downarrow}p < .01$ when compared to U-19. $^{\backslash}p < .01$ when compared to national category.

Discussion

This study demonstrates the technical-tactical performance profile of blocking and court defence depending on attack tempo at various age groups and categories of competition in men's volleyball. As the category increases, there is a significant increase in block and court defence for first and second tempo spikes and a significant decrease in these actions for third tempo spikes, with or without contact with the ball. Regarding performance, only the block and court defence for third tempo spikes showed increased efficiency (block points and digs which allow a team to set up their counterattack).

An increase in contacted blocks when progressing to higher categories may be related to players´ anthropometric development and physical abilities (Grgantov *et al.*, 2006). Physical improvements would restrain the spike; thus increasing the percentage of contacted blocks. However, players´ development may not be enough to prevent a decline in the percentage of contacted digs which occur when the ball avoids a block and heads toward the opponent's court. When comparing blocks and digs, the percentage of ball contacts for digs is greater than the percentage of ball contacts for blocks throughout all categories. This could be related to a shortage of time to set up a block depending on how close one is to the opponent's spike. Thus, the proximity of blockers to the spike would hinder their perception and interception of the ball and its path, while defenders would have more time to identify and respond to it (Selinger & Ackerman-Blount, 1985).

An increase in blocks and digs for first and second tempo spikes (contacted and non-contacted) demonstrates that the higher the category, the higher the speed of play. This is positively affected by an improvement in reception and court defense performance which occurs in higher ages and categories of competition (García-Alcaraz, Palao, & Ortega, 2014; Grgantov *et al.*, 2006). An increase in the speed of the game may reduce the time available for defensive actions, thus limiting both the number of players who may block (Afonso, Mesquita, & Palao, 2005) and the defensive moves (Afonso *et al.*, 2005, 2010; Selinger & Ackermann-Blount, 1985). This limitation of perception and execution on defensive actions is intended to counteract the increase in the height of the net (FIVB, 2008), the increase in the height of the players, and the development of players´ physical abilities (e.g. jump, speed, etc.) (Grgantov *et al.*, 2006), which are variables that may favour the performance of defensive actions when progressing to higher categories.

Regarding the performance of the block and court defence, there was a significant improvement in performance for slow attacks when analysing higher categories. This may be related to the amount of time available for defenders to execute their defensive actions. Previous studies have demonstrated that a shortage in time determines players´ defensive moves (Afonso *et al.*, 2010; Afonso *et al.*, 2005; Selinger & Ackermann-Blount, 1985), thus limiting the execution of a cohesive block (Bergeles & Nikolaidou, 2011) and the number of blockers (Afonso *et al.*, 2005). On the other hand, an increase in time for slow attacks fosters anticipation, decision-making, and players´ moves when blocking and defending. This is because slow attack times are related to low-performance receptions (Papadimitriou, Paschali, Sermaki, Mellas, & Papas, 2004), which limit the options for attacking and determine the setting zone, thus promoting the set-up of a block with a larger number of players (Afonso *et al.*, 2005). An improvement in performance of court defence in slow attacks may also be due to the relationship between court defence (i.e. the second line of defence) and the block (i.e. the first line of defence). Increasing the number of blockers (Afonso *et al.*, 2005), or setting up a more cohesive block (Bergeles & Nikolaidou, 2011), reduces the number of trajectories of attack aimed at areas not covered by defenders, thus facilitating the performance of court defence.

The significant improvement in performance of blocks and court defence for slow attacks may explain the significant decrease in the percentage of blocks and digs contacted in slow attacks. Regarding the block, this decline would be related to the spiker´s performance, particularly in one´s ability to avoid getting blocked. Thus, the increase in training and players´ experience as they progress to higher categories would improve their ability to spike. In contrast, temporal limitations of the block in fast attacks would be an advantage for spikers, who may perform better when attacking against this limited block. In this regard, Rocha and Barbanti (2004) found an increase in the attack´s efficacy when the ball contacts the block, although the attack tempo is not specified. As for defence, a significant increase in the percentage of contacted digs in fast attacks (first and second tempo) may be related to a decrease in the number of blockers (Afonso *et al.*, 2005), which promotes the increase in the number of balls headed toward diggers.

These results present the performance profile of blocking and court defence according to attack tempo in various categories of competition. The data provide reference values which may be useful when setting training and competition objectives for the various categories. Due to the relationship between defensive actions and attack tempo and between attack tempo and performance in previous actions (i.e. reception/defence and set) (Eom & Schutz, 1992), there is a need for further research on the effect of these variables on block and court defence performance. Thus, the attack that is set up upon receiving the ball is different in terms of offensive actions that are set up from a team's defence, mainly due to the setter's location and the spikers' availability to counterattack as quickly as possible (Castro & Mesquita, 2010). Variables such as spike direction distance between the point where the spiker hits the ball and the blocker positions his hands, ball speed, number of blockers, defence area, player role, set momentum, etc., may also need further analysis.

Conclusions

The results of this study show changes in the performance of the block and court defence depending on various age groups and competition level. When progressing to higher categories, there is a significant increase in the percentage of contacted blocks and digs with no ball contact, a significant increase in the percentage of defensive actions (i.e. blocks and digs) contacted in quick attacks (i.e. second and first tempo), and a significant improvement in performance in slow attacks (i.e. third tempo). These data may contribute to developing a technical-tactical performance profile of blocking and court defence in various categories of competition. These values may help to develop training programs, assess performance in competition, and expand knowledge about variables that describe performance. Nevertheless, the complex interaction of defensive actions with other game variables, such as attack time, attack zone, height of block, etc., requires further study which would fulfil a gap in current knowledge of performance variables.

References

Afonso, J., & Mesquita, I. (2011). Determinants of block cohesiveness and attack efficacy in high-level women's volleyball. *European Journal of Sport Science, 11*(1), 69-75.

Afonso, J., Mesquita, I., & Palao, J.M. (2005). Relationship between the tempo and zone of spike and the number of blockers against the hitters. *International Journal of Volleyball Research, 8*(1), 19-23.

Afonso, J., Mesquita, I., Marcelino, R., & Da Silva, J.A. (2010). Analysis of the setter's tactical action in high-performance women's volleyball. *Kinesiology, 42*, 82-89.

Anguera, M.T. (2003). Diseños observacionales en la actividad física y el deporte: estructura, alcance y nuevas perspectivas. In A. Oña, & A. Bilbao (Eds.), *II Congreso Mundial de Ciencias de la Actividad Física y el Deporte: Deporte y Calidad de vida* (pp. 253-282). Granada (Spain): Gráficas Alhambra.

Bergeles, N., & Nikolaidou, M E. (2011). Setter's performance and attack tempo as determinants of attack efficacy in Olympic-level male volleyball teams. *International Journal of Performance Analysis in Sport, 11*(3), 535-544.

Castro, J.M., & Mesquita, I. (2010). Analysis of the attack tempo determinants in volleyball's complex II: A study on elite male teams. *International Journal of Performance Analysis in Sport, 10*(3), 197-206.

Castro, J.M., Souza, A., & Mesquita, I. (2011). Attack efficacy in volleyball: Elite male teams. *Perceptual and Motor Skills, 113*(2), 395-408.

Costa, G., Caetano, J., Neiva, N., Junqueira, G., Afonso, J., Costa, P., & Mesquita, I. (2011). Determinants of attack tactics in youth male elite volleyball. *International Journal of Performance Analysis in Sport, 11*(1), 96-104.

Eom, H. J., & Schutz, R.W. (1992). Statistical analyses of volleyball team performance. *Research Quarterly for Exercise and Sport, 63*(1), 11-18.

FIVB (2008). Reglas oficiales del voleibol [Official volleyball rules]. Retrieved from www.rfevb.com.

García-Alcaraz, A., Palao, J.M., & Ortega, E. (2014). Perfil de rendimiento técnico-táctico de la recepción en función de la categoría de competición en voleibol masculino. *Kronos, 13*(1). Retrieved from http://g-se.com/es/journals/kronos/articulos/perfil-de-rendimiento-tecnico-tactico-de-la-recepcion-en-funcion-de-la-categoria-de-competicion-en-voleibol-masculino-1706

Grgantov, Z., Katic, R., & Jankovic, V. (2006). Morphological characteristics, technical and situation efficacy of young female volleyball players. *Collegium Antropologicum, 1*, 87-96.

Hughes, M.D., & Daniel, R. (2003). Playing patterns of elite and non-elite volleyball. *International Journal of Performance Analysis in Sport, 3*(1), 50-56.

Malina, R.M., & Bouchard, C. (1991). *Growth, maturation, and physical activity*. Champaign, IL: Human Kinetics.

Palao, J. M., Santos, J.A., & Ureña, A. (2007). Effect of the manner of spike execution on spike performance in volleyball. *International Journal of Performance Analysis in Sport, 7*(2), 126-138.

Papadimitriou, K., Paschali, E., Sermaki, I., Mellas, S., & Papas, M. (2004). The effect of the opponents' serve on the offensive actions of Greek setters in volleyball games. *International Journal of Performance Analysis in Sport, 4*(1), 23-33.

Rocha, C., & Barbanti, V.J. (2004). Analysis of factors that influence the attack in high level male volleyball. *Brazilian Journal of Physical Education and Sport, 18*(4), 103-114.

Selinger, A., & Ackermann-Blount, J. (1985). *Arie Selinger's power volleyball*. New York: St. Martin Press.

Stamm, R., Stamm, M., & Thomson, K. (2005). Role of adolescent female volleyball players' psychophysiological properties and body build in performance of different elements of the game. *Perceptual and Motor Skills, 101*, 108-120.

Stanganelli, L.C.R., Dourado, A.C., Oncken, P., Mançan, S., & Costa, S.C. (2008). Adaptations on jump capacity in Brazilian volleyball players prior to the under-19 world championship. *Journal of Strength and Conditioning Research, 22*(3), 741-749.

Stone, J. (2002). Digging and ball control. In D. Shondell, & C. Reynaud (Eds.), *The volleyball coaching bible* (pp. 163-176). Champaign, IL: Human Kinetics.

Author's note

Antonio García-de-Alcaraz is affiliated with the Department of Sports, Faculty of Physical Activity and Sport Sciences, Polytechnic University of Madrid, Spain.

Enrique Ortega is affiliated with the Department of Physical Activity and Sport, Faculty of Sport Sciences, University of Murcia, Spain.

José M. Palao is affiliated with Department of Health, Exercise Science and Sport Management. University of Wisconsin, Parkside, United States.

Corresponding author

Antonio García de Alcaraz Serrano
Facultad de Ciencias de la Actividad Física y del Deporte, INEF. Departamento de Deportes. C/ Martín Fierro, 7, Spain.
Email: antoniogadealse@gmail.com

10

The global reality of the Paralympic Movement: Challenges and opportunities in disability sports

Eliane Mauerberg-deCastro
Debra Frances Campbell
Universidade Estadual Paulista "Júlio de Mesquita Filho," Rio Claro, SP, Brasil

Carolina Paioli Tavares
Universidade Estadual de Ponta Grossa, Ponta Grossa, PR, Brasil

Abstract—The purpose of this study was to briefly illustrate some of the challenges and realities of national and international Paralympic sports. The *elite disabled athlete* paradigm is still not widely known in the world of regular sports competitions. The winning elite disabled athletes are restricted to a few countries, including the U.S., Canada, Germany, China, and Australia, with limited distribution of disability sport opportunities in other countries. This tendency for the success of a minority of countries reflects global problems of social vulnerability in accessibility (e.g., in dismantling the stigma of disability), political vulnerability (e.g., representative organizations of sports for the disabled do not fully pratice the philosophy of "sport for all"), and economic vulnerability (e.g., lack of opportunities for training, assistive sports technology, and sponsorships). Furthermore, elite Paralympic athletes have become veterans. For example, the participation of Brazilian elite athletes in the 1984 Paralympics marked the beginning of a new generation of athletes (approximately 16%) who returned to the Games in 1988. In both 2008 and 2012, nearly 28% of total participants were Brazilian veterans. Although this picture reveals longevity of athletes in the sport, there are many limitations in sports accessibility, often due to geographical centralization of opportunities in large urban centers. Yet, today, the world of Paralympic sport has been transformed into a sports spectacle, thanks to the exceptional performance of some athletes, to the technology of mass communication, and to the support of audiences during the Games. These sport "superstars" offer the world new images and new constructs of "ability." While this forum has helped to bring attention to these "heroes," other Brazilian athletes (and from other countries as well) are still waiting for their opportunities. Indeed, worldwide, young blind individuals, those in wheelchairs, amputees, or simply the uncoordinated, expect to play, run, swim, and take part in the international model of "sport for all." They expect sports opportunities to be a part of their daily lives, an option for rehabilitation and the preservation of health, and a basic human right.

Keywords: Paralympic games, disability sports, Paralympic Movement

Introduction

Since the 1940s, people with disabilities have been using sport as a therapeutic tool to overcome health complications, prevent secondary disabilities, and to survive. Experiences with survival include preventing premature death and dealing with society's stigma. These experiences also have helped athletes with disabilities construct a new dimension in the paradigm of "overcoming limits in sports"[1,3]. However, across cultures around the world, elite athletes with disability have a common reality that includes restricted access to assistive technology and specific sports equipment, limited media coverage and lack of sponsorships, ethical issues and doping, sports injuries, and provisions for retirement, among others. Also, their voices are often silent and are seldom part of the decision-making process in sports organizations. The diversity of competencies required for effective leadership in sports organizations and a traditional "medical model" approach in many nations toward disability pose the risk that the disability sports environment will continue to be patronizing[4]. Such patronizing attitudes typically lead to segregation[4,5].

Worldwide organizations have attempted to be sensitive to issues of segregation in order to protect human rights. Leading international human rights organizations, such as the *World Programme of Action Concerning Disabled Persons*, for example, have endorsed practices of inclusion of individuals with disability in the arena of sports, in particular during school activities[6]. However, many countries and societies around the world have not completely abandoned the institutional model in education[4,7,8]. Therefore, in such countries the presence of students and athletes with disability in inclusive settings is rare. Even rarer is the presence of teachers and coaches with disability, whether in an initiation or high-performance setting. As a result, athletes with disability tend to be alienated with respect gaining knowledge and opportunities related to becoming professionals in the business of sport.

Over the past several decades the Paralympic games as a global event, and the International Paralympic Committee (IPC)

as a global organization, helped to create forums for popularizing *disability sports*[1] among the general population. Using mass and social media, and employing advocacy strategies for human rights and inclusion, as well as international campaigns for health promotion through sports, IPC has helped to expand the ordinary sports viewer's notions of sports performance and entertainment. This, in turn, has helped to empower people with disability in the role of athlete, coach, administrator, and business person, even though the IPC is a non-profit entity, as are many other disability sports organizations.

In addition to promoting sports excellence, the IPC's strategic plan 2015-2018 includes vital issues that need to be addressed to guarantee the success of the Paralympic Movement, as well as to detect potential problems areas [9]. These include fostering representation and liaison by people with disability and institutional partners (e.g., the United Nations); democratic access to sports by all (e.g., the Agitos program); economic challenges in various world regions (e.g., branding sports and sustainable funding); fame, ethics, and doping; health and sports injuries; and retirement and sports career transitions.

Our purpose here is to summarize major accomplishments in the history of the Paralympic Movement—both successes and shortcomings. Also, we hope to provide an overview of some of the issues that inspire the IPC's current strategic plan, and to contextualize these, in particular with regard to the Brazilian Paralympian Movement.

From survival to high performance: The winners and the legacy

Engagement of disabled people in sport activities is commonly acknowledged as a vital protocol in their rehabilitation. Health professionals have become accustomed to using sport as a key therapeutic tool for rehabilitation, for the prevention of health problems, and to reduce the rate of mortality.

Disability sports emerged with the return home of casualties from First and Second World Wars[2]. Practice of physical exercise was officially identified in hospitals in North America and Europe in the early 20th century, primarily as a division of physical medicine and rehabilitation[10]. However, the sports paradigm in medical rehabilitation inside of hospitals was inspired by the neurologist, Dr. Ludwig Guttmann, who in 1944 developed a competitive "dressing exercise," known as Ward X, within the facilities of the Stoke Mandeville Hospital in Buckinghamshire, England[11]. Four years later, coinciding with the opening day of the Olympic Games in London, an archery competition took place in the hospital. In 1950, this event marked the creation of the Stoke Mandeville Festival of Sport. In 1952, these games became international in scope and a hallmark for the future Paralympic Games, which began in 1960, in Rome.

For individuals who become disabled, engaging in sports can be a strategy for post-hospital survival. Disability sports help participants create defenses against the effects of secondary disabilities or health impairments (e.g., atrophy, infections, osteoporosis, significant orthopedic disorders), more common in these patients than in the general population[5]. Also, engaging in sports can provide opportunities for people with disabilities to experience a sense of empowerment, and to achieve excellence in sport performance.

Accustomed to extreme challenges, today's Paralympic athletes often exhibit spectacular performances of sporting ability, making the Paralympic Games the second largest sports event in the world (Figure 1), and an extraordinary phenomenon of diversity. However, the elite disability sport paradigm is still unknown in the world of regular sport competition, and the tradition of participation in elite disability sport is still reserved for a few disabled athletes and, for decades, to a few countries. In fact, it wasn't until after the early 1990s that more than half of the world's countries began participating in the Paralympic Games. In 2012, 84% of countries worldwide attended the event, in contrast with 1960, when only 12% of the world's countries were represented at the Games. Advances in sport science, training, assistive technology, and modernization of the functional classification system[3] that replaced the medical model,

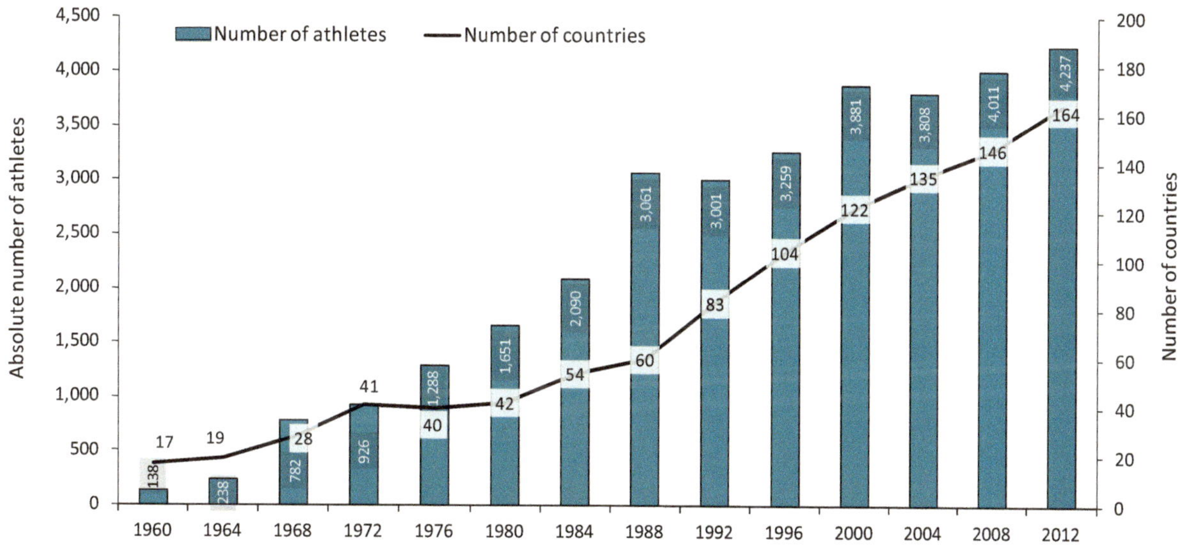

Figure 1. Global participation (athletes and countries) in the Paralympic Games, from 1960 until 2012[9].

all have increased the volume of participants globally, although the number of winning nations continues to be relatively small.

Winning results for disabled elite disabled athletes are still restricted to a few countries such as the U.S., Canada, Germany, China, and Australia, who have received between 9% and 29% of all medals, in all Paralympic Games. Brazil won 2.8% of the Paralympic sports medals in its best campaign in London (7th place), in 2012, against first-ranked China's 15.2%. The U.S. has attended all of the events since 1960, and has won First Place in eight out of a total of 16 Games over the past 52 years. The total amount of medals throughout the U.S.'s history of participation is 2,066, from a total of 18,877 (11%). China has the next best performance. Since its first participation in 1984, China has ranked First Place three times, with a total of 783 medals (5% of total medals from 1984 to 2012). Brazil has accumulated 228 medals since 1972 (1.3 % of all medals). Figure 2 shows the number of countries that have collected the majority of medals in contrast with countries that have won less than five medals. The success of the winning countries (an average of seven countries, with a minimum of two medals and a maximum of 14) reflects the earnings of an average of 818 medals (nearly 61% of the total medals awarded since 1960). Between 1972 and 1984, the number of participating countries has been stable, but with a very rapid and linear increase in number of medals, even though the top

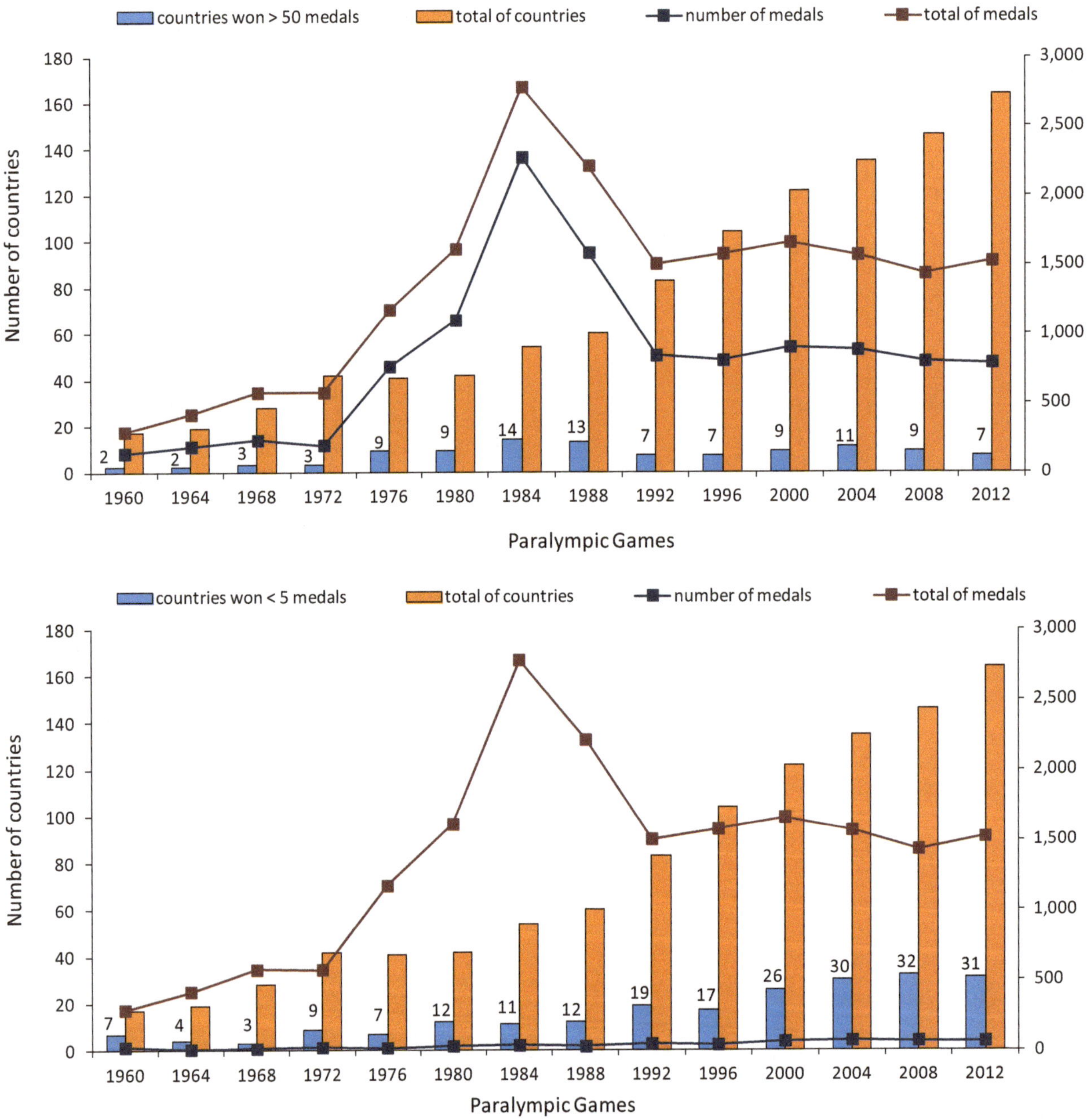

Figure 2. Total number of medals, and countries that have participated in the Paralympic Games since 1960. Contrast between the number of countries that have won more than 50 medals (top), and the countries that have won less than five medals (bottom)[9].

winners continue to come from only a relative few countries (e.g., Italy, U.S., Germany, Australia, and China). In 1992, the number of medals declined nearly by half.

Restrictions on the number of modalities by the IPC (currently 25 for summer events, and six for winter events) have limited the number of available medals. Insertions of sports are assessed by the IPC based on worldwide participation (i.e., countries and continents), quadrennial competition agenda, compliance with an athlete classification system, anti-doping program, rules and regulations, and evidences of sport attractiveness to audiences[12]. The other factor for limiting number of medals was the improvement of a functional classification system (i.e., the system determines the functional potential of athletic performance)—in opposition to the medical classification system (i.e., assessment of disability limitations in each sport class)—which was first used in 1992. These factors have been the most instrumental in stabilizing the volume of medals.

The number of countries that have earned no medals since 1960 has increased with the number of participating countries. In the last edition of the games, the proportions started to level, after 1996, between winners of some medals and participants with no medals. In 2012, 54% of the participating countries did not win any medals (Figure 3).

Officially, the International Olympic Committee (IOC) does not recognize the medal table method that ranks countries at the Olympic Games, as members believe this prompts injustice to smaller countries, along with presenting other philosophical issues related to the Olympic movement. However, the employment of countries' medal rankings is

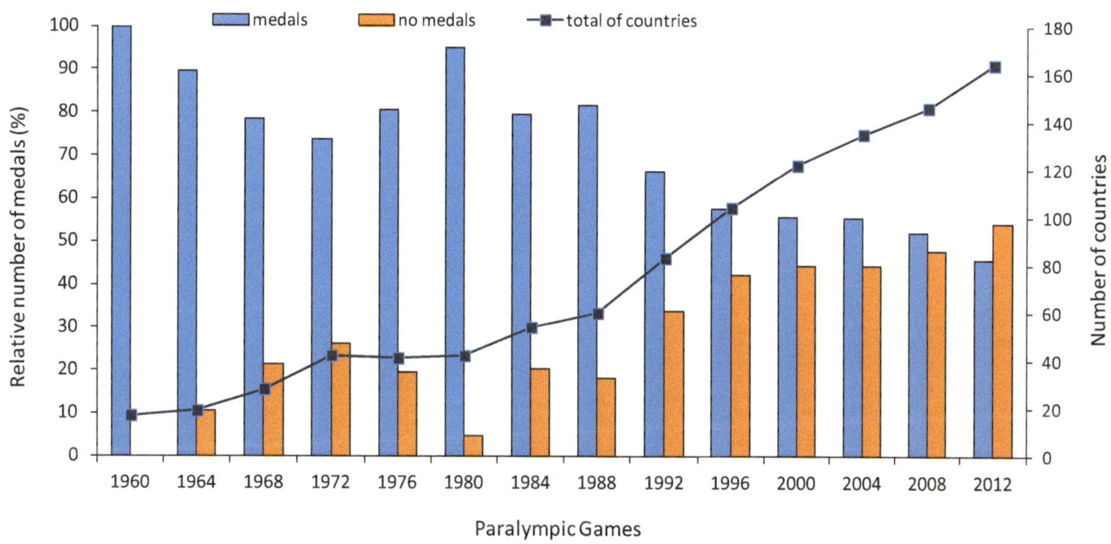

Figure 3. Contrast between countries that have participated in the Paralympic Games since 1960 that have won medals and countries that have won no medals[9].

used here for the purpose of acquiring information about athletes' performances in the Games, some recorded as early as 1908[13].

The discrepancy between the few winning countries and the remaining countries around the world reflects global problems of accessibility of people with disability to opportunities in sports. Many social structures in different societies around the world still struggle to dismantle the stigma of disability. Also, economic vulnerability affects a large number of countries, which results in lack of opportunities for training, poor or no assistive sports technology, the absence of professionals to integrate rehabilitation into the sports environment, as well as invisibility to sponsorship, among other factors[14] .

The Brazilian scenario

The Brazilian Paralympic scenario started in 1972, in Heidelberg (then West Germany), when, among the 40 participating countries, Brazil ranked in the 32nd position. In the 2012 London Summer Paralympic Games, Brazil had climbed to seventh position among the 164 participating nations. Extraordinary results such as those achieved by swimmer Daniel Dias, who won six Gold medals and broke five world records, brings a sharp contrast with performances by nondisabled Brazilian Olympic athletes. He is considered the greatest Brazilian Paralympic medalist (15 medals in total)[15]. Daniel paired his success with Alan Fonteles, double amputee (class T44), who completed the "100 meter" in 10.75 seconds, and the "200 meter" in 21.45 seconds. These results are not far from those of non-disabled athlete Usain Bolt during the 2012 Olympic Games: 9.58 seconds in the "100 meter," and 19.19 seconds in the "200 meter"[16].

It seems unrealistic to compare the performance of Olympic and Paralympic athletes, due in part to the number of classes in disability sport competitions. However, in its short history with the Paralympic Games, Brazil, for example, has been successful in raising its status in the general classification rank (7th place in London). In the most recent Olympic Games in London, Brazil received 17 medals and was ranked in 14th place. Throughout the history of Brazil's participation in a total of 22 Olympic games, athletes have returned home with 125 medals (26 Gold, 35 Silver and 64

Bronze medals), according to the Brazilian Olympic Committee[17]. On the other hand, throughout their 11 editions of Paralympic participation, Brazilian athletes have brought home a total of 237 medals[18]. Figure 4 depicts the relationship between number of Brazilian athletes, earned medals, and classification positions throughout the Paralympic Games since 1972. After the Games in Greece, the number of Brazilian athletes who represented the country nearly doubled relative to those in previous Games. Note that the general classification rank has steadily approached those of the top countries since the 1996 Paralympic Games in Atlanta.

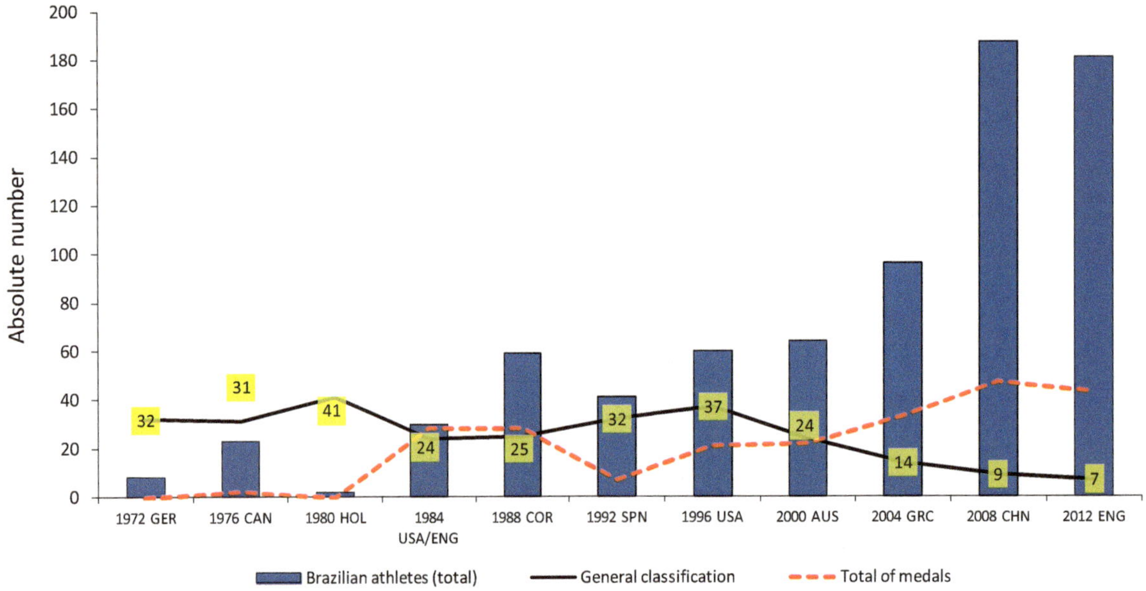

Figure 4. Absolute number of participant Brazilian athletes, earned medals, and general classification position in the Paralympic Games, from 1972 until 2012 (source: IPC, 2015a).

Implementing and maintaining disability sports

A major characteristic of disability sports is its association with rehabilitation. And, while exercise programs can help individuals with disability improve health and function, quite often these individuals seek social affiliation, personal affirmation, and self-empowerment through sports. Therefore, it is common to observe in athletes with disability a rapid climb to the elite sports in national and international scenarios. However, only limited opportunities for competitions exist, with a small number of eligible athletes for competitions as compared to those in regular sports, and only a very few of these reach the top or become elite athletes. Yet, the engagement of disabled athletes in national and international competitions may take as short as six months to two years from their start in the practice of sport, according to a review by Brazuna and Mauerberg-deCastro[19]. Therefore, athletes' rapid rise and longevity in the sport are two other dominant characteristics of disability sports.

Aware of how opportunities for healthy living could positively affect Chinese citizens with disability, in 2014, the Chinese Central Government implemented key projects to provide rehabilitation services throughout many regions of China. These projects now provide 7.5 million disabled individuals with age- and condition-appropriate, long-term specialized therapeutic protocols for all areas of disability and health challenges. Also, early detection of disability has become a part of these efforts, with rehabilitation integrated into sports. The national plan, supervised and administered by the China Disabled Persons' Federation (CDPF) and commissioned by the Government of China, attempts to cover wide areas of the lives of people with disability, including education, employment, sports, and rehabilitation. In 2014, the CDPF coordinated 800 sports events involving people with disability, and the training of 11,000 fitness coaches to work in disability sports. The number of provincial sports training bases now totals 234 countrywide. The CDPF serves as China's official National Paralympic Committee.

China, now a leading nation in the Paralympic Games, continuously invests in new developments in disability sports, and constantly reveals an extraordinary number of new elite athletes. Some countries like Brazil, however, continue to rely on a limited number of athletes who are members of a long-lasting, early generation of athletes. The elite Brazilian Paralympic athletes that have achieved success now are veterans. Of the 181 athletes who went to London in 2012, approximately 22% were athletes who had participated in previous Games, and 7% had participated in more than two Games. Although the 1984 Paralympics had fewer Brazilian athletes, their participation marked the beginning of a new generation of athletes (16%) that returned to the next games. In 2008 and 2012, 24% and 22% respectively were Brazilian veteran athletes (Figure 5). Although this picture reveals longevity of athletes in the sport—which is unusual when compared to non-disabled athletes[4], there are many limitations in sports accessibility, predominantly because of geographical centralization of opportunities in large urban centers.

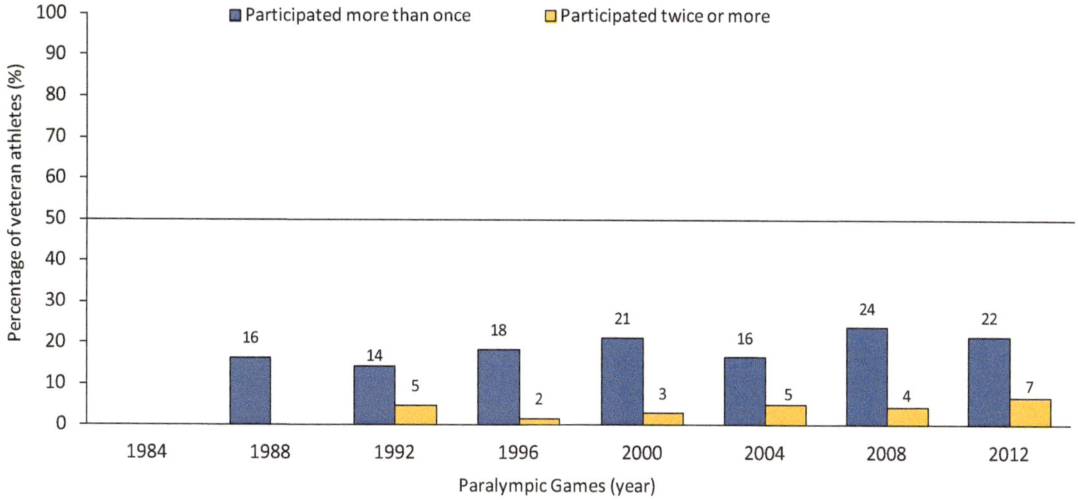

Figure 5. Veteran Brazilian Paralympic athletes returning more than once, and more than twice, to the Games. Participation from 1984 until 2012. (These data are subject to inaccuracies, as the precise number of athletes is unknown, especially in the early years of the Games. Some of the athletes' names were misspelled or omitted from the IPC database)[9].

The Brazilian veteran athletes who participated in the Paralympic Games the most times are Ádria dos Santos and Antonio Tenório da Silva, at five times each, competing for 16 years at the Paralympic level since 1996. Typically, longevity of the athletic career is desirable — which also is true for non-disabled athletes. Yet, Brazil is a large country geographically, and athletes must congregate in large urban centers, where most training and sports practice opportunities are located. This requires many athletes to move from their hometowns to participate in training and to receive assistive care, as rehabilitation is part of the training protocol. The long-term commitment to moving away from families and friends, as well as to compliance with goals and training seasons, also depend on resources from sponsorships and government grants.

Government agencies in some societies, such as in Brazil, for example, show confusion about how to implement "*sport for all*," therefore setting disability sport within a marginalized, elitist, non-democratic context. Even many organizations whose goal is to represent sports for the disabled haven't yet successfully constructed a widespread tradition of implementing sports opportunities to individuals with disability. Outstanding sports programs are commonly located in large cities. Often, partnerships between universities and organizations/institutions interested in sports programs are vehicles through which people with disability find opportunities for practicing a sport. Since the number of universities is limited, and most opportunities happen within urban centers, many young (future) athletes with disability from other geographic locations will never explore such opportunities.

Fame and achievements: Ethics (or lack of) in the Paralympic Movement

Although "heroism" and "sportsman" are common descriptors granted to disabled athletes who become part of the elite cadre in the sport scenario, the world of Paralympic sports competition is not immune to scandal, corruption, and illicit means for achieving success. In fact, in Paralympic sports, the discussion of ethics involves an "ambiguity of expectations" related to the concepts of *inclusion* and *accessibility*. Santamaria and Mazzeo[20] explored this ambiguity in relation to the prevalence of doping in sport. These authors observed that doping negatively affects the image of the sport industry and represents a serious threat to the health of the athlete. Yet, the act of winning increases the probability that an athlete will be rewarded with sponsorships, fame, and money. Therefore, many athletes are willing to take risks, even participating in unethical activities such as doping. Athletes with disabilities, too, are part of this problem.

In the 2000 Summer Paralympics, the Spanish basketball team, in the class of intellectual disabilities, was disqualified after winning the Gold medal. None of the athletes were intellectually disabled. The incident showed the fragility of the classification system and the weak eligibility criteria for athletes with intellectual disability. The result was the suspension of intellectual disability from the Paralympics, which returned only in 2012.

The Paralympic Games have been relatively free of scandal, but many disabled athletes have been caught violating the Anti-Doping Code[21]. In 2015, the Portuguese Paralympic Committee launched its educational campaign about doping that targeted athletes with disabilities. With the intention to "promote and protect the integrity of sport and the health of athletes," the IPC, along with the international federations and national Paralympic committees, organized the IPC Anti-Doping Code[22].

According to Van de Vliet[23], an incidence of only 1% of violations of the anti-doping rules in the Paralympic Movement has been reported. Violations usually are detected and recorded during competition. Since 2000, a total of 60 violations were registered by the International Paralympic Committee. Of these, 37 were detected in weightlifting, which is four times the incidence of any violation in the next sport modality, athletics.

Annually, since 2007, the IPC anti-doping test results are publicly exposed and, once investigation confirms an athlete's doping test failure, the IPC reveals the athlete's identity and reason for disqualification. In 2004, a Brazilian weightlifter was permanently banned for using methasterone metabolite[22]. The athlete's banning figures alongside two other athletes in this category of severity. The list of names of athletes who are currently serving limited bans to participate in the year 2015 includes at least 15 athletes from various countries.

The IPC 2007 statistical report of violations of the Doping Code from the sample of 288 athletes detected 15 violations ranging from "atypical results" to "confirmed violations." Statistics from the Beijing Games, including doping tests conducted outside of and during competitions, showed that the number of tested athletes increased to 1,155, with 32 violations. Once a violation is detected, the process of an athlete's defense begins before the Committee makes a final decision. In 2011, a Brazilian weightlifter was suspended for two years for violating the Anti-Doping Code. Again in 2012, another Brazilian weightlifter was suspended for nine months. Weightlifting, as mentioned above, is among the sports whose athletes most often violate the anti-doping code. Of the sanctions for the seven total violations in 2010, four were for weightlifters. In 2011, the number was again four (out of seven) weightlifters. In 2012, for a total of eight penalties, six were given to weightlifters. In 2013, seven of the ten penalties went to weightlifters, and, in 2014, eight of eleven penalties were given to weightlifters[22].

Another problem is that, like many of today's athletes, Paralympic athletes use dietary supplements. Pipe and Ayotte[24] claimed that contaminated nutritional supplements have a huge potential for resulting in positive doping tests, and this reality is one of the main concerns of coaches and athletes. Countless supplements available in the market are contaminated with steroids and stimulants that are prohibited by the Anti-Doping Code. Furthermore, athletes with disabilities often depend on the chronic use of medications associated with complications that arise from their health conditions. This situation obfuscates the work of the Anti-Doping Committee and creates the need for each athlete to update their biological profile with the IPC by a licensed physician.

Another controversial doping practice in the Paralympic world is called "boosting." This practice, performed by spinal cord-injured athletes with lesions above the 6th vertebra, is the deliberate induction of chest pain or discomfort in the body areas below the lesion. The result, in addition to increased blood pressure in contrast to a low heart rate, is an improvement in circulation of the muscles. Boosting is the deliberate self-induction of autonomic dysreflexia, in which systolic blood pressure raises up to 180 mmHg or above. The potential risk is a stroke, intracranial hemorrhage, and death. Despite this, some athletes run these risks, because they believe they can improve athletic performance by up to 15%. Treated separately from other forms of doping, boosting began to be monitored during the Games in Sydney 2000[21]. Between 2007 and 2009, the IPC used a questionnaire to investigate the practice of boosting in 93 high-level athletes, wheelchair users, in the class T6 or above. The results showed that almost 50% of these athletes believed that the practice is more or less dangerous, yet more than 16% had used the practice in competitions, and 79% had experienced spontaneous autonomic dysreflexia[25].

The controversial world of sport as practiced by athletes with disabilities includes social, political, and ethical dilemmas, and, of course, health concerns. Maintaining good health is one of the central goals associated with the rehabilitation of the disabled individual. However, ironically, the cost may be the result of another aspect of vulnerability in the world of disability sports: secondary disabilities associated with sports injuries.

Athletes have left their marks on Paralympic sports: But, at what cost?

New performance records in Paralympic sports are increasingly and gradually gaining the attention of fans, at least during media coverage of the Games. Although the Paralympic cycle is four years, and even though Winter Paralympics is alternated—making a two-year gap between the Summer and Winter Games, the Summer Games have become the most prestigious. While national and international competitions do take place, athletes predominantly prepare their training seasons to meet this Paralympic event.

Training routines have conditioned athletes for high-performance sports, and to respond quickly to the demands of competition seasons, including opportunities to win medals, they push their physical limits in an intense regime of training[19]. However, they also are more exposed to injuries and, consequently, to increased risk of suffering additional disability conditions, particularly from chronic injuries.

Survey13, administered in London in 2012, and which relates to the incidence of sports injuries in Paralympic athletes, is the most detailed study on the problem or sports injuries by the IPC, according to Webborn and Emery[26]. These authors summarize the findings: 3,565 athletes (84% of the participating athletes) of 160 delegates (98% of the countries' delegates of the games) responded to a questionnaire related to injuries that occurred during training and competition in 20 sports. The results showed that a total of 49,910 athletes per day were monitored globally. During the London Games, a total of 539 athletes suffered 633 injuries. The global injury rate was 12.7 injuries per 1,000 athletes. In the same study, the injury rate was similar among male and female athletes. Pre-Games injury rates in women were higher than during the competitions. Higher rates of injury were found in older athletes for sports such as football 5 (22.4 per 1,000 injuries). In general, 51.5% of lesions were primary acute traumatic injuries. The most common injury (percentage of total injuries) occurred in the shoulder (17.7%), followed by wrist/hand (11.4%), elbow (8.8%), and knee (7.9%). The 2012 London/ IPC study identified major differences between sports, and it highlighted the need for longitudinal studies rather than those limited exclusively to a Paralympic season.

One of the earliest studies on incidence of injury in athletes with disabilities was conducted by Curtis and Dillon[27]. Of 128 wheelchair athletes interviewed, all reported suffering at least one injury since they began their sport. Some had accumulated as many as 14 injuries. A total of 93 athletes reported 291 injuries.

The most common injuries involved soft tissues (33%), bed sores (18%), and skin lacerations (17%). In these cases, many of the athletes never sought medical treatment.

As in the past, many athletes with disabilities come from limited economic conditions; others reside in countries that do not provide forms of treatment or prevention. Chronic problems arising from repeated injuries can lead to more serious consequences over time. For example, athletes who use wheelchairs may develop weakness and numbness in the hands, or carpal tunnel syndrome (CTS). Constant trauma and compression of the heel of the hand for each stroke in the act of pushing the wheelchair may reduce the functionality of the upper limbs and increase incidence of vertebral herniations. Obtaining appropriate diagnoses and treatment are not always feasible due to lack of resources and, sometimes, lack of recognition that there is a problem. The problem becomes more serious when it occurs in regions affected by disability, such as paralyzed areas that lack sensation.

Health education programs for preventing disabilities must be offered to disabled athletes, particularly to those who come from poorer regions or low socio-economic backgrounds. Athletes should be trained to inspect their bodies using various strategies, especially if they can't see injuries (blind athletes) or feel the affected area (paralyzed athletes). Athletes should be able to recognize the demands of their training protocols—through routine and constant performance assessments, and, therefore, know how to differentiate normal signs of fatigue from signals of a body damaged by exercise. Sports injuries that become a routine in the life of a disabled athlete can prematurely end his or her athletic career, and lead to the early retirement of elite athletes[28].

Does empowerment through disability sports preclude success in business?

There is no question that elite (non-disabled) athletes who win and earn medals gain much popularity and financial opportunities—often making them millionaire sports figures. Sport is big business, producing billions of dollars in revenues. According to Forbes[29], the sports industry in the North American market—driven by major professional leagues such as Major League Soccer, as well as by intercollegiate sports—is a growth industry. The industry, which produced $ 53.6 billion in 2012, is expected to produce $ 67.7 billion in 2017, marking an annual growth rate of 4.8%. Sport is a hugely profitable business, and athletes no longer play for fun. They now are paid professionals.

Olympic athletes, especially males, naturally attract private sector companies for sponsorships, investments, and to represent their brands. While such athletes typically reach celebrity status through their association with certain brands and transition into having long, successful careers, Paralympic athletes mostly attract the attention of charitable investors or of government funding. Media coverage typically grants visibility to disabled athletes only for the period in which their winning appears relevant, which commonly is tied to a particular Paralympic season. The Paralympic Games, the most important competition in the world for disabled athletes, occurs every four years. The news cycle for Paralympic athletes, therefore, allows some athletes simply to fall into anonymity for what could be considered a very long period of time for an athlete. Despite this, during the past two Games, some Paralympic athletes, Brazilian Alan Fonteles, for example, have gained notoriety, and have captured the attention of the media as well as of private investors. Currently, Fonteles earns a salary of 60,000 reais (+- US$ 17,000), according to Globo.com[30]. Yet, his earnings are astronomically less than the earnings of professional athletes like Anderson Varejão, who plays basketball in the NBA and earns $10 million per year[31]. For elite athletes with disability, sport as a career and a means for living is highly unpredictable, and presents a very uncertain future.

In Brazil, for example, the lack of public and private sector funding for disability sports led to the creation of the Agnelo Piva Law, in 2001[5]. Two percent of federal lottery prize money is budgeted to the Brazilian Olympic Committee (85%), and to the Brazilian Paralympic Committee (15%). This incentive has allowed the Brazilian Paralympic Committee (CPB) to deploy new projects, one of which was the establishment of a *permanent training team*. Also, elite athletes began to receive scholarship incentives and prize money for each medal they win. Scholarships last for four years, typically until the next Paralympic event.

With a mission to "promote the universal access of disabled people to the practice of sports in its various levels," the CPB[32] created a program for the development of new athletes in the school system, the Paralympic School Club. As a consequence, since 2006, the CPB annually organizes the School Paralympic games, designed for middle- and high school students throughout Brazil. In 2012, 1,200 athletes from 24 states gathered in the city of São Paulo to compete in one of the largest national games for students with disabilities[33]. For comparison, the most recent school games for non-disabled students (called Youth School Games, or "Jogos Escolares da Juventude"), founded in 1969[34], had 3,000 participants.

Although government agencies have begun to invest in new young people with disability so that they may engage in sports, access to training and the professional quality of coaches and other sports professionals are limited. For the athletes already established in the national and international sport scenarios, coaches and sports professionals are from various backgrounds, often with only hands-on experience and quite often far removed from training methods based on science.

Additionally, the disability sports area is administered and led primarily by non-disabled people. With few funded positions, individuals committed to disability sports typically are volunteers for non-profit or government funded organizations[35,36]. This structure and the volunteer function are not so common in the world of general sports, which are increasingly oriented toward financial profit. Also, athletes and sports professionals who have a disability rarely are employed to participate in or coach regular sports. The biased attitudes of non-disabled individuals toward professionals with disability tend to make them focus on limitations caused by the disability condition, not on competencies. Disability sports are generally conceived within the context of philanthropy, and people with disability, whether athletes or sports professionals, are expected to be "recipients of opportunities" granted by the non-disabled world.

Indeed, individuals with disability historically have been dismissed from participating in decision-making policies, as well as having been ignored when voicing their choices in a variety of contexts (e.g., education, sports, family affairs, and work force, among others). James Charlton and his South-African colleagues, Michael Masutha and William Rowland[37], began to advocate the need for scholars and international organizations to recognize a new paradigm that they termed, "Nothing about us without us." Their concerns about people with disabilities' invisibility and lack of power resulted in new policies that helped to increase the presence of peers with disability, who acted as liaisons during important decisions about disability issues, whether in sports, education, research, and for professional organizations. In 2004, United Nations Enable action adopted the theme, "Nothing about Us without Us," with the purpose of providing an opportunity for "active involvement and participation of persons with disabilities in the planning of strategies and policies that affect their lives." The United Nations Convention on the Rights of Persons with Disabilities, adopted by the United Nations General Assembly in December 2006, endorsed inclusive sports as a critical component of global disability rights.

Many individuals with disability gained respect, access, and became representative stakeholders in sports organizations, such as with Sir Philip Craven becoming the current president of the IPC executive board, and members at large such as Ann Cody, Duane Kale, John Petersson, and Todd Nicholson. In the United Kingdom, the English Federation of Disability Sports[38] created the *Inspire to Lead Project,* alongside the Sports Leaders UK, Youth Sport Trust, and Sport England, to provide people with disability with leadership and volunteer opportunities. Since the Paralympic games, the *Inspire to Lead Project* has recruited and trained over 120 young disabled people to develop qualifications in sports leadership. The governing board of the EFDS also includes members with disability, such as Dr. Philip Friend, and Fran Williamson. Similarly, Disabled Sports USA includes members with disability on their board of directors, such as Executive Director Kirk Bauer and President Robert Meserve. The China Disabled Persons' Federation (CDPF), the official organization recognized by the IPC, has two chair members with disability, Mr. Li Zhijun and Mr. Liu Zaijun. Each has, respectively, visual impairment and hearing impairment[39].

The Brazilian Paralympic Committee (CPB), in 2009 created the Counsel of Athletes, whose president, Ms. Simone Rocha, holds a chair on the Board of Directors to represent peer athletes' expectations and views about the activities of the Paralympic Movement. The counsel is formed by seven members, who are expected to come from various geographic regions in Brazil to advocate for diverse needs.

Media coverage (especially TV and social media) of the Paralympic games has helped to expand its exposure to audiences worldwide, educating them about a multitude of abilities in athletic performance, in many sports modalities. The games in London and Beijing were viewed by 3.8 billion people, according to IPC President Sir Philip Craven[40]. Such visibility helps to break stereotypes and challenge archaic, hegemonic social paradigms. Unfortunately, with regard to job opportunities in sports or in more general areas, professionals with disability have been underemployed; their personal perspectives about disability have not necessarily been considered an asset in their skill set. More recently, however, individuals with disability have become important contributors to sport organizations due to their ability to help with real-world strategic planning.

Breaking stereotypes is not an easy task for anyone. When it comes to disabled athletes' participation in a non-disabled world of sport, controversy often raises more restrictions than opens opportunities. For example, the eligibility of disabled athletes to participate in the Olympics can raise questions about the assistive and sport technology that athletes with disability rely on.

Mass media have only recently begun to give visibility to athletes with disabilities in the Olympic sport scenario. However, disabled athletes who have participated in the past in the Olympics have done so mostly in silence. In the 2012 London Olympics, the world looked at this phenomenon when Oscar Pistorius[5] marked the history of the sport of track and field as the first bilateral amputee to compete with Olympic athletes. Yet, athletes with disabilities have participated in the Olympic Games since 1904 (Table 1).

Table 1. Athletes with disabilities who participated in the Olympic Games.

Year	Athlete	Disability condition	Modality	Result
1904	George Eyser (USA)	One-leg amputee	Gymnastic	3 Gold medals, 2 Silver and 1 Bronze
1928-1936	Olivér Halassy (Hungary)	One-leg amputee	Water polo	2 Gold medals, 1 Silver
1952	Lis Hartel (Denmk)	Polio	Women's equestrian	1 Silver medal
1984	Neroli Fairhall (New Zealand),	Paraplegia	Women's bow arrow	-
1996	Paola Fantato (Italy)	Polio	Women's bow arrow	-
2004–2008	Marla Runyan (USA)	Legal blindness	Women's 1,500 m track	8th place in the finals
2008	Natalie du Toit (South Africa)	One-leg amputee	Swimming	Qualified for the Olympic Games in Beijing
2008	Natalia Partyka (Polan)	One-hand/wirst amputee	Table tennis	Qualified for the Olympic Games in Beijing
2012	Dong Hyun (South Corea)	Legal blindness	Bow arrow	Record in 2012 and Bronze medal for his team
2012	Oscar Pistorius (South Africa)	Two-leg amputee	100 m, 200 m, and 400 m tracks	Qualified for the Olympic Games in London

Source: Wallechinsky and Loucky: http://www.wired.com/2012/08/11-disabled-olympians/.

Leaving the sport competition scenario: a bleak future?

Disability sport's history has been constructed by a few athletes who, themselves, had limited opportunities in their athletic careers. Athletes with disability became elite because of their and their families' personal investments. Disability sport provides individuals with a means to compete against oneself; to compete against one's own disability, against society's stereotypes. When individuals with disability become athletes, they develop new meaning through a new lifestyle. It is a lifestyle that increases chances for survival and, above all, provides a context for empowerment that comes from within. In actuality, they gain little from the sports marketplace. Therefore, these athletes rarely transition to retirement with societal or institutional support. Figure 6 depicts the implications of participating in disability sports on an athlete's life. The implications of leaving disability sport are well documented in the literature.

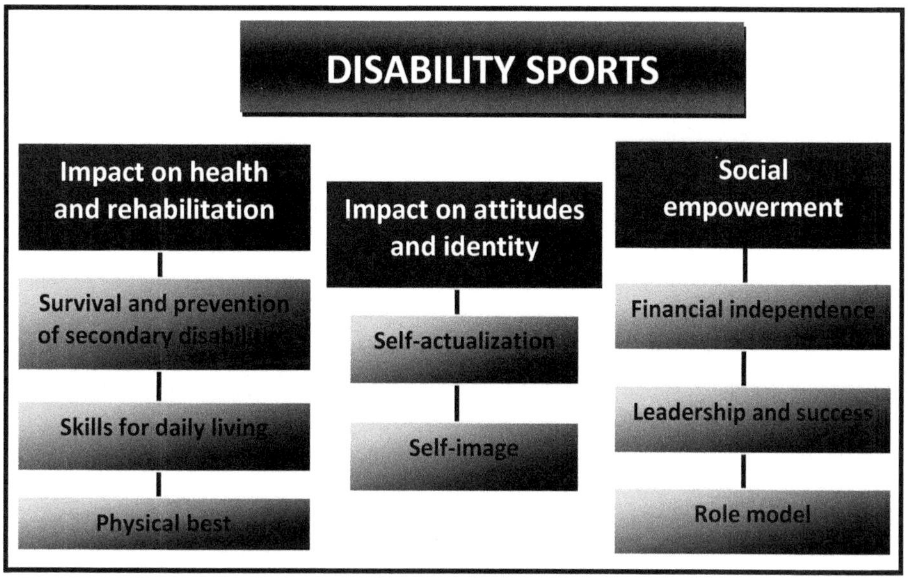
DISABILITY SPORTS
Impact on health and rehabilitation
Survival and prevention of secondary disability
Skills for daily living
Physical best
Impact on attitudes and identity
Self-actualization
Self-image
Social empowerment
Financial independence
Leadership and success
Role model

Figure 6. Implications of disability sports in an athlete's life.

Various societies worldwide provide financial support or *disability pensions* from health insurance agencies or from government agencies. Some athletes receive early retirement and, although the monetary amount is often below poverty standards, disabled people have free time. Time availability increases chances for sport commitments. However, many athletes come from modest families and rarely have the opportunity to become acquainted with international cultures. For some, sport participation can present such opportunities[41].

Because sport participation often gives people with disability a new sense of life, athletes who leave the world of competition report feeling that they have lost something, beginning with leaving a circle of friends. They perceive that leaving the sport affects their physical competence, health, and their personal identity[42]. However, disabled athletes typically have not made plans for the time when they will have to leave the sports world. Nor have their financial resources allowed them to make plans for the future.

In 2013, the Brazilian Paralympic Committee launched the program, "Heroes of disability sports" (i.e., "Heróis do Paradesporto")[43]. Nominated by the CPB and the Federal Lotteries, former athletes with disabilities who are now advocating for the Paralympic Movement receive a financial grant for 12 months (renewable). Recently Ádria Rocha Santos, Antônio Delfino, and Luiz Cláudio Pereira joined the program as ambassadors of the movement[43]. However, this is an important initiative, since there is no official program to guide or help athletes in retirement. Some examples of successful transition to retirement include swimmer Fabiana Sugimori, who attended four Paralympic Games, class S11 for the blind. She was sponsored by the Loterias Caixa throughout her career and became a tenured employee of the bank Caixa Econômica Federal. Swimmer Clodoaldo Silva is another example of financial success. His outstanding performance in the Athens Games in 2004, where he won six Gold medals, gave him notoriety and fame. Clodoaldo has several sources of income, thanks to his popularity. He is constantly invited to lecture and discuss his experiences as a disabled athlete[44].

Although rare, the retirement of Olympic athletes can provide an opportunity for the application of knowledge to Paralympic sports. The Brazilian runner Joaquim Cruz, Gold medal winner of the 800 m track event during the 1984 Olympic Games in Los Angeles, is today one of the coaches of Paralympic athletes from the United States. In Brazil, the volleyball player Amauri, member of the generation Volleyball Silver in the 1980s, currently lends his expertise to the development of sitting volleyball[45].

In an attempt to change this situation of uncertainty in the sporting careers of disabled athletes, in April 2015, the Ministry of Sports reactivated the National Commission of Athletes. The Commission is coordinated by former athletes Lars Grael (president), basketball player Hortência (vice president), and

Anderson Lopes (secretary and representative of Paralympic athletics). The main issues of discussion include the athlete's career transition to retirement, support for former athletes in financial difficulty, and new guidelines on the Brazilian law of incentive to sport. Officially, this is the first time that issues of retirement of both Olympic and Paralympic athletes have been under the administration of the Ministry of Sports and the Olympic and Paralympic Committees[46].

Conclusions

In 2016, Brazil will host the 15th Paralympic Games in Rio de Janeiro. The IPC president, Sir Philip Craven, expects that the Games will show the best performances by athletes in the history of sports for the disabled. Over 176 countries will compete in 23 sports in an attempt to break the 251 records set in London, in 2012. Again, we will witness the "power of the human spirit," according to Sir Philip[47].

The Paralympic Movement of the IPC is perhaps one of the most effective human rights organizations due its ability to direct society's attention to critical issues related to disability and sports. The potential of sports for the disabled lies not just in its ability to provide audiences with spectacular events, but also as a means for improving human dignity and to help improve our understanding of the value of diversity. The consequences of the success of the Movement worldwide encompass areas of health and sport promotion, visibility of disability, the popularization of Paralympic sports, the scientific development of sport sciences in regard to athletes with disability, sports injuries, doping, sports periodization, physiological adaptation to exercise, the biomechanics of disability, and assistive technology, among others[1,40].

Yet, today, the world of the Paralympic sport has been transformed from relative obscurity into a spectacle, thanks to the participation of exceptional athletes, to the technology of mass communication, and to changing views and the support of society. These sport "superstars" offer the "ordinary world" their unique visibility and new concepts of ability. While some of these heroes have already been celebrated, many future Brazilian athletes are still waiting for their opportunities. Young blind individuals, those in wheelchairs, amputees, or simply the uncoordinated, are spread throughout the cities and countryside of Brazil, and expect, above all, to play, run, swim, and take part in the international model of "sport for all." They expect sports opportunities to be a part of their daily lives, an option for rehabilitation, for the preservation of health, and a human right.

For the Paralympic athletes, sports define their identities, often damaged by pre-conceptions about the "perfect" or "efficient" body[19]. Sports provide a sense of competence and responsibility and, in the disabled world, become part of the history of a community. The sense of political responsibility that the sport environment offers to athletes also generates opportunities for becoming role models and for improving leadership skills. Leadership implies rigid adherence to the ethics and moral values of *Olympism*. Unfortunately, ethics and moral values often are corrupted by the same heroes who stumble over the temptation of a "medal at any cost."

As for government organizations and society, inclusion and accessibility have financial implications: the development of policies based on human rights. The realities of the athletes of the past inspire the achievements of the athletes of today. However, diversity in the meaning of athletic achievement—whether earning medals or breaking records—is not the only legacy for future generations. The meaning of success of the Paralympic movement, both locally and globally, should not be solely weighed in statistics about economic impact on host countries or on sport performance excellence. Instead, the success of the Paralympic Movement should be measured beyond the sports arenas, to where people with disability have been inspired to seek long-term quality of life through the practice of sports.

Endnotes

[1] According to DePauw and Gavron[48], the term disability sports indicates sports that are designed for or specifically practiced by athletes with disabilities. Disabled World (2004) expanded this concept to include adaptive sports or parasports.

[2] Yeo et al.[49], based on statistics from the 1980s, revealed that life expectancy after spinal cord injury still is 1/5 of that of the general population. The years after World War II marked a period in which the majority of spinal cord injury victims died within the first two years of hospitalization due to sepsis and infections aggravated by prolonged immobilization. Survivors still showed high mortality rates: 4-5 times higher after the first and second decades from time of injury.

[3] The functional classification system is a system used to determine which categories of competition an athlete is likely to encounter adversaries with similar disability conditions. The system uses medical data of impairment and impairment on sport performance (i.e., sport specific). The sport classes include athletes that are equally challenged by a disability in order to make the competition a fair situation[40].

[4] Among veteran Olympic athletes, Miraildes Maciel Mota, known as Formiga, is a Brazilian football player for the women's national football team, who participated five times in the Olympic Games (1996, 2000, 2004, 2008, and 2012). Volleyball player Hélia Rogério de Souza Pinto, known as Fofão, participated five times in the Olympics (1988, 1992, 1996, 2004, and 2008). The Brazilian athlete with the highest number of Olympic appearances was the sailor Torben Grael (1984, 1988, 1992, 1996, 2000, and 2004). Hugo Hoyama (table tennis), Rodrigo Pessoa (equestrian), Oscar (basketball), Robert Scheidt (sailors) are medalists who participated in five Olympic Games[50,51].

[5] Oscar Pistorius, after being convicted of the murder of his girlfriend Reeva Steenkamp, in 2014, will not compete in any Paralympic Games for at least 5 years (length of sentence), according to The Guardian[52]. However, his sports career is likely to end as, on

December 3, 2015, South Africa's Court of Appeal in Bloemfontein overruled Judge Masipa's sentence of manslaughter and convicted Pistorius of murder. He will return to court to be sentenced again to a longer jail sentence[53].

References

1. Blauwet C, Willick SE. The Paralympic Movement: Using Sports to Promote Health, Disability Rights, and Social Integration for Athletes with Disabilities. Physical Medicine Rehab. 2012; 4:851-856.
2. Gold JR, Gold MM. Access for all: The rise of the Paralympic Games. Journal of the Royal Society for the Promotion of Health 2007; *127*(3), 137–141.
3. Steadward R. Integration and sport in the Paralympic movement. Sports Sci Rev. 1996; 5(1):26-41.
4. Mauerberg-deCastro E. Theory and practice in adapted physical education. The disability rights paradigm in synchrony with complex systems concepts. In. Ennis C. (ed.). Routledge Handbook of Physical Education Abingdon: Francis & Taylor 2016; pp 201-222.
5. Mauerberg-deCastro E. Atividade Física Adaptada (Adapted Physical Activity). Ribeirão Preto: Novo Conceito, 2011.
6. UN *World programme of action concerning disabled persons*. 2010. Available from: http://www.un.org/disabilities/default.asp?id=23 (accessed on August 23, 2014).
7. Mushoriwa, T. A study of attitudes of primary school teachers in Harare towards the inclusion of blind children in regular classes. Brit J Special Education, 2001; 28: 142-147.
8. Wong DKP. Do contacts make a difference? The effects of mainstreaming on student attitudes towards people with disabilities. Res Develop Disabil. 2008; 29:70-82.
9. IPC. Strategic Plan 2015 to 2018. 2015. Available from: https://www.paralympic.org/sites/default/files/document/150619133600866_2015_06%2BIPC%2BStrategic%2BPlan%2B2015-2018_Digital.pdf, (accessed on May 5, 2016).
10. Medical College of Wisconsin. History of Physical Medicine and Rehabilitation. 2015. Available from: http://www.mcw.edu/physicalmedicine/history.htm (accessed on June 6, 2015)
11. The Institute Guttmann. History. 2015. Available from: http://www.guttmann.com/en/history (accessed on April 13, 2016).
12. IPC. IPC Governing Board approves first 16 sports to be included in the Tokyo 2020 Paralympic Games. 2014. Available from: https://www.paralympic.org/news/ipc-governing-board-approves-first-16-sports-be-included-tokyo-2020-paralympic-games (accessed on May 25, 2016)
13. IOC. Documents. Olympic Movement. 2016. Available from: http://www.olympic.org/documents-reports-studies-publications (accessed on May 25, 2016).
14. Hums MA, Moorman AM, Wolff EA. The Inclusion of the Paralympics in the Olympic and Amateur Sports Act: Legal and Policy Implications Governing Bodies for Integration of Athletes with Disabilities into the United States Olympic Committee and National. J Sport a Social Issues, 2003;*27*:261.
15. Laureus. Second Laureus Award for Paralympic great Daniel Dias. 2013. Available from: http://www.laureus.com/news/second-laureus-award-paralympic-great-daniel-dias (accessed on May 6, 2015).
16. Williamson L. Sparks fly as blade stars go for Rio double after Oliveira steals the show with new world record at Olympic Stadium. *MailOnline*. 2013. Available from: http://www.dailymail.co.uk/sport/othersports/article-2380447/Alan-Oliveira-steals-new-world-record-Olympic-Stadium.html#ixzz3dAI7JOHZ (accessed on May 7, 2015).
17. COB. Dados relevantes do Brasil em Jogos Olímpicos (Relevant data from Brazil in the Olympic Games). 2016. Available from: http://www.cob.org.br/pt/time-brasil/brasil-nos-jogos (accessed on April 6, 2016);
18. IPC. IPC Historical Results Database. 2015. Available from: https://www.paralympic.org/results/historical (accessed on May 5, 2016).
19. Brazuna MR, Mauerberg-deCastro E. A Trajetória do Atleta Portador de Deficiência Física no Esporte Adaptado de Rendimento. Uma Revisão da Literatura (The trajectory of the athlete with physical disability in the elite adapted sport. A review of the literature). Motriz J, 2001; *7*(2):115-123.
20. Santamaria S, Mazzeo F. Ethical issues and doping in Olimpic and Paralympic Games. Sport Medicine Journal, no. 40, 2014. Available from: http://www.medicinasportiva.ro/SRoMS/english/Journal/No.40/Ethical-issues-doping-Olimpic-Paralympic-Games-full.html (accessed on June 12, 2015).
21. IPC. IPC Position Statement on autonomic Dysreflexia and Boosting, Section 2, Chapter 4.33, 2009. Available from: http://www.paralympic.org/sites/default/files/document/141113170443787_2014_10_13%2BSec%2Bii%2Bchapter%2B4_3_Position%2BStatement%2Bon%2BAutonomic%2BDysreflexia%2Band%2BBoosting.pdf 2009 (accessed on June 13, 2015).
22. IPC. Annual anti-doping statistics. 2015. Available from: https://www.paralympic.org/sites/default/files/document/140408122808010_2013_Annual%2BStatistics%2BAD_Final.pdf (accessed on May 5, 2016).
23. Van de Vliet P. Antidoping in Paralympic Sport. Clin J Sport Medicine, 2012; *22* (1):21-25.
24. Pipe A, Ayotte C. Nutritional Supplements and Doping. Clin J Sport Medicine, 2012; *12*:245–249.
25. Bhambhani Y, Mactavish J, Warren S, Thompson WR, Webborn A, Bressan E, *et al.* . Boosting in athletes with high-level spinal cord injury: knowledge, incidence and attitudes of athletes in Paralympic sport. Disability Rehab, 2010; *32* (26):2172-2190.
26. Webborn N, Emery C. Descriptive Epidemiology of Paralympic Sports Injuries. Paralympic Sports Medicine Sci, 2014; *6*:S18-S22.
27. Curtis KA, Dillon DA. Survey of wheelchair athletic injuries: common patterns and prevention. Paraplegia 1985; *23*:170-175.
28. Wheeler GD, Steadward RD, Legg D, Hutzler Y. Campbell E. Johnson A. Personal investment in disability sport careers: an international study. Adapted Physical Activity Quarterly 1999; *16*(3):219-237
29. Forbes. "*Thanks to media, sports industry growth is set to accelerate*". 2013. Available from: http://www.forbes.com/sites/tomvanriper/2013/11/13/thanks-to-mediasports-industry-growth-set-to-accelerate/ (accessed on November 13, 2013).

30. Globo.com. Alan Fonteles. 2013. Available from: http://globoesporte.globo.com/atleta/alan-fonteles.html (accessed on November 13, 2014).
31. Veja. Varejão renova com Cleveland e receberá US$ 30 milhões (Varejão renews contract with Cleveland and will receive $ 30 million). 2014. Available from: http://veja.abril.com.br/noticia/esporte/varejao-renova-com-cleveland-e-recebera-us-30-mi/ (accessed on June 11, 2015).
32. CPB. Paraolímpicos da Silva (Paralympics' Silva). 2015. Available from: http://www.cpb.org.br/paraolimpicos-da-silva/ (accessed on April 11, 2015).
33. CPB. Paralimpíadas escolares (School Paralympics) 2012. Available from: http://www.cpb.org.br/categoria/paralimpiadas-escolares/ (accessed on June 6, 2013).
34. Brasil. Jogos Escolares da Juventude. Histórico (The Youth School Games). Ministério do Esporte. 2013. Available from: http://www.esporte.gov.br/ (accessed on June 6, 2013).
35. Alexiou H. Developing young disabled people through sports leadership and volunteering. English Federation of Disability Sport East Midlands. 2009.
36. Fitzgerald H, Lang M. A Review of the Literature on Volunteering, Disability and Sport. English Federation of Disability Sport (East Midlands), The Carnegie Research Institute, Leeds Metropolitan University. Leeds: Carnegie Hall, 2009.
37. Charlton JI. Nothing About Us Without Us: Disability Oppression and Empowerment. University of California Press. ISBN 0-520-22481-7 1998. Available from: http://books.google.com/books?id=ohqff8DBt9gC&lpg=PA3&pg=PA3#v=onepage&q&f=false (accessed on June 22, 2010).
38. English Federation of Disability Sports (EFDS, 2012). Inspire to lead. Available from: http://www.efds.co.uk/resources/past_programmes/581_inspire_to_lead (accessed on April 11, 2016).
39. CDPF. China Disabled Persons' Federation (CDPF). 2016. Available from: http://www.cdpf.org.cn/englishold/ (accessed n April 6, 2016).
40. IPC. Classification. 2015. Available from: https://www.paralympic.org/classification (accessed on June 2, 2015).
41. Hopper CA. Socialization of wheelchair athletes in sports. Doctoral dissertation, University of Oregon, Eugene; 1984.
42. Wheeler G, Malone L, Van Vlack S, Nelson E, Steadward R. Retirement from Paralympic sport: A pilot study. Adapted Physical Activity Quarterly, 1996; *13*(4): 382-399.
43. CPB. Ádria Santos e Antonio Delfino entram para a galeria dos Heróis do Paradesporto (Ádria Santos and Antonio Delfino enter the gallery of para-sports heroes). 2014. Available from: http://www.cpb.org.br/adria-santos-e-antonio-delfino-entram-para-a-galeria-dos-herois-do-paradesporto/ (accessed on June 14, 2015).
44. Lancenet. Líbero Fabi pede a criação de projeto para ajudar atletas aposentados (Libero Fabi calls for the creation of a project to help retired athletes). 2012. Available from: http://www.lancenet.com.br/minuto/Libero-Fabi-criacao-atletas-aposentados_0_773322855.html (accessed on June 14, 2015).
45. Brasil. Como os atletas paralímpicos buscam patrocínio e encerram a carreira (How Paralympic athletes seek sponsorship and make career transition) - Bloco 4. 2012. Available from: http://www2.camara.leg.br/camaranoticias/radio/materias/REPORTAGEM-ESPECIAL/411061-COMO-OS-ATLETAS-PARALIMPICOS-BUSCAM-PATROCINIO-E-ENCERRAM-A-CARREIRA.html (accessed on June 14, 2015)
46. Brasil. Logo após tomar posse, Comissão Nacional de Atletas promove primeira reunião (Soon after taking office, National Commission of athletes promotes first meeting). 2015. Available from: http://www.brasil2016.gov.br/pt-br/noticias/logo-apos-tomar-posse-comissao-nacional-de-atletas-promove-primeira-reuniao (accessed on June 14, 2015).
47. Rio 2016 Paralympic Games. IPC president predicts record-breaking performances at Rio 2016 Paralympic Games. 2016. Available from: https://www.rio2016.com/en/paralympics/news/ipc-president-predicts-record-breaking-performances-at-rio-2016-paralympic-games (accessed on June 2, 2016).
48. DePauw K, Gavron S. Disability Sport. 2nd ed. Champaign, IL: Human Kinetics, 2005.
49. Yeo JD, Walsh J, Rutkowski S, Soden R, Craven M, Middleton J. Mortality following spinal cord injury. *Spinal Cord*, 1998; 36: 329-33.
50. Torben Grael. Biography. nd. Available from: http://torben-grael.com/biography.php (Accessed on June 10, 2015).
51. Robertscheidt. O Robert é o maior atleta Olímpico individual do Brasil de todos os tempos (Robert is the most successful Olympic athlete of all time in Brazil). nd. Available from: http://www.robertscheidt.com.br/site_test.asp (Accessed on June 10, 2015).
52. The Guardian. Oscar Pistorius unlikely to run for South Africa again, says sports minister. 2014. Available from: http://www.theguardian.com/sport/2014/oct/23/oscar-pistorius-south-africa-sports-minister-reeva-steenkamp (accessed on June 1, 2015).
53. BBC News. *Oscar Pistorius trial: 10 key moments*. 2015. Available from: http://www.bbc.com/news/world-africa-29018522 (accessed on May 16, 2016).

Corresponding author

Eliane Mauerberg-deCastro
Department of Physical Education.
Laboratory of Action and Perception,
São Paulo State University
(Universidade Estadual Paulista)
Av. 24-A, 1515, Bela Vista
Zip code:13506-900
Rio Claro, SP, Brazil
Email: mauerber@rc.unesp.br

11

Respiratory muscle strength and aerobic performance of wheelchair basketball players

Raphael N. Pereira
Marcos Fabio R. Abreu
Camila B. Gonçalves
Universidade Metodista de Piracicaba, Piracicaba, Brasil

Wilson Flávio S. Corrêa
Clube dos Deficientes Físicos do Pará – "All Star Rodas", Pará, Brasil

Daniel R. Mizuhira
Associação dos Amigos Paradesportistas de Piracicaba, Piracicaba, Brasil

Marlene A. Moreno
Universidade Metodista de Piracicaba, Piracicaba, Brasil

Abstract—The respiratory system has been described as a limiting factor in the performance of athletes. Therefore, the objective of this study was to evaluate the relationship between the respiratory muscle strength (RMS) and aerobic performance of wheelchair basketball players (WCBPs). We evaluated 19 male WCBPs who were divided into two groups: trunk control group (TCG) and without trunk control group (WTCG). All participants underwent a pulmonary function test, evaluation of maximal inspiratory (MIP) and expiratory (MEP) pressures, and an aerobic performance test. The MIP of both groups and the MEP values of TCG exceeded the predicted values for age and gender. No differences were observed in the MIP and aerobic performance between the groups although a difference was observed in the MEP values. Positive correlations were observed between MIP/MEP and the aerobic performance for both groups. These results suggested that the overall RMS of this group of WCBPs fell within or above the predicted values. Hence, the study concluded that RMS can positively influence the aerobic performance of WCBP.

Keywords: respiratory muscles, adapted physical activity, athletic performance, breathing tests

Introduction

Respiratory muscle strength is an important variable for evaluating the respiratory health of people with disabilities, especially in subjects who have some form of muscle dysfunction generating trunk instability. Apart from being related to postural control, trunk muscles are responsible for the rib cage motion and the pressure difference that ensures proper air flow in and out of the lungs during the breathing process. A dysfunction in this process could predispose the subject to develop some pulmonary diseases such as atelectasis and pneumonia[1]. In view of the respiratory alterations and their aggravation resulting from a sedentary lifestyle, participation in physical activity and sports has been encouraged as a means of health promotion among people with disabilities[2].

Meanwhile, the respiratory system has also been described as a limiting factor in the aerobic performance of highly-trained athletes. These limitations are related to increased respiratory work, exercise-induced arterial hypoxemia, respiratory muscle fatigue, and dyspnea[3]. The increase in respiratory rate, tidal volume, and minute volume; particularly in sustained exercises that exceed 85% of the maximal oxygen uptake (VO_2 max)—generates a greater metabolic demand on the inspiratory muscles, especially in the diaphragm, and can lead to muscle fatigue in some cases[4].

The increase in the inspiratory muscle work during physical exercises also generates a greater activation of metaboreflex. The major activation of this reflex leads to specific adaptations in the blood flow circulation, which cause the redirection of peripheral blood flow from the limbs to the diaphragm and other inspiratory muscles[5]. Therefore, the exacerbation of this mechanism could decline the exercise performance of well-trained subjects[6,7].

In search of strategies to improve aerobic performance, specific inspiratory muscle training programs have been developed, the aims of which are to postpone or prevent inspiratory muscle fatigue and reduce the blood flow redirection from the limb muscles[8]. However, divergent results have been found with regards the effectiveness of this strategy of training among wheelchair athletes[9-11].

Thus far, only one study has reported the behavior of respiratory muscle strength (inspiratory and expiratory) in wheelchair basketball players (WCBPs)[12]. However, this study only reported the respiratory muscle strength of paraplegic athletes without assessing subjects with other types of disabilities.

Thus, considering the importance of respiratory muscle strength to the exercise performance of athletes and the relevance of evaluating the respiratory health of people with disabilities, the aims of this study are to (1) evaluate the respiratory muscle strength and the aerobic performance of WCBPs and (2) compare the obtained values of inspiratory muscle strength (IMS) and expiratory muscle strength (EMS) with the predicted values by equation. Moreover, the respective relationships between IMS and EMS and the aerobic performances of these subjects are also assessed.

Methods

Study design

This is a clinical trial with an observational and cross-sectional design.

Participants

Thirty-one male WCBPs were considered for participation, of which 19 were eventually selected. Inclusion criteria were as follows: male and training for WCB for more than one year. Exclusion criteria included smoking and/or the presence of cardiovascular, respiratory, motor or cognitive alterations that make it impossible to perform the research procedures.

WCB training sessions took place three to five times per week for 3–5 h each and included physical training and coaching on techniques and tactics. The training involved stretching and resistance exercises as well as cardiovascular resistance; the WCB resistance training focused on the arm, shoulder, and trunk musculature.

Apart from physical training, the athletes were involved in technical and tactical training specific to WCB. Approximately 60% of the sessions were dedicated to practice games and tactical positioning, while 40% of the sessions focused on specific activities, such as shooting, passing, and obstacle courses.

The participants were divided into two groups according to functional classification score, as suggested by the International Wheelchair Basketball Federation (IWBF): without trunk control group (WTCG, N = 12, functional classification from 1.0 to 2.5) and with trunk control group (TCG, N = 07, functional classification from 3.0 to 4.5) (Figure 1). The IWBF functional classification for group division was chosen because this process also indirectly evaluated some respiratory muscle functions. Some of these muscles also acted as postural muscles (e.g., sternocleidomastoid, trapezius [upper fibers], pectoralis minor, serratus anterior and posterior superior, and rib lifters muscles). The characteristics of the participants and the etiologies of their respective disabilities are described in Table 1.

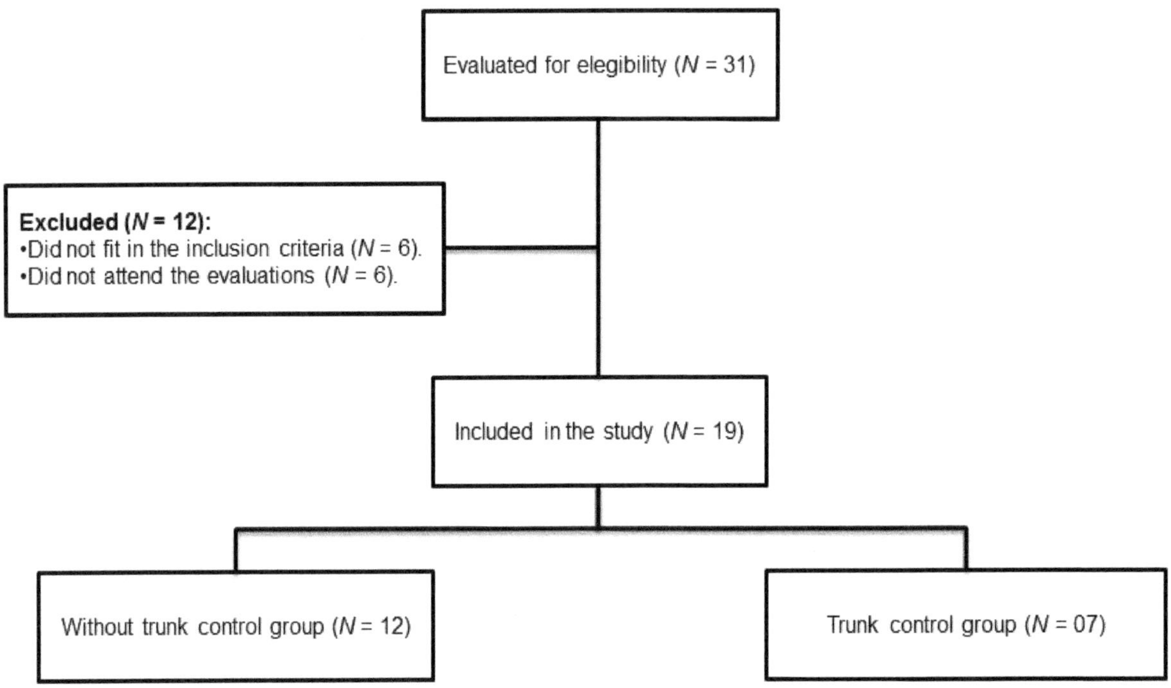

Figure 1. Flowchart presenting sample loss in the study.

Table 1. Characteristics of the subjects.

		WTCG	TCG	p value
N		12	7	
Age (years)	**Mean**	31.67	30.00	0.64
	SD	8.15	6.06	
Body mass (kg)	**Mean**	65.41	68.99	0.64
	SD	16.16	14.90	
Height (m)*	**Mean**	1.59	1.55	0.90
	SD	0.17	0.24	
Time of disability (years)	**Mean**	17.23	22.67	0.31
	SD	10.14	11.69	
Training experience (years)	**Mean**	5.14	7.91	0.21
	SD	4.67	4.74	
Training volume (hours/week)	**Mean**	23.50	18.00	0.45
	SD	10.32	11.22	
IWBF basketball classification		1.0 – 2.5	3.0 – 4.5	
Etiology of physical disabilities				
SCI (T4–L5)		7	1	
Spina bifida		2	1	
Polio		1	1	
Congenital malformation		1	2	
Unilateral amputation		0	2	
Arthrogryposis multiplex		1	0	

Note. WTCG = without trunk control group; TCG = with trunk control group; IWBF = International Wheelchair Basketball Federation; SCI = spinal cord injury; (T4–L5) = level of SCI; p value = comparison between WTCG vs. TCG; * non-parametric data. (Data presented as mean and standard deviation [SD]).

All participants were informed about the study's relevance and procedures. After agreeing to participate, they were asked to sign an informed consent form. This study was approved by the research Ethics Committee of the involved institution (protocol number 57/13).

Procedures

All subjects underwent a 48-hour period of rest (without training) prior to the evaluation protocol. An interview was conducted to collect data about the volunteers' health and to verify their eligibility. After this interview, the evaluation protocol was carried out on two consecutive days. On the first day, the respiratory variables were evaluated with a pulmonary function test and maximal respiratory pressure measurements (inspiratory and expiratory). On the second day, (24 h after the first evaluation procedures) we assessed the participants' aerobic performance by using the 12-minute aerobic test for wheelchair users.

Pulmonary function test

The pulmonary function tests were carried out with a spirometer (Easy one, ndd Medizintechnik AG, Zurich, Switzerland) according to the American Thoracic Society (ATS) guidelines for technique, acceptability, and reproducibility[13]. The device was calibrated before each test according to the manufacturer's instructions. Spirometric variables were recorded and expressed in body temperature and pressure as well as saturated conditions.

The measurement protocol was as follows. First, we carefully described the procedures to them, after which the subjects rested for 10 min. The examination then began with the subjects seated upright (90° hip flexion angle) in their own wheelchair with their heads in neutral position and wearing a nose clip to avoid air leakage through the nostrils. The mouthpiece was correctly placed over each subject's mouth to avoid air leakage.

The force vital capacity (FVC) maneuver was carried out. For this maneuver, the subjects were instructed to maximally inspire and then exhale completely with maximum effort. The participants were verbally encouraged to exhale forcibly until the end of the maneuver. Expiration was interrupted after 6 s.

Each maneuver was carried out until three acceptable and two reproducible curves were obtained without exceeding eight attempts. During the maneuvers, real-time graphics of the curves were shown to them, indicating whether they met the acceptance criteria proposed by the ATS[13].

The tests were superimposed automatically in the equipment, which made it easier to verify their reproducibility. Thus, after the acceptance criteria were fulfilled, the curves were classified according to reproducibility, with the maximal differences for FVC and FEV_1 in the two best curves (i.e., 5% or 150 mL) being considered for analysis. Tests that exceeded these limits were excluded. The curves were analyzed by using two evaluators, and those considered technically inappropriate were excluded from the analysis. After the acceptability and reproducibility criteria were met, the highest values of the studied variables were recorded.

The absolute values were obtained based on spirometric tests and the percentages of the predicted values for age and gender of both groups for FVC and the volume exhaled during the first second of a forced expiratory maneuver (FEV_1). Based on the equations for healthy subjects, which were developed by previous study for use as guidelines in pulmonary function tests, equations were used to predict normal values so as to verify the presence of ventilator dysfunctions and thus characterize the population[14].

Respiratory muscle strength

The respiratory muscle strength values were obtained by measuring maximal inspiratory and expiratory pressures (MIP and MEP) with an analog manometer (Ger-ar®, São Paulo, Brazil) scaled in cmH_2O with an operational limit of ± 300 cmH_2O.

MIP and MEP were measured from residual volume (RV) and total lung capacity (TLC), respectively. Each subject was asked to sit in an erect position (90° hip flexion). A nose clip was used to prevent air leakage through the nostrils; a rigid plastic mouthpiece that was connected to the manometer was also used. The entire protocol was conducted in the presence of a trained evaluator. At least five maximal maneuvers were performed, of which three had to be acceptable and reproducible (difference of less than 10%); a one-minute rest interval was given between each maneuver. The inspiratory and expiratory efforts had to be sustained for at least one second, and the highest values obtained were recorded for subsequent analysis[15]. The maximal predicted respiratory pressures were calculated in absolute values and percentages for each volunteer using equations[15].

Aerobic performance test

To evaluate each participant's aerobic performance, the 12-minute test for wheelchair users was conducted in a covered multisport court. A rectangle measuring 25 × 15 meters (m) was marked on the court. A total of 12 cones were placed on the rectangular space: four cones were placed at each corner and the remaining eight cones were spaced every 2 m, forming a rectangle with a perimeter of 75.32 m. Figure 2 shows the test area.

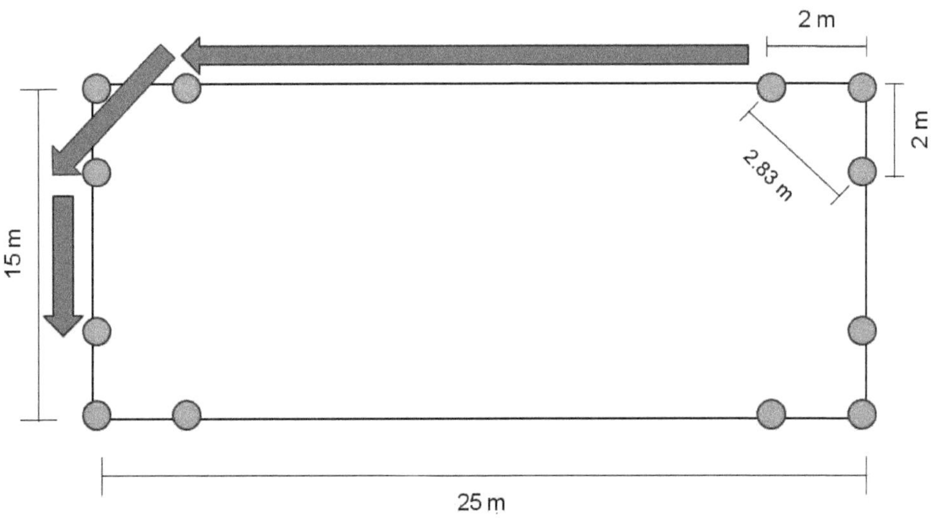

Figure 2. Test area for the 12-minute aerobic test.

The participants' resting cardiopulmonary variables were checked before conducting the test. Blood pressure (BP) was measured with the auscultation method, heart rate (HR) with a Polar RS800CX® heart rate monitor (Polar Electro Co.Ltda. Kempele, Oulu, Finland), and peripheral oxygen saturation (SpO_2) with pulse oximetry (Solmedica MD300C1 oximeter, Beijing Choice Eletronic Tech. Co., Ltd.). Subjective perception of effort was measured by using the Borg scale (CR-10).

After completing these procedures, the test was initiated, during which the participants were instructed to follow the marked track, turn strategically to maintain velocity, and cover the greatest distance possible within 12 min. The test began and ended with a beep, and standardized verbal encouragement was given each minute by the same evaluator (e.g., "2 min have passed and you are doing very well, keep it up").

At the end of the test, in addition to calculating the total distance covered, the previously mentioned cardiopulmonary variables were measured again. The estimated VO_2max reached was then calculated according to a previous method[16].

Statistical analysis

The statistical procedures were carried out using Bioestat v.5.0. The Shapiro-Wilk test was conducted to analyze the normality of the data distribution. Student's t-test was used for parametric data, and the Mann-Whitney test was used to compare non-parametric data.

To measure the effect size, Cohen's d was calculated by using the Effect Size Generator 2.3 software (Swinburne University of Technology, Center for Neuropsychology, Melbourne, Australia). The threshold values for effect size statistics were 0.2, 0.5, and 0.8 for small, medium, and large effect sizes, respectively[17].

Pearson's linear correlation coefficient was used to analyze the relationship between variables. All results were described as means and standard deviation, and the significance level adopted for all analyses was 5%.

Results

Table 2 presents the relative and absolute values of the spirometric variables. Neither of the groups presented restrictive or obstructive pulmonary disease. In both groups, values that were over 80% of the predicted were found for all variables. A small effect size was found for small to FEV_1/FVC; medium to FVC (L), FEV_1 (L), and FEV_1 (%); and large to FVC (%) comparisons.

Table 3 shows the obtained and predicted MIP and MEP values. It is noteworthy that both groups showed MIP values above the predicted ones, both with large effect size. Regarding

MEP, the values obtained in the TCG were significantly higher than the predicted values, with large effect size. Meanwhile, the WTCG presented no significant difference for this variable and showed medium effect size for this comparison.

Table 2. Absolute and relative values obtained from the pulmonary function test.

		WTCG	TCG	Difference (%)	p value	Effect size
FVC (L)	Mean	3.95	4.52	12.61	0.27	0.56
	SD	1.10	0.92			
FVC (%)	Mean	96.25	130.71	26.36	0.07	0.82
	SD	24.36	52.75			
FEV_1 (L)	Mean	3.26	3.68	11.41	0.30	0.54
	SD	0.91	0.63			
FEV_1 (%)	Mean	93.42	121.86	23.34	0.19	0.78
	SD	18.51	48.24			
FEV_1/FVC	Mean	0.84	0.82	2.38	0.47	0.30
	SD	0.08	0.05			

Note. WTCG = without trunk control group; TCG = with trunk control group; p value = comparison between WTCG vs. TCG; FVC = forced vital capacity; FEV_1 = forced expired volume after 1 second. (Data presented as mean and standard deviation [SD]).

Table 3. Comparison between obtained and predicted values of maximal inspiratory and expiratory pressures in both groups.

	Group		Obtained (cmH_2O)	Predicted (cmH_2O)	Difference (%)	p value (Obtained vs. Predicted)
MIP	WTCG	Mean	157.50	129.97	17.48	0.04
		SD	40.82	6.52		
	TCG	Mean	180.00	131.30	27.06	0.04
		SD	49.75	4.84		
MEP	WTCG	Mean	166.25	139.35	16.18	0.19
		SD	66.34	6.60		
	TCG	Mean	237.14	141.00	40.54	0.002
		SD	50.57	4.90		

Note. MIP = maximal inspiratory pressure. MEP = maximal expiratory pressure. WTCG = without trunk control group. TCG = with trunk control group. P value = comparison between Obtained vs. Predicted values of MIP and MEP. (Data presented as mean and standard deviation [SD]).

Table 4 presents the comparisons of obtained values for maximal respiratory pressure and the variables of the aerobic performance test. Significant difference was found only between MEP values, which had a large effect size. The other variables showed small (MIP; Δ Diastolic blood pressure; Final SpO_2), medium (Δ Systolic blood pressure and Final Borg scale), and large effect sizes (Δ Heart rate and VO_2 max).

Table 4. Comparison of respiratory pressure obtained values and of the 12-minute aerobic test result between the two groups.

		WTCG	TCG	Difference (%)	p value	Effect size
Obtained MIP (cmH_2O)	Mean	157.50	180.00	12.50	0.30	0.49
	SD	40.82	49.75			
Obtained MEP (cmH_2O)	Mean	166.25	237.14	29.89	0.03	1.20
	SD	66.34	50.57			
Distance covered (m)	Mean	2055.81	2275.55	9.66	0.09	0.88
	SD	261.91	238.69			
Δ Heart rate	Mean	102.33	88.71	13.31	0.08	0.84
	SD	13.24	18.58			
Δ SBP (mmHg)*	Mean	30.00	39.29	23.64	0.42	0.52
	SD	12.06	22.07			
Δ DBP (mmHg)	Mean	- 9.17	- 6.43	29.88	0.73	0.17
	SD	18.81	11.80			
Final SpO_2 (%)*	Mean	97.75	97.86	0.11	0.87	0.18
	SD	0.75	0.38			
Final Borg scale (0–10)*	Mean	8.83	9.43	6.36	0.22	0.65
	SD	1.03	0.79			
VO_2 max (ml/kg/min)	Mean	26.94	31.00	13.10	0.09	0.88
	SD	4.83	4.40			

Note. MIP = maximal inspiratory pressure; MEP = maximal expiratory pressure; WTCG = without trunk control group; TCG = with trunk control group; Δ Heart rate = variation in the heart rate values before and after the exercise test; Δ SBP = variation in the systolic blood pressure values before and after the exercise test; Δ DBP = variation in the diastolic blood pressure values before and after the exercise test; SpO2 = peripheral oxygen saturation at the end of the test; VO_2 m_{ax} = maximal oxygen uptake; p value = comparison between WTCG vs. TCG; * non-parametric data. (Data presented as mean and standard deviation [SD]).

Regarding the correlations between distance covered in the aerobic performance test and the maximal respiratory pressures, the WTCG showed positive correlations for both MIP ($r = 0.60$; $R^2 = 0.36$; $p = 0.04$) and MEP ($r = 0.35$; $R^2 = 0.12$; $p = 0.36$). At the same time, the TCG showed positive correlations for MIP ($r = 0.71$; $R^2 = 0.50$; $p = 0.07$) and MEP ($r = 0.51$; $R^2 = 0.26$; $p = 0.24$). These data are presented in Figure 3.

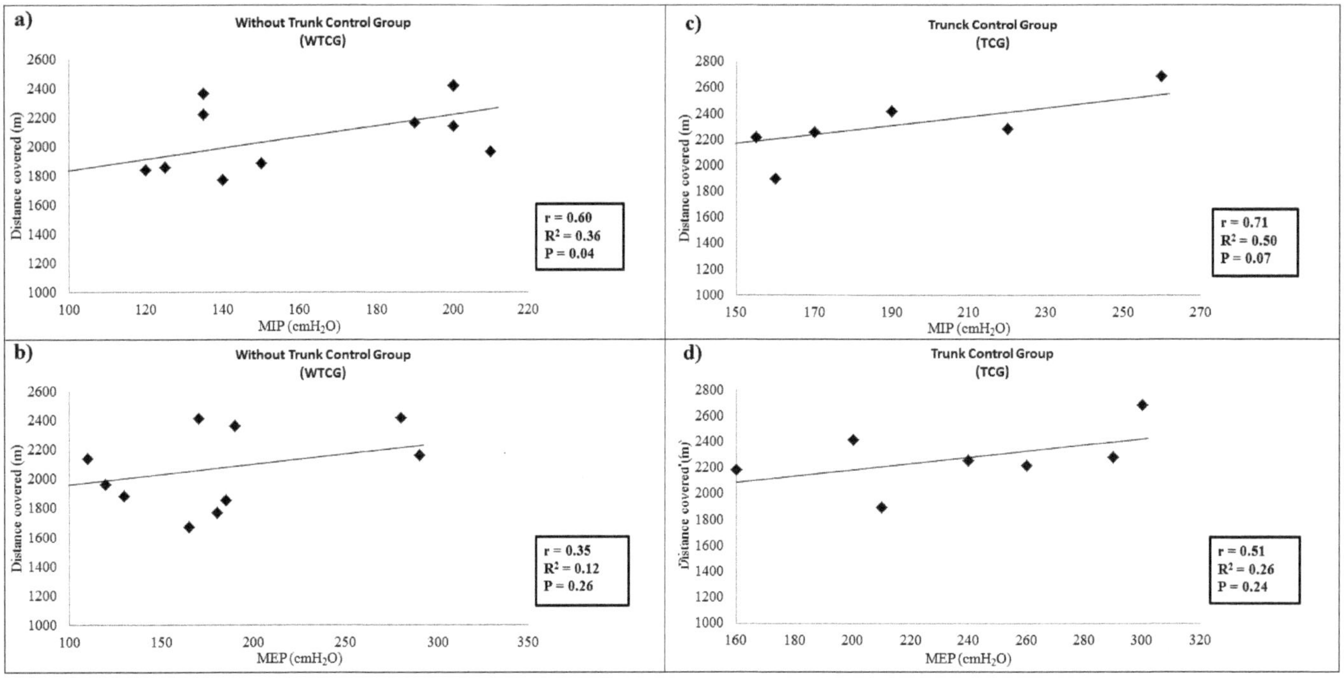

Figure 3. Correlations between the distances covered in the aerobic performance test and the maximum inspiratory pressure (MIP) and maximum expiratory pressure (MEP).

a) Correlation between the distances covered and MIP in the WTCG; b) Correlation between the distances covered and MEP in the WTCG; c) Correlation between the distances covered and MIP in the TCG; d) Correlation between the distances covered and MEP in the TCG.

Discussion

The pulmonary function test revealed that both groups did not present ventilatory disorders. Several authors have indicated the relevance of spinal cord injury (SCI) in decreased pulmonary function resulting from alterations in the mechanics of respiratory muscles[1,12,18,19]. In addition, evidence showed a decline in the pulmonary function of subjects with SCI, which they attributed to higher body mass index, lower inspiratory muscle strength, and declined levels of physical fitness[20]. In another study, it was demonstrated values of 2.67 ± 0.83 and 3.10 ± 1.10 L for FVC at the baseline of intervention and control groups of sedentary subjects with SCI, respectively; they also reported FEV_1 values of 2.11 ± 0.68 and 2.18 ± 0.75 L for these two groups[21]. In the present study, we found values that exceeded those reported in the abovementioned studies.

Regarding Paralympic athletes without SCI, only a single study has reported the pulmonary function of these subjects at the baseline[22]. It was found values of 4.74 ± 0.77 L for FVC and 4.10 ± 0.68 L for FEV_1 at the baseline of a group of highly trained subjects from the Swiss Paralympic team with single-limb amputation or blindness. These values are almost similar to the variables reported in the present study. However, caution must be taken when comparing these data, because in the present study, we investigated subjects who trained in just one specific sport modality whereas Osthoff[22] did not specify the sports modality of their volunteers.

These findings suggest that the WCB regular training could preserve the pulmonary function of the present study's subjects. Indeed, WCBPs make ample use of the upper limb and trunk muscles both for wheelchair propulsion and for throwing the ball during the matches[23-25]. Some of these muscles involved in the stabilization, positioning, and execution of upper limb; trunk movements also act as the accessory muscles facilitating the inspiratory and expiratory processes. Therefore, the training of these muscles during the WCB practice may have helped prevent alterations in respiratory mechanics and, consequently, in the pulmonary function of these subjects, especially in those who had SCI.

In the present study, the level of the participants' SCI fell between T4 and L5. According to the literature, this should indicate a reduced functioning of the intercostal muscles, which have innervations originating in the spinal roots from T1 to T11[1]. According to De Troyer[26], alterations in intercostal muscle function may lead to decreased IMS and consequent decreases in thoracic expansibility. However, in the current study, the obtained MIP values were higher than the predicted values, and similar values were obtained in both groups.

The literature features few studies on the effects of wheelchair sports training on respiratory muscle strength. Furthermore, the majority of these studies evaluated only subjects with SCI. Goosey-Tolfrey[9] found lower MIP and MEP values at the baseline in their study (MIP = 75.4 ± 33.3 cmH_2O and MEP = 69.4 ± 21.0 cmH_2O for the intervention group; MIP = 74.5 ± 27.3 cmH_2O and MEP = 60.4 ± 18.3 cmH_2O for the control group) when they analyzed competitive WCBPs with SCI, post-polio, or spina bifida. However, recently, it was reported obtained values of MIP similar to those predicted by equation in tetraplegics who trained in wheelchair rugby (MIP = 113.7 ± 35.5) and paraplegics who trained in WCB (MIP = 112.2 ± 23.3)[12]. In that same study, however, the subjects showed MEP values that were lower than the predicted ones (MEP = 73.7 ± 20.7 cmH_2O for the wheelchair rugby athletes group [tetraplegics]; MEP = 105.6 ± 34.3 cmH_2O for the WBC group [paraplegics]).

Regarding the respiratory muscle strength, several authors investigated its comportment in able-bodied trained subjects and showed values that are below those reported in the present study. One study found values of 129.1 ± 16.5 cmH_2O for the MIP at the baseline when they studied the effects of inspiratory muscle training in 17 competitive male rowers[27]. More recently, it was reported baseline values of 115 ± 26 and 117 ± 30 cmH_2O for the MIP of the experimental and control group, respectively, in 16 club-level competitive swimmers[28].

The findings of the present study are in agreement with those described by Moreno[12] and could also be attributed to the previously described training of the accessory muscles during the WCB practice. Moreover, some of scapular girdle muscles act in upper limb movement and stabilization and serve as accessory muscles in the forced inspiration process[23-25,29]. The constant utilization of these muscles during the WCB training may have resulted in adaptations in their functions and morphologies, which culminated in a greater capacity to generate force.

Regarding MEP behavior, the obtained values were higher than the predicted values only in the TCG. This group's obtained values were higher than those of the WTCG. The natural process of expiration does not require muscular activity and only requires a difference between the pulmonary and external pressures. However, during forced expiration, muscles located in the thoracic (pectoralis major) and trunk (abdominals) regions actively assist the increase of expiratory flow and the deflation of the lungs[30,31]. Maintaining abdominal muscle functionality is linked with preserving trunk control. The maintenance of trunk control is one of the most important behaviors in the IWBF functional classification. Greater trunk stabilization and angular movements (flexion, extension, lateralization, and rotation) generate greater functional classification scores[32]. Therefore, we suggest that the TCG had better trunk control and stabilization owing to their higher functional classification scores. For this reason, this group's MEP values exceeded the predicted ones and were even higher than the WTCG values. This may be attributed to the fact that the TCG had better abdominal muscle function and strength. It should be noted that the obtained WTCG MEP values were not lower than the predicted values, even though 7 of the 12 volunteers in this group had SCI between T4 and L5, suggesting the possible functional impairment of the abdominal muscles. These finding may also be attributed to the regular training of WCBPs, as previously suggested by Moreno[12].

Additionally, similarities in distance covered and VO_2 max were observed in the aerobic test results of the two groups. Leicht,[33] detected a mean VO_2peak of 24.5 mL/kg/min for a group of disabled athletes with high SCI (quadriplegics), 34.9 mL/kg/min for a group of disabled athletes with low SCI (paraplegics), and 42 mL/kg/min in a group of disabled athletes with no SCI and greater trunk control. These findings indicate that a smaller group of muscles utilized during exercise generates lower oxygen uptake, considering that the VO_2 max value takes into account the supply, transportation, and the muscular capacity to extract the oxygen.

Our findings agree with other results presented in the literature. Franklin[16] observed a VO_2 max of 22 $mL/kg^{-1}/min^{-1}$ in a heterogeneous group of 30 wheelchair users (25 paraplegics, two with polio, and three amputees) who practiced sports regularly. The distance covered by these individuals in the 12-minute aerobic test ranged from 0.64 to 1.79 miles (1029.68 to 2880.73 meters). Using a multi-stage test, Vanderthommen[34] evaluated the aerobic physical performance of a heterogeneous group of wheelchair users who practiced sports and found a VO_2peak of 25.3 mL/kg/min. used an adaptation for wheelchair users of the multistage Léger and Boucher test and found a VO_2peak of 2.05 l/min^{-1}.

The literature has suggested that SCI type (partial or complete) and level can lead to reductions in the muscle mass that are activated during exercise and to alterations in the activation of the autonomous nervous system. In turn, these culminate in decreased aerobic capacity, with lower levels being observed in individuals with high SCI (quadriplegics) than in subjects with lower SCI (paraplegics)[33]. However, no differences in aerobic performance between the groups were observed in the present study. This finding may be due to the fact that the TCG had fewer participants (n = 7) than the WTCG.

The relationships found in both groups between MIP and distance covered in the aerobic performance test showed a positive and strong correlation, in which 36% and 50% of aerobic performance test results were influenced by IMS in the WTCG and TCG, respectively. The overloads imposed on inspiratory muscles during an intense exercise activity can limit the aerobic performance of highly trained athletes as well as healthy non-athletes[7,8,36]. Thus, the positive relationships founded between IMS and distance covered in the aerobic performance test may be related to the lower activation of the metaboreflex induced by the work of the inspiratory muscles. Considering that stronger muscles have a lower oxygen demand, the volunteers who presented better inspiratory muscle performances probably had lower oxygen demands from these muscles during the test, which led to lower amounts of required local blood flow. This mechanism may have optimized the blood flow distribution to the active muscles of the trunk and upper limbs, which in turn, reduced the pH imbalance caused by the exercise. This, in turn, led to decreased muscle fatigue and sensation of dyspnea, which culminated in better results on the aerobic test.

MEP was also positively correlated with distance covered in the aerobic performance test for both groups with a moderate strength. Moreover, it is important to note that 26% and 24% of the WTCG and TCG aerobic performance test results, respectively, were influenced by EMS. For wheelchair users, apart from abdominal muscles being use in the forced expiratory process[30] these muscles are also associated with greater efficiency in wheelchair propulsion[37,38]. Thus, the relationship found between EMS and aerobic performance may have been due to the greater activation of the abdominal muscles and better trunk control, which probably led to higher MEP values and better mechanical efficiency in wheelchair propulsion.

We did not find in the literature other studies that correlated IMS and/or EMS with the aerobic performance of wheelchair athletes. Thus, comparing our results with those of previous studies must be done with caution. Some others limitations were found and should be mentioned. The heterogeneity of the volunteers and the small sample size, particularly in the TCG, could have influenced the results. First, we have to take into account the difficulty of finding the specific population being studied study (WBCPs). Nevertheless, the inclusion and exclusion criteria were rigorously followed to minimize possible bias, and all eligible volunteers participated in the study were included. We propose that future studies try to have a higher number of participants and divide the volunteers according the respective etiologies of their disabilities.

We also have to highlight the fact that the equations used to obtain the predicted values for the respiratory variables were developed for individuals without disabilities, and that no similar equations could be found, which can be adapted for people with physical disabilities. Furthermore, evaluating the metabolic variables and the redirection of blood flow during the aerobic performance test could have better clarified the findings of this study.

The choice of the aerobic performance test could also be questioned. An ergospirometry test is often considered the gold standard test in evaluating the athlete's aerobic performance. However, owing to the lack of necessary equipment to perform this test, the field test was chosen because of the daily practice of the athletes and because of their specificity with the sport modality that was studied. We must also consider that the equation used to obtain the VO_2max values took into account the distance covered by the athlete in this test. Moreover, the correlations analysis was also based on the distance covered because this variable can significantly predict physical capacity in field tests.

The lack of a reproducibility evaluation of the aerobic performance test can also be described as a limitation of the present study. The repetition of the test procedures by the subjects generated better results because of the learning effect. Unfortunately, because of the hard training routine of the athletes, we could not accomplish the second test to avoid this learning bias.

In conclusion, neither of the studied groups presented pulmonary alterations of restrictive or obstructive origin, and the inspiratory and expiratory muscle strengths were within or above the values predicted for age and gender. There were no significant differences in the inspiratory muscle strength or aerobic performance between the groups; however, the expiratory muscle strength of the TCG was greater than that of the WTCG, which could be attributed to greater trunk control and use of abdominal muscles in the former.

In addition, there were positive correlations between the maximal respiratory pressures and the distance covered in the aerobic performance test for both groups. These findings demonstrate that respiratory muscle strength is related to the aerobic performance of these WCBPs.

References

1. Winslow C, Rozovsky J. Effect of spinal cord injury on the respiratory system. Am J Phys Med Rehabil *2003*; *82*(10): 803-14.
2. Scelza WM, Kalpakjian CZ, Zemper ED, Tate DG. Perceived barriers to exercise in people with spinal cord injury. Am J Phys Med Rehabil 2005; *84*: 576-83.
3. Wells GD, Norris SR. Assessment of physiological capacities of elite athletes & respiratory limitations to exercise performance. Paediatr Respir Rev, 2009; *10*(3): 91-8.
4. Johnson BD, Babcock MA, Suman OE, Dempsey JA. Exercise-induced diaphragmatic fatigue in healthy humans. J Physiol *1993; 460*: 385-405.
5. St Croix CM, Morgan BJ, Wetter TJ, Dempsey JA. Fatiguing inspiratory muscle work causes reflex sympathetic activation in humans. *J Physiol* 2000; *529*: 493-504.
6. Aaron EA, Seow KC, Johnson BD, Dempsey JA. Oxygen cost of exercise hyperpnea: implications for performance. J Appl Physiol *(1985),* 1992*;* *72*(5): 1818-25.
7. Dempsey JA, McKenzie DC, Haverkamp HC, Eldridge MW. Update in the understanding of respiratory limitations to exercise performance in fit, active adults. Chest 2008*; 134*(3): 613-22.
8. McConnell AK, Lomax M. The influence of inspiratory muscle work history and specific inspiratory muscle training upon human limb muscle fatigue. J Physiol 2006; *577*(Pt 1): 445-57.
9. Goosey-Tolfrey V, Foden E, Perret C, Degens H. Effects of inspiratory muscle training on respiratory function and repetitive sprint performance in wheelchair basketball players. Br J Sports Med 2010*; 44*(9): 665-68.
10. Litchke LG, Russian CJ, Lloyd LK, Schmidt EA, Price L, Walker JL. Effects of respiratory resistance training with a concurrent flow device on wheelchair athletes. J Spinal Cord Med 2008*; 31*(1): 65-71.
11. Vergès S, Flore P, Nantermoz G, Lafaix PA, Wuyam B. Respiratory muscle training in athletes with spinal cord injury. Int J Sports Med 2009*; 30*(7): 526-32.
12. Moreno MA, Zamunér AR, Paris JV, Teodori RM, Barros RM. Effects of wheelchair sports on respiratory muscle strength and thoracic mobility of individuals with spinal cord injury. Am J Phys Med Rehabil, 2012; 91(6): 470-77.
13. Miller MR, Hankinson J, Brusasco V, Burgos F, Casaburi R, Coates A, *et al.* Standardisation of spirometry. Eur Respir J, 2005; 26(2): 319-38.
14. Pereira CAC. Diretrizes para Testes de Função Pulmonar. J Pneumol 2002*; 28*(suppl 3): 1-82.
15. Neder JA, Andreoni S, Lerario MC, Nery LE. Reference values for lung function tests. II. Maximal respiratory pressures and voluntary ventilation. Braz J Med Biol Res 1999*; 32*(6): 719-27.
16. Franklin BA, Swantek KI, Grais SL, Johnstone KS, Gordon S, Timmis GC. Field test estimation of maximal oxygen consumption in wheelchair users. Arch Phys Med Rehabil, 1990*; 71*(8): 574-78.
17. Cohen J. Statistical Power Analysis for the behavioural science. 2nd Edition, Lawrence Earlbaum Associates, 1988.
18. Aarabi B, Harrop JS, Tator CH, Alexander M, Dettori JR, Grossman RG, *et al.* Predictors of pulmonary complications in blunt traumatic spinal cord injury. J Neurosurg Spine 2012; 17(1 Suppl): 38-45.

19. West CR, Campbell IG, Shave RE, Romer LM. Resting cardiopulmonary function in Paralympic athletes with cervical spinal cord injury. Med Sci Sports Exerc 2012; 44(2): 323-29.
20. Postma K, Haisma JA, de Groot S, Hopman MT, Bergen MP, Stam HJ, *et al*. Changes in pulmonary function during the early years after inpatient rehabilitation in persons with spinal cord injury: a prospective cohort study. Arch Phys Med Rehabil 2013; 94(8): 1540-46.
21. Postma K, Haisma JA, Hopman MT, Bergen MP, Stam HJ, Bussmann JB. Resistive inspiratory muscle training in people with spinal cord injury during inpatient rehabilitation: a randomized controlled trial. Phys Ther 2014; 94(12): 1709-19.
22. Osthoff M, Michel F, Strupler M, Miedinger D, Taegtmeyer AB, Leuppi JD, *et al*. Bronchial hyperresponsiveness testing in athletes of the Swiss Paralympic team. BMC Sports Sci Med Rehabil 2013; *5*(1):7.
23. Kulig K, Newsam CJ, Mulroy SJ, Rao S, Gronley JK, Bontrager EL, *et al*. The effect of level of spinal cord injury on shoulder joint kinetics during manual wheelchair propulsion. Clin Biomech (Bristol, Avon) 2001; 16(9): 744-51.
24. Mulroy SJ, Farrokhi S, Newsam CJ, Perry J. Effects of spinal cord injury level on the activity of shoulder muscles during wheelchair propulsion: an electromyographic study. Arch Phys Med Rehabil 2004; 85(6): 925-34.
25. Sinnott KA, Milburn P, McNaughton H. Factors associated with thoracic spinal cord injury, lesion level and rotator cuff disorders. Spinal Cord 2000; *38*(12): 748-53.
26. De Troyer A, Estenne M, Vincken W. Rib cage motion and muscle use in high tetraplegia. Am Rev Respir Dis, 1986; 133(6): 1115-9.
27. Griffiths LA, McConnell AK. The influence of inspiratory and expiratory muscle training upon rowing performance. Eur J Appl Physiol 2007; 99(5): 457-66.
28. Kilding AE, Brown S, McConnell AK. Inspiratory muscle training improves 100 and 200 m swimming performance. Eur J Appl Physiol 2010; 108(3): 505-11.
29. De Troyer A, Kirkwood PA, Wilson TA. Respiratory action of the intercostal muscles. Physiol Rev, 2005; *85*(2): 717-56.
30. Campbell EJ, Green JH. The expiratory function of the abdominal muscles in man; an electromyographic study. J Physiol,1953; 120(3): 409-18.
31. McKenzie DC. Respiratory physiology: adaptations to high-level exercise. Br J Sports Med 2012; 46(6): 381-84.
32. Perriman D. Official player classification manual. 2010; *International Wheelchair Basketball Federation*. Available from http://www.iwbf.org/_OLD_JULY_2013/images/!!!Classification/2010-2014 [acessed in July 19, 2013].
33. Leicht CA, Bishop NC, Goosey-Tolfrey VL. Submaximal exercise responses in tetraplegic, paraplegic and non spinal cord injured elite wheelchair athletes. Scand J Med Sci Sports 2012; 22(6): 729-36.
34. Vanderthommen M, Francaux M, Colinet C, Lehance C, Lhermerout C, Crielaard JM, *et al*. A multistage field test of wheelchair users for evaluation of fitness and prediction of peak oxygen consumption. J Rehabil Res Dev 2002; *39*(6): 685-92.
35. Vinet A, Le Gallais D, Bouges S, Bernard PL, Poulain M, Varray A, *et al*. Prediction of VO(2peak) in wheelchair-dependent athletes from the adapted Léger and Boucher test. Spinal Cord 2002; 40(10): 507-12.
36. Romer LM, Lovering AT, Haverkamp HC, Pegelow DF, Dempsey JA. Effect of inspiratory muscle work on peripheral fatigue of locomotor muscles in healthy humans. J Physiol, 2006; *571*(Pt 2): 425-39.
37. Rodgers MM, Keyser RE, Gardner ER, Russell PJ, Gorman PH. Influence of trunk flexion on biomechanics of wheelchair propulsion. J Rehabil Res Dev 2000; *37*(3): 283-95.
38. Yang YS, Koontz AM, Triolo RJ, Mercer JL, Boninger ML. (2006). Surface electromyography activity of trunk muscles during wheelchair propulsion. Clin Biomech (Bristol, Avon), 2006; *21*(10): 1032-41.

Corresponding author

Marlene Aparecida Moreno, PhD, Postgraduate program in physical therapy, Methodist University of Piracicaba, Rodovia do Açúcar Km 156, Taquaral, Piracicaba, SP
Email: ma.moreno@terra.com.br

12

Effects of water ingestion throughout exercise and recovery on cardiac autonomic modulation during and after exercise

Isadora Lessa Moreno
Universidade Federal de São Paulo, São Paulo, SP, Brasil

Luiz Carlos Marques Vanderlei
Franciele Marques Vanderlei
Carlos Marcelo Pastre
Universidade Estadual Paulista "Julio de Mesquita Filho", Presidente Prudente, SP, Brasil

Luiz Carlos de Abreu
Faculdade de Medicina do ABC, Santo André, SP, Brasil

Celso Ferreira
Universidade Federal de São Paulo, São Paulo, SP, Brasil

Abstract—Purpose: To analyze the effects of water intake on heart rate variability (HRV) during and after exercise. Methods: Thirty-one young males performed three different procedures: I) a maximal exercise test to determine the load for the protocols; II) the control protocol (CP); III) the experimental protocol (EP). The protocols comprised 10 minutes at rest, 90 minutes of treadmill exercise (60% of VO_2 peak), and 60 minutes of recovery. No rehydration beverage consumption was allowed during the CP. During the EP, the participants were given water every 15 minutes, being that the amount of water to be ingested by each volunteer was divided over the time of exercise and recovery. For the analysis of HRV data, time and frequency domain indices were investigated in the following moments (M): M1 (5 minutes final of rest), M2 (25–30 minutes of exercise), M3 (55–60 minutes of exercise), M4 (85–90 minutes of exercise), M5 (5–10 minutes of recovery), M6 (15–20 minutes of recovery), M7 (25–30 minutes of recovery), M8 (40–45 minutes of recovery), and M9 (55–60 minutes of recovery). Results: There was no statistically significant difference between the groups that were examined during the exercise. HRV values for the CP and EP at the end of the exercise period were as follows SDNN (5.95±1.89 vs 6.89±2.11); RMSSD (3.29±0.78 vs 3.39±0.95); HF [nu] (24.06±14.26 vs 19.10±11.94); LF [nu] (75.93±14.26 vs 80.89±11.94); HF [ms^2] (0.90±1.16 vs 0.94±0.89); LF [ms^2] (4.65±5.94 vs 5.35±5.09); and LF/HF ratio (4.64±3.15 vs 6.95±5.57). HRV values for the CP and the EP at the end of the recovery period were as follows: SDNN (39.63±19.63 vs 49.95±17.79); RMSSD (21.63±15.55 vs 36.43±22.73); HF [ms^2] (285.51±392.27 vs 699.29±699.66); LF [nu] (74.55±13.25 vs 61.19±19.27); and HF [nu] (25.44±13.25 vs 38.8±19.27). Conclusion: The hydration with water was not enough to significantly influence the linear HRV indices during exercise; however, it promoted faster recovery of these variables after exercise.

Keywords: exercise, rehydration solutions, autonomic nervous system, heart rate

Introduction

The process of dehydration occurs when fluid loss is not compensated by the ingestion of fluid, which in turn will lead to a deterioration of temperature regulation, performance, and health. Ensuring adequate fluid intake before, during, and after exercise can improve performance and reduce the problems associated with heat[1-4].

Efficient hydration ensures the ideal conditions for the practitioner to maintain their physical capability to provide proper functioning of the homeostatic processes required by exercise[5].

From a physiological standpoint, studies have shown the benefits of water intake during and/or after exercise. A previous study subjected ten individuals to ingestion of water immediately after a 30-minute cycling exercise at a workload representing 80% of anaerobic threshold. They showed that water consumption accelerated cardiac vagal reactivation after exercise; however, no significant influence on heart rate (HR) and blood pressure responses was observed[6]. In another study, the participants were subjected to a protocol of hydration during and after exercise: the results showed minimal changes in systolic blood pressure (SBP) and diastolic blood pressure (DBP) and a smaller increase in HR during exercise[7]. The results showed better HR recovery and faster return of SBP and DBP and better performance of pulse oxygen saturation and respiratory rate. Peçanha, Paula-Ribeiro, Campana-Rezende,

Bartels, Marins, de Lima[8] evaluated the effects of water intake on the parasympathetic recovery after high-intensity exercise in active young individuals and found that water accelerates post-exercise vagal reactivation.

Although studies have shown that water intake (the method of hydration most commonly used) before or during exercise is beneficial to cardiac autonomic responses post-exercise, it is not known what is the effect of water intake performed repeatedly throughout the exercise and recovery period on these responses. In addition, the studies did not evaluate these responses for an extended recovery time. Therefore, our purpose was to evaluate the effects of hydration protocols on autonomic modulation of the heart in young people during and post-exercise. We hypothesized that hydration with water during exercise and recovery may attenuate autonomic changes induced by exercise and accelerate recovery. To test this hypothesis, we assessed linear indices of heart rate variability (HRV) in young men with and without water intake (Vittalev, Spaipa, Brazil).

Methods

Participants

Thirty-one healthy, young male volunteers (21.5±1.8 yrs) were investigated. All were active according to the International Physical Activity Questionnaire (IPAQ)[9]. These volunteers had no damaging habits such as smoking or alcohol consumption, were not taking medications that influence cardiac autonomic activity, and were not diagnosed with any cardiovascular, metabolic or endocrine disorder. No volunteers were excluded during the course of the experiment. Every individual signed a consent letter and was informed of the procedures and objectives of the study. The study's procedures were all approved by the Research Ethics Committee of the Federal University of São Paulo –UNIFESP (Number 0861/11).

Experimental design protocol

For all visits, volunteers were instructed to avoid consuming caffeine 24 h before the procedures, to consume a light fruit-based meal 2 h before the tests, to have a good night's sleep (7–8 h), to avoid strenuous physical exercise the day before the test and to wear appropriate and comfortable clothes (shorts, shirt, shoes, and socks) for physical exercise.

The clinical trial was based on previous studies[10,11]. Participants reported to the laboratory three days per week, at an interval of 48 hours between visits. An incremental test was applied during the first visit, which was performed on a treadmill (Super ATL, Inbrasport, Brazil) according to the Bruce protocol[12]. To establish the baseline, volunteers were allowed to rest in a standing position on the mat before the test began. Once the test started, verbal encouragement was used in an attempt to obtain a maximum physical effort; the test was interrupted by voluntary exhaustion. To determine oxygen consumption (VO_2), expired gases were analyzed using a regularly calibrated metabolic analyzer (VO*2000*, Medical Graphics, St Paul, MN, USA). The VO_2 peak was taken to be the highest VO_2 achieved in the test. The HR reached at 60% of VO_2 peak was used to determine the exercise intensity for the protocols, considering that gastric emptying is considerably disturbed at intensities above 70% of VO_2 peak[13].

In subsequent visits, called control (CP) and experimental (EP) protocols, volunteers were allowed to rest in the supine position for 10 minutes, followed by 90 minutes of exercise (60% of VO_2 peak), and 60 minutes of recovery. Volunteers were not given any fluids to drink during the CP; however, during the EP they were given water (Vittalev, Spaipa, Brazil) containing bicarbonate (62.49 mg/L), calcium (7.792 mg/L), carbonate (3.91 mg/L), chloride (0.09 mg/L), strontium (0.343 mg/L), fluorid (0.05 mg/L), magnesium (0.340 mg/L), potassium (1.485 mg/L), sodium (16.090 mg/L), and sulfate (0.18 mg/L). Water intake was administered in 10 equal portions at regular intervals of 15 minutes from the fifteenth minute of exercise until the end of the recovery. They were given water at temperatures between 15 and 22°C. The amount of water administered was based on the difference in body weight before and after the CP, therefore the CP was always realized before the EP—there was no randomization. This technique indicates that 1 g reduction in body weight is equal to 1 mL of fluid reduction[14].

The protocols were performed in a room under environment temperatures (26.0±2.3°C) and humidity (55.1±10.4%) between 3 p.m. and 6 p.m. to avoid circadian variations. To ensure the condition of initial hydration all the volunteers drank water (500 mL) at one time 2 h before both protocols[1]. Body weight (digital scale Plenna, TIN 00139 MÁXIMA, Brazil), and height (stadiometer ES 2020, Sanny, Brazil) were measured in all the subjects upon their arrival at the laboratory. The heart monitor was then strapped on each subject's thorax over the distal third of the sternum. The HR receiver (Polar Electro S810i, Kempele, Finland) was placed on the wrist for beat-to-beat HR measurements and for HRV analysis.

HR was analyzed at the following periods: final 10 minutes of rest; after 30, 60, and 90 minutes of exercise; after 5, 10, 20, 30, 40, 50, and 60 minutes of recovery.

The volunteers remained at rest in the supine position for 10 minutes and immediately their axillary temperature (thermometer BD Thermofácil, China) was measured. Subsequently, the participants performed a treadmill exercise (60% of VO_2 peak) for 90 minutes and were then allowed to rest in the supine position for 60 minutes for recovery. Axillary temperature was checked again immediately following exercise; the volunteers' nude weight was measured again at the end of the recovery period.

Urine was collected and analyzed (10 Choiceline, Roche®, Brazil) at the end of the EP and after measurement of final body weight. Urine density was used as a marker for hydration level[15].

Heart rate variability indices analysis

HRV was recorded beat-to-beat through the monitoring process (Polar Electro S810i) at a sampling rate of 1000 Hz. During the period of higher signal stability, verified of visual form, an interval of 5 minutes was selected, and series with more than 256 RR intervals were used for analysis, following digital filtering complemented by manual filtering to eliminate premature ectopic beats and artifacts. Only series with more than 95% sinus rhythm were included in the study[16,17]. To analyze HRV in the frequency domain, we used the low (LF) and high frequencies (HF) spectral components in normalized units (nu) and absolute (ms^2), and the LF/HF ratio, which represents the relationship between low and high frequencies[16]. We considered the following range: LF, 0.04–0.15 Hz and HF, 0.15–0.4 Hz. The spectral analysis was calculated using the Fast Fourier Transform algorithm[18]. Analysis in the time domain was performed by means of SDNN (ms) (standard deviation of normal-to-normal RR intervals) and RMSSD (ms) (root-mean square of differences between adjacent normal RR intervals in a time interval)[16].

HRV indices were analyzed at the following moments: M1 (final 5 minutes rest); M2 (25–30 minutes after exercise); M3 (55–60 minutes after exercise); M4 (85–90 minutes after exercise); M5 (5–10 minutes of recovery); M6 (15–20 minute recovery); M7 (25–30 minute recovery); M8 (40–45 minute recovery) and M9 (55–60 minute recovery). Series with more than 256 RR intervals were used for analysis[16]. We used Kubios HRV version 2.0 software to analyze these indices[19].

Statistical Analysis

Gaussian distribution of the data was verified using the Shapiro-Wilks test. For comparisons between protocols (control vs. experimental) and moments (M1, M2, M3 and M4 during exercise and M1 vs. M5, M6, M7, M8, M9 during recovery) two-way repeated measures analysis of variance was applied, followed by the Bonferroni post-test for parametric distributions or Dunn's post-test for non-parametric data. The repeated measures data were checked for sphericity violation using Mauchly's test and the Greenhouse-Geisser correction was conducted when sphericity was violated. Significance level was set at $p < 0.05$ for all tests. SPSS (version 13.0) software (SPSS Inc., Chicago, IL, USA) was used for statistical analysis.

The sample size calculation was done considering how variable the RMSSD index. The magnitude of assumed significant difference was 12 ms, considering a standard deviation of 16 ms, with alpha risk of 5% and beta of 80%, and the sample size resulted in 28 young. Considering possible sample loss, adds up 10% to sample size calculated, totaling 31 young.

Results

The anthropometric characteristics of the participants and their responses obtained during the incremental test are described in Table 1. Table 2 shows data regarding body mass and temperature in the CP and the EP. We observed weight loss in the CP (Table 2). The percentage of body weight loss in the CP was 2.0±0.6%, while in the EP it was 0.1±0.8%. The average consumption of water was 1.4±0.5 L in the EP. The density of urine (1.017±0.004 g/mL) evaluated at the end of the EP confirms that the volume of solution intake was sufficient to maintain the participants at euhydrated status[15]. Body temperature behaved similarly in both protocols, increasing significantly at the end of the exercise (Table 2).

Table 1. Subject characteristics.

Variables	Mean ± Standard Deviation	Minimum/ Maximum
Anthropometric data	21.5 ± 1.8	[18 – 25]
Age (yr)	72.6 ± 11.5	[53.8 – 95.3]
Body mass (kg)	1.70 ± 0.10	[1.60 – 1.90]
Height (m)	23.0 ± 2.8	[16.8 – 28.1]
BMI (kg/m^2)		
Incremental test	3.3 ± 0.6	[2.0 – 5.1]
VO_{2peak} ($L.min^{-1}$)	160.7 ± 10.7	[139 – 179]
HR (bpm) at 60% VO_{2peak}		
VO_{2peak} relative to body mass ($L.min^{-1}$ / Kg)	0.047 ± 0.007	[0.027 – 0.058]

Legend: yr, years; kg, kilograms; m, meters; BMI, body mass index; VO2peak, peak oxygen consumption; HR, heart rate; bpm, beats per minute; L.min-1, liter per minute.

Table 2. Values of body mass and temperature in control and experimental protocols.

Variable	Moment	Control protocol	Experimental protocol
		Mean ± Standard Deviation Median [minimum–maximum]	
Body mass (kg)	Before the protocol	73.0 ± 11.6 * (72.9) [54.7 – 96.1]	73.1 ± 11.4 (73.2) [53.5 – 96.6]
	After the protocol	71.6 ± 11.3 (71.0) [53.6 – 94.2]	73.0 ± 11.5 (72.6) [53.5 – 97]
	Δ (%)	2.0 ± 0.6	0.1 ±0.8
	Before exercise	36.4 ± 0.5 # (36.5) [35 - 38]	36.5 ± 0.4* (36.5) [35 – 36.9]
Body temperature (ºC)	After exercise	37.2 ± 0.5 (37.2) [35.5 - 38]	37.0 ± 0.5 (37.0) [36.0 – 38.0]

Legend: kg, kilogram; °C, degrees Celsius; Δ, delta; %, percentage. *Value with a significant difference compared with after the exercise (Student t test of paired data; p < .05); #value with a significant difference compared with after the exercise (Wilcoxon test; p < .05);

Figure 1 shows HR values during exercise (Figure 1a) and recovery (Figure 1b). During exercise, we observed the effect of moment ($p < 0.001$) on HR; however, there was no effect among protocols ($p = 0.31$) and in the moment and protocol interaction ($p = 0.29$). In both protocols, we noted that HR was significantly increased at 30, 60, and 90 minutes of exercise compared to rest, however, although not significant, the increase was lower in the EP. In the recovery period, we observed the effects of moment ($p < 0.001$), and moment and protocol interaction ($p = 0.006$)

on HR; there was no effect among protocols ($p = 0.081$). In the CP, a significant decrease was observed when comparing all minutes of recovery at rest, while in the EP it was only observed in the 1, 3, 5, 7, 10, and 30 minute. In the EP, after 40 minutes of recovery the HR did return to baseline.

Figures 2 and 3 show the behavior of HRV indices in time and frequency domains, respectively, during exercise. There was a moment effect for the time domain indices (SDNN and RMSSD; $p < 0.001$). No effects were observed between the protocols (SDNN, $p = 0.66$; RMSSD, $p = 0.94$) and in the moment and protocol interaction (SDNN, $p = 0.91$; RMSSD, $p = 0.88$). We noted that SDNN (ms) and RMSSD (ms) were significantly decreased at M2, M3, and M4 of exercise in both the CP and EP compared to M1 (rest). Moreover, there was a decrease in the SDNN (ms) for the CP at M2 of exercise compared to M4 of exercise.

Likewise, we observed a moment effect in all indices in the frequency domain ($p < 0.001$). No effects were observed for those indices between the protocols [LF (ms^2), $p = 0.50$; HF (ms^2), $p = 0.72$; LF (nu), $p = 0.63$; HF (nu), $p = 0.63$; LF/HF, $p = 0.31$]. There were no interactions between moment and protocol [LF (ms^2), $p = 0.53$; HF (ms^2), $p = 0.71$, LF (nu), $p = 0.64$; HF (nu), $p = 0.64$, LF / HF, $p = 0.87$]. Regarding the comparison between moments, we observed that LF (ms^2), HF (ms^2), and HF (nu) were significantly higher at M1 (rest) compared to M2, M3, and M4 of exercise in both the CP and the EP. LF (nu) and LF/HF were significantly lower at M1 compared to M2, M3 and M4 of exercise in both the CP and the EP. Moreover, LF (ms^2) was significantly higher at M2 of exercise compared to M4 of exercise in the CP, while HF (ms^2) was significantly higher at M2 of exercise compared to M4 of exercise in the EP.

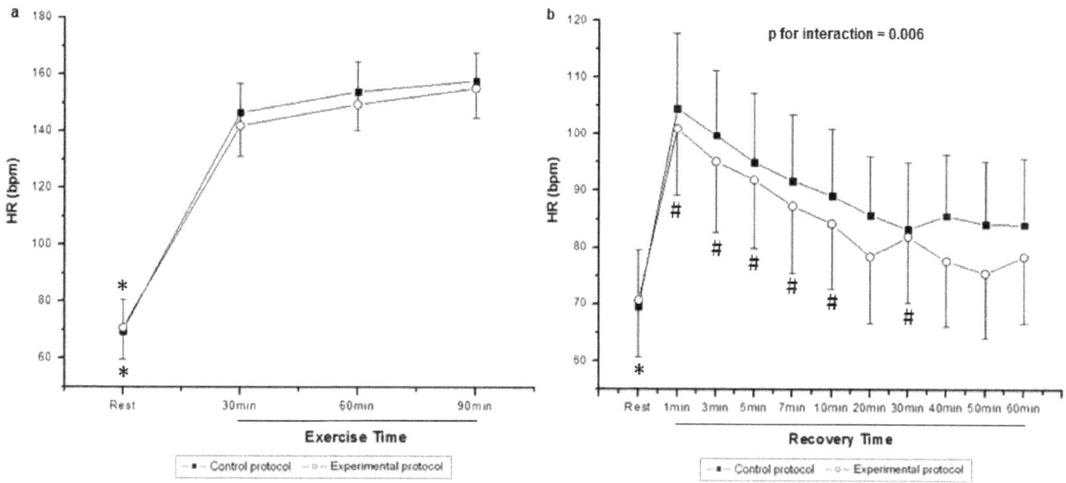

Figure 1. Values are mean ± standard deviation. Heart rate (HR) during (a) exercise and (b) recovery, and the comparison in control and experimental protocols; *Different from all the times of exercise and recovery ($p < 0.05$); #Different from M1 ($p < 0.05$); HR, heart rate; bpm, beats per minute.

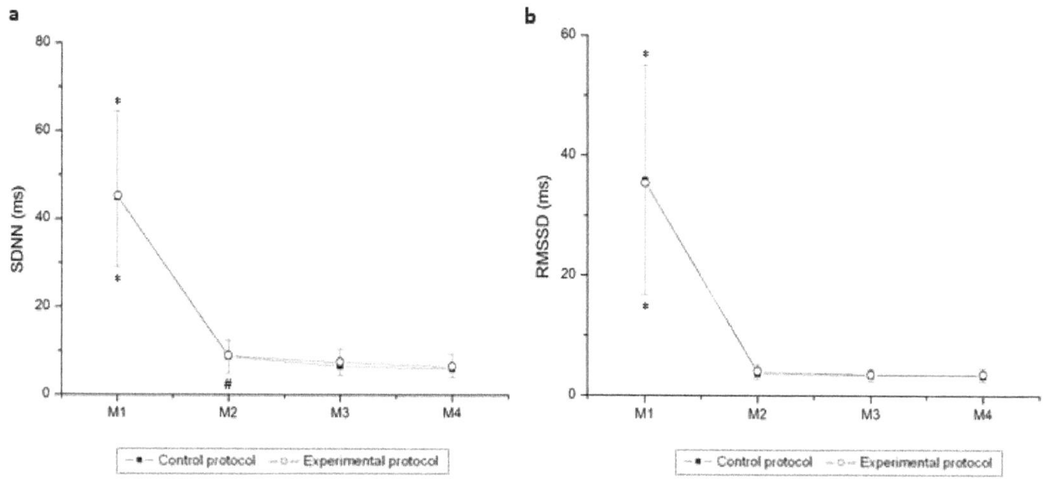

Figure 2. Values are mean ± standard deviation. (a) SDNN and (b) RMSSD during exercise and the comparison in control and experimental protocols. Final 5 minutes of rest (M1) and minutes of exercise: 25–30 (M2), 55–60 (M3), 85–90 (M4). *Different from M2, M3, and M4 ($p < 0.05$). #Different from M4 in the CP ($p < 0.05$); SDNN, standard deviation of the mean of all normal RR intervals; RMSSD, square root of the mean squared differences between successive normal RR intervals; M, moment; ms, milliseconds.

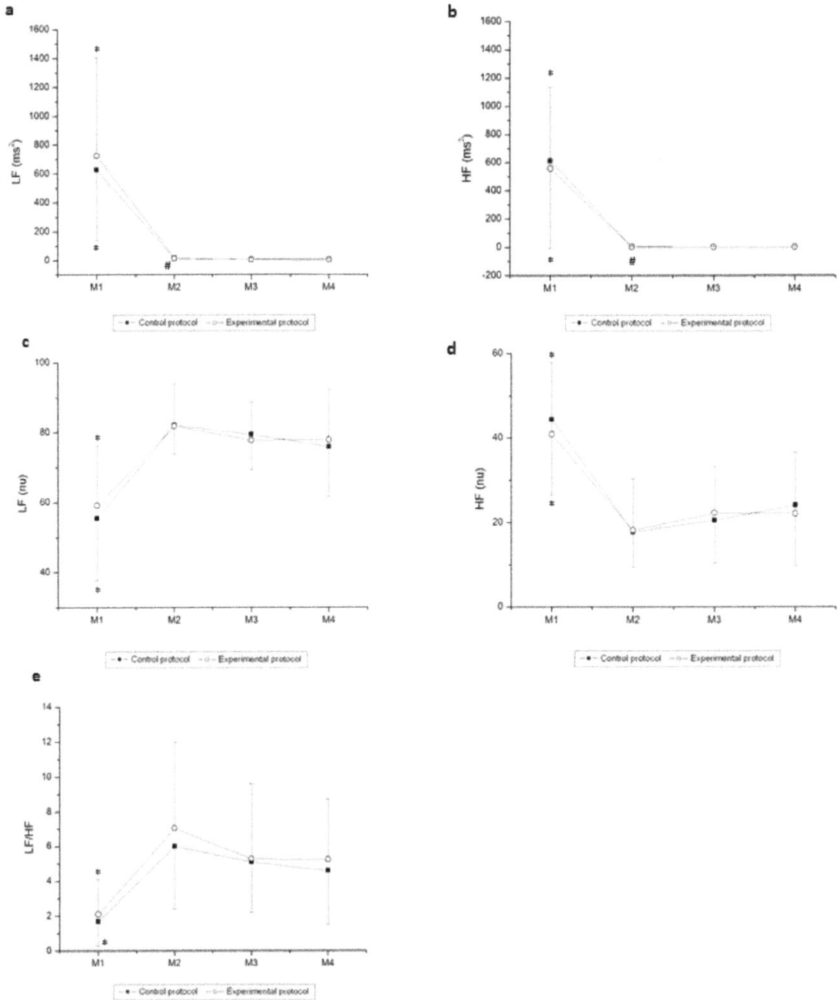

Figure 3. Values are mean ± standard deviation. (**a**) LFms², (**b**) HFms², (**c**) LFnu, (**d**) HFnu, and (**e**) LF/HF during exercise and the comparison in control and experimental protocols. Final 5 minutes of rest (M1) and minutes of exercise: 25–30 (M2), 55–60 (M3), 85–90 (M4). *Different from M2, M3, and M4 ($p < 0.05$); #Different from M4 in the CP (LF ms²) and the EP (HF ms²) ($p < 0.05$); LF, low frequency; HF, high frequency; M, moment; ms, milliseconds; nu, normalized units.

Figures 4 and 5 present the behavior of the HRV index in the time and frequency domains, respectively, during recovery. In relation to the time domain indices, we observed moment effects in the analyzed indices and interactions between moment and protocol (SDNN and RMSSD, $p < 0.001$). Effect of the protocol on RMSSD (ms) ($p = 0.04$) was observed, but not observed for the SDNN ($p = 0.12$). Regarding the comparison of the SDNN (ms) index between recovery and rest, it was significantly reduced at M5, M6, M7, M8, and M9 of recovery compared to M1 (rest) in the CP, while it was significantly decreased at M5 compared to M1 (rest) in the EP. Regarding RMSSD (ms), it was significantly reduced at M5, M6, and M7 of recovery compared to M1 (rest) in the EP, whereas it was significantly decreased at M5, M6, M7, M8, and M9 of recovery compared to M1 (rest) in the CP.

In relation to the frequency domain, moment effect was observed in all indices analyzed ($p < 0.001$). Effects were observed for those indices between the protocols [HF (ms²), $p = 0.03$; LF (nu), $p = 0.03$; HF (nu), $p = 0.03$], except for the LF/HF ratio ($p = 0.18$) and LF (ms²) ($p = 0.87$). Interactions between moment and protocol were observed for those indices [HF (ms²), $p = 0.002$; LF (nu), $p = 0.004$; HF (nu), $p = 0.004$], except for the LF/HF ratio ($p = 0.62$) and LF (ms²) ($p = 0.96$).

The LF (ms²) index was reduced at M5 and M6 of recovery compared to M1 (rest) in the CP while it was significantly decreased at M5 of recovery compared to M1 (rest) in the EP. HF (ms²) was significantly reduced at M5, M6, M7, and M8 of recovery compared to M1 (rest) in the CP, while it was significantly decreased at M5 and M6 of recovery compared to M1 (rest) in the EP. In relation to LF (nu), it was significantly increased at M5, M6, M7, M8, and M9 of recovery compared to M1 (rest) in the CP, whereas it was significantly increased at M5 of recovery compared to M1 (rest) in the EP. HF (nu) was significantly reduced at M5, M6, M7, M8, and M9 of recovery compared to M1 (rest) in the CP while it was significantly lower at M5 of recovery compared to M1 (rest) in the EP. LF/HF ratio was significantly higher at M5, M6, M7, M8, and M9 of recovery compared to M1 (rest) in the CP and significantly increased at M5 of recovery compared to M1 (rest) in the EP.

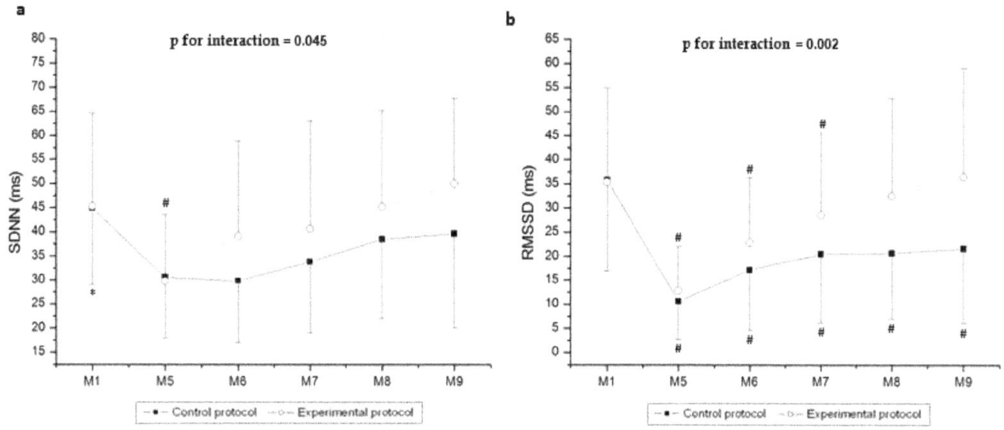

Figure 4. Values are mean ± standard deviation. (**a**) SDNN and (**b**) RMSSD during recovery and the comparison in control and experimental protocols. Final 5 minutes of rest (M1) and minutes of recovery: 5–10 (M5), 15–20 (M6), 25–30 (M7), 40–45 (M8), 55–60 (M9). *Different from M5, M6, M7, M8, and M9 ($p < 0.05$); #Different from M1($p < 0.05$); SDNN, standard deviation of the mean of all normal RR intervals; RMSSD, square root of the mean squared differences between successive normal RR intervals; M, moment; ms, milliseconds.

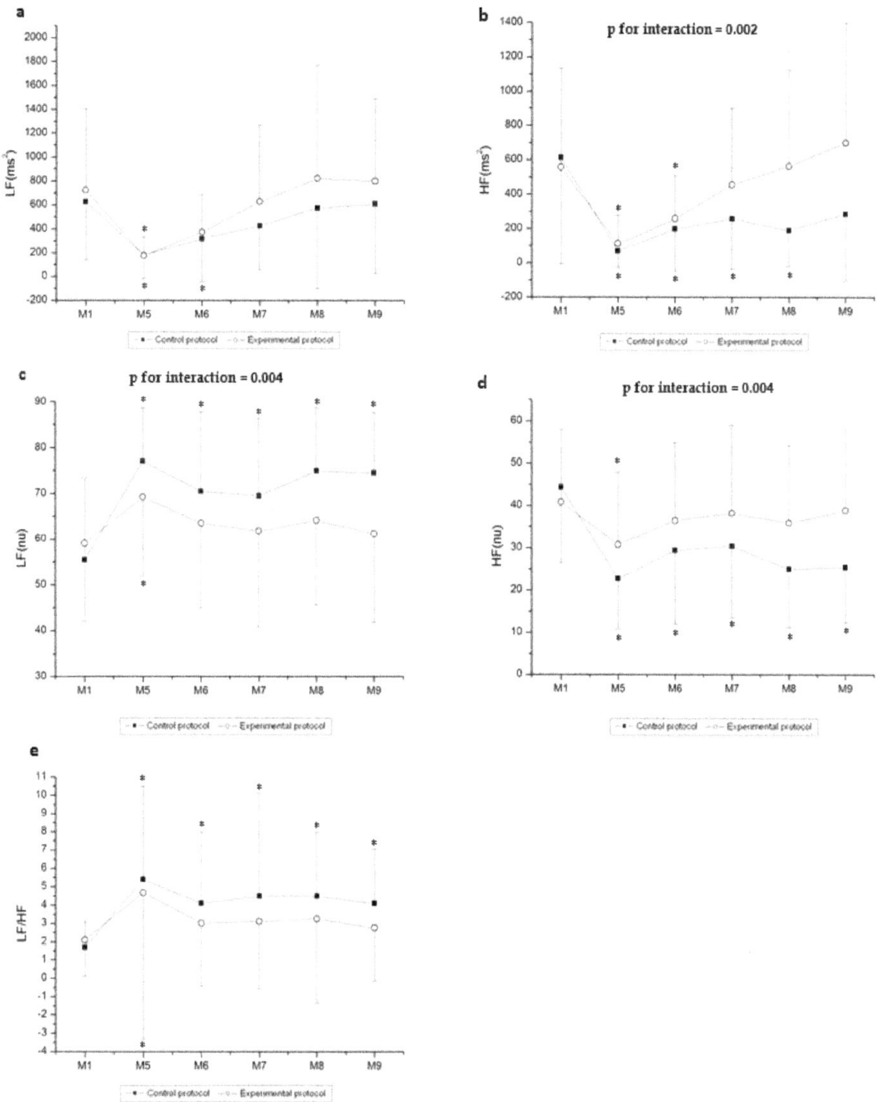

Figure 5. Values are mean ± standard deviation. (**a**) LFms², (**b**) HFms², (**c**) LFnu, (**d**) HFnu, and(**e**) LF/HF during recovery and the comparison in control and experimental protocols. Final 5 minutes of rest (M1) and minutes of recovery: 5–10 (M5), 15–20 (M6), 25–30 (M7), 40–45 (M8), 55–60 (M9). *Different from M1 ($p < 0.05$); LF, low frequency; HF, high frequency; M, moment; ms, milliseconds; nu, normalized units.

Discussion

The results obtained in this study show that the hydration protocol, despite having produced generally smaller changes in the HRV indices, failed to significantly influence these variables during exercise. However, water intake during the recovery period induced significant changes in cardiac autonomic modulation, promoting faster recovery of HRV indices.

It is well known that the loss of fluids through sweating, is the fundamental mechanism of heat dissipation during exercise, resulting in decreased plasma volume (PV)[20]. An early study observed that loss of 2.1% of body weight resulted in an average reduction of 5.2% in PV[21]. Despite PV not being rated in this study, we observed a loss of 2.0±0.6% of body weight when participants were not hydrated. Additionally, a study suggested that the reduction in stroke volume in participants dehydrated during exercise of moderate intensity is associated with a reduction in blood volume and an increase in HR and body temperature[22]. In our study, body temperature exhibited similar behavior in both protocols—which was also reported by Horswill, Stofan, Lovett and Hannasch[23]—and were not observed significant differences in HR during exercise when water was administered to volunteers in comparison to the CP.

Regarding to cardiac autonomic modulation, no significant interaction of the hydration protocol on the HRV indices analyzed was observed despite the predominance of sympathetic modulation on vagal tone during exercise. The RMSSD (ms) and HF (nu) indices, reflecting predominantly parasympathetic drive[24], decreased during exercise, although they exhibited higher, but not significant values, when water was administered to volunteers in comparison to CP. The reduction in PV resulting from the loss of body weight during exercise is responsible for reducing vagal modulation in dehydrated individuals[25-27], and possibly influenced by the lower values of RMSSD (ms) and HF (nu) in the non-hydrated condition.

Reduction in global HRV is expected during exercise[28] as well as increase in HR, stroke volume, cardiac output, and SBP, to supply the metabolic requirements. These mechanisms may explain the increased in LF (nu) index during exercise, that is predominantly modulated by sympathetic modulation, and also the increase in LF/HF ratio, reflecting the sympathovagal balance.[11] Accordingly, the increase in the spectral indices suggests a sympathetic activation during exercise at low and moderate intensities[29]. Similarly, it was reported reduced SDNN (ms), RMSSD (ms) and HF and increased LF during exercise in individuals subjected to 8 minutes of the step test at 70% of the maximal potency[30].

During exercise, as a consequence of reduced cardiac vagal modulation, the reduction of global HRV is accompanied by a decrease in absolute power (ms^2) of the spectral components[31]. This behavior was also observed in the present study: LF (ms^2) and HF (ms^2) indices decreased during exercise compared with the rest, regardless of the administration of water. The literature indicates that both spectral indices decreased according to exercise intensity[32]. Therefore, we expected minimal changes to be observed in these indices due to the work load maintenance during exercise in our study.

It is important to note that during exercise other aspects, such as central command, mechanoreflex, and metaboreflex stimuli are probably more potent than hydration to influence the changes in autonomic modulation, which could also justify the absence of changes observed during exercise between protocols.

When the recovery period is analyzed, the hydration protocols promoted faster HR recovery (40 minutes post-exercise) compared with the condition in which no rehydration fluid was offered, as evidenced by the significant interaction between time and protocols on this parameter. Significant interaction between time and protocols was also observed after supplying water at the beginning and at 15, 35 and 55 minutes of exercise for 16 participants[33]. They found that from the tenth minute of recovery, HR in the poorly hydrated condition was significantly higher (100±4 bpm) until the end of the experiment compared to well-hydrated condition (90±4 bpm).

According to Hendrickse and Triger[34], the function of volume retention by the sympathetic system is checked by the reciprocal activity of the vagal system, which promotes diuresis of salt and water. Yun, Lee, and Bazar[35] suggest that hydration reduces the sympathetic drive to maintain volume and increases the parasympathetic impulse to promote diuresis. Additionally, the modulation of baroreceptors during gastric distension may be another factor that promotes reduction of sympathetic modulation due to a secondary effect of increased vagal afferent modulation[35]. A previous study reported that the ingestion of 500 mL of water caused a bradycardic response followed by an increase in cardiac vagal modulation[36]. These factors may have influenced the pattern of HR response observed in this study when water was administered as well as the behavior of HRV indices.

The indices that reflect the predominance of vagal modulation, RMSSD (ms), HF (ms^2) and HF (nu) showed a gradual increase and rapid recovery, observed in around 40 minutes when the participants were hydrated with water. In contrast, complete recovery of these indices in hypohydrated individuals was not observed. Additionally, a significant interaction between time and protocol was observed for all these indices, which suggests better recovery after exercise in the hydrated condition.

Similarly, the indices that reflect predominantly sympathetic modulation, LF [ms^2] and LF [nu], also recovered better in the EP, especially the LF [nu] index which at 15 minutes post-exercise returned to the baseline. Despite the LF [ms^2] index having shown similar behavior in both protocols, the LF index [nu] revealed a significant interaction between time and protocols, suggesting faster recovery after exercise in the hydrated condition and thus sympathetic predominance in hypohydrated individuals.

Therefore, it is suggested that the process of water deficit, closely associated with the practice of physical activity resulting in 2% loss of body weight observed in the CP of this study, altered the osmotic balance and favored the predominance of post-exercise sympathetic outflow in hypohydrated individuals[37].

The LF/HF ratio confirms the sympathetic predominance in hypohydrated individuals in the recovery period. Despite the lack of significant interaction between time and protocols being observed, the sympathetic-vagal balance was lower in the EP compared to CP, with recovery of this index being observed, at 15 minutes, in the hydrated condition. Indeed, hydration can reduce the sympathetic-vagal ratio by reducing sympathetic modulation through modulation of cardiovascular baroreceptors[35]. Accordingly, the rapid post-exercise cardiac vagal reactivation observed when 500 mL of water were ingested after 30 minute submaximal exercise, was caused mainly by osmotic mechanisms which, mediated by stimulation of osmosensitive structures in the gastrointestinal tract or in the circulation portal, potentially influenced cardiac vagal modulation[6].

In this study, the hypohydrated state also reduced overall HRV after exercise. Significant interaction was observed between moments and protocols for SDNN [ms], suggesting better post-exercise recovery of these indices in the hydrated condition, and given that at 15 minute post-exercise the return of this index to baseline was observed. This response confirms the influence of hydration status on post-exercise cardiac autonomic stability.

This study has some limitations. The minimum interval between the execution of the CP and the EP was adhered to; however, some collections were completed over a period longer than a week, which may hinder the interpretation of the variables studied. Another important aspect refers to the use of supine rest and recovery conditions, considering that this exercise was performed in the upright position. Although we chose to compare rest and exercise in different positions, we believed that the modifications produced in the parameters during exercise were not influenced by the postural change. However, in addition to being more tolerable for the volunteer, the choice of the supine position during the recovery period has not impaired the results because the parameters were compared to a baseline, with participants in the same position. Finally, the absence of randomization between protocols can be influenced the results, however, for the dynamic correct of trial was necessary to accomplish firstly the CP to determine the loss of body mass and based on these data suggest the amount of water to be consumed in the hydration protocol.

However, the results of this study reinforce the importance of hydration when performing physical exercise to promote a better response in cardiac autonomic modulation. In sports scope, a faster recovery of the autonomic modulation indicates that the autonomic nervous system of the individual quickly is ready to receive a new stimulus, while in the clinical scope, a better recovery of the autonomic modulation may be important to prevent or reduce cardiovascular events after exercise such as cardiac arrhythmias, decreased or increased blood pressure, pulmonary hyperventilation increasing body pH and an excessive production of metabolites[38,39]. As a future perspective, investigating the influence of water intake over exercise and recovery on sodium concentration and PV can bring better knowledge of this hydration protocol.

Conclusion

In young participants, hydration with small amounts of water ingested throughout exercise and recovery did not change autonomic regulation during the exercise, but accelerated autonomic recovery measured by HRV indices in the time and frequency domains.

References

1. Hernandez AJ, Nahas RM. Dietary changes, water replacement, food supplements and drugs: evidence of ergogenic action and potential health risks. Rev Bras Med Esporte. 2009;15: 3-12.
2. Moreno IL, Pastre CM, Papoti M, Vanderlei LCM. Efeitos da reposição hidroeletrolítica sobre parâmetros cardiorrespiratórios em exercício e recuperação. Motriz. 2012; 18:165-175.
3. Rodriguez NR, DiMarco NM, Langley S. Nutrition and athletic performance. Med Sci Sports Exerc. 2009; 41: 709-731.
4. Sawka MN, Burke LM, Eichner ER, Maughan RJ, Montain SJ, Stachenfeld NS. American college of sports medicine position stand. Exercise and fluid replacement. Med Sci Sports Exerc. 2007; 39: 377-390.
5. Montain SJ. Hydration recommendations for sport 2008. Curr Sports Med Reports. 2008; 7;187-192.
6. Vianna LC, Oliveira RB, Silva BM, Ricardo DR, Araújo CG. Water intake accelerates post-exercise cardiac vagal reactivation in humans. Eu J Appl Physiol. 2008; 102: 283-288.
7. Moreno IL, Vanderlei LC, Pastre CM, Vanderlei FM, Abreu LC, Ferreira C. Cardiorespiratory effects of water ingestion during and after exercise. Int Arch Med. 2013; 6: 35.
8. Peçanha T, Paula-Ribeiro M, Campana-Rezende E, Bartels R, Marins JC, de Lima JR. Water intake accelerates parasympathetic reactivation after high-intensity exercise. International J Sport Nutr Exerc Metab. 2014; 24: 489-496.
9. Naugle KM, Riley JL. Self-reported physical activity predicts pain inhibitory and facilitatory function. Med Sci Sports Exerc. 2014; 46:622-629.
10. Moreno IL, Pastre CM, Ferreira C, Abreu LC, Valenti VE, Vanderrlei LCM. Effects of an isotonic beverage on autonomic regulation during and after exercise. J Society Sports Nutr. 2013; 10:2-11.
11. Vanderlei FM, Moreno IL, Vanderlei LCM, Pastre CM, Abreu LC, Ferreira C. Comparison of the effects of hydration with water or isotonic solution on the recovery of cardiac autonomic modulation. Int J Sport Nutr Exerc Metab. 2015; 25:145-153.
12. Shah BN. On the 50th anniversary of the first description of a multistage exercise treadmill test: re-visiting the birth of the 'Bruce protocol'. Heart. 2013; 99:1793-1794.
13. Costill DL, Sparks KE. Rapid fluid replacement following thermal dehydration. J Appl Physiol. 1973; 34:299-303.
14. Von Duvillard SP, Braun WA, Markofski M, Beneke R, Leithäuser R. Fluids and hydration in prolonged endurance performance. Nutrition. 2004; 20:651-656.
15. Armstrong LE, Pumerantz AC, Fiala KA, Roti MW, Kavouras SA, Casa DJ, Maresh CM. Human hydration indices: acute and longitudinal reference values. Int J Sport Nutr Exerc Metab. 2010; 20:145-153.
16. Task Force of the European Society of Cardiology of the North American Society of pacing electrophysiology. Heart rate variability standards of measurement, physiological interpretation and clinical use. Circulation. 1996; 93: 1043-1065.
17. Godoy MF, Takakura IT, Correa PR. The relevance of nonlinear dynamic analysis (Chaos Theory) to predict morbidity and mortality in patients undergoing surgical myocardial revascularization. Arq Ciências Saúde. 2005; 12: 167-171.

18. Corrêa PR, Catai AM, Takakura IT, Machado MN, Godoy MF. Heart rate variability and pulmonary infections after myocardial revascularization. Arq Bras Cardiol. 2010; 95: 448-456.
19. Tarvainen MP, Niskanen JP, Lipponen JA, Ranta-aho PO, Karjalainen PA. Kubios HRV – A software for advanced heart rate variability analysis. *In:* 4th European Conference os the International Federation for Medical and Biological Engineering, Sloten JV, Verdonck P, Nyssen M, Haueisen J, editors. 2008, pp. 1022-1025.
20. Sawka MN, Young AJ. Physiological systems and their responses to conditions of heat and cold. *In:* Tipton CM, Sawka MN, Tate CA, Terjung RL, editors. ACSM`s Advanced Exercises Physiology. Baltimore: Lippincott, Williams & Wilkins; 2006. p. 535-63.
21. Maughan RJ, Leiper JB, Shirreffs SM. Restoration of fluid balance after exercise induced dehydration: effects of food and fluid intake. Eur J Appl Physiol. 1996; 73: 317-325.
22. González-Alonso J, Mora-Rodríguez R, Coyle EF. Stroke volume during exercise: interaction of environment and hydration. Am J Physiol: Heart Circ Physiol. 2000; 278:H321–H330.
23. Horswill CA, Stofan JR, Lovett SC, Hannasch C. Core temperature and metabolic responses after carbohydrate intake during exercise at 30 degrees C. J Athletic Training. 2008; 43:585-591.
24. Vanderlei LCM, Pastre CM, Hoshi RA, Carvalho TD, Godoy MF. Basic notions of heart rate variability and its clinical applicability. Rev Bras Cirurgia Cardiovascular. 2009; 24:205-217.
25. González-Alonso J, Mora-Rodríguez R, Below PR, Coyle EF. Dehydration markedly impairs cardiovascular function in hyperthermic endurance athletes during exercise. J Appl Physiol. 1997; 82: 1229-1236.
26. Crandall CG, Zhang R, Levine BD. Effects of whole body heating on dynamic baroreflex regulation of heart rate in humans. Am J Physiol: Heart Circ Physiol. 2000; 279:H2486-2492.
27. Charkoudian N, Halliwill JR, Morgan BJ, Eisenach JH, Joyner MJ. Influences of hydration on postexercise cardiovascular control in humans. J Physiol. 2003; 552, 635-44.
28. Alonso DO, Forjaz CLM, Rezende LO, Braga AM, Barretto AC, Negrão CE, Rondon MU. Heart rate response and its variability during different phases of maximal graded exercise. Arq Bras Cardiol. 1998; 71:787-792.
29. Mendonca GV, Fernhall B, Heffernan KS, Pereira FD. Spectral methods of heart rate variability analysis during dynamic exercise. Clin Auton Res. 2009; 19:237-245.
30. Javorka M, Zila I, Balhárek T, Javorka K. Heart rate recovery after exercise: relations to heart rate variability and complexity. Braz J Med Biol Res. 2002; 35:991-1000.
31. Perini R, Veicsteinas A. Heart rate variability and autonomic activity at rest and during exercise in various physiological conditions. Eur J Appl Physiol. 2003; 90:317-325.
32. Sandercock GRH, Brodie DA. The use of heart rate variability measures to assess autonomic control during exercise. Scand J Med Sci Sports. 2006; 16:302-313.
33. Saat M, Tochihara Y, Hashiguchi N, Sirisinghe RG, Fujita M, Chou CM. Effects of exercise in the heat on thermoregulation of Japanese and Malaysian males. J Physiol Anthropol Appl Human Sci. 2005; 24:267-275.
34. Hendrickse MT, Triger DR. Vagal dysfunction and impaired urinary sodium and water excretion in cirrhosis. Am J Gastroenterol. 1994; 89:750–757.
35. Yun AJ, Lee PY, Bazar KA. Clinical benefits of hydration and volume expansion in a wide range of illnesses may be attributable to reduction of sympatho-vagal ratio. Med Hypotheses. 2005; 64:646-650.
36. Routledge HC, Chowdhary S, Coote JH, Townend JN. Cardiac vagal response to water ingestion in normal human subjects. Clin Sci. 2002; 103:157-162.
37. Scrogin KE, Grygielko ET, Brooks VL. Osmolality: a physiological long-term regulator of lumbar sympathetic nerve activity and arterial pressure. Am J Physiol. 1999; 276: R1579-R1586.
38. Brum PC, Forjaz CLM, Tinucci T, Negrão CE. Adaptações agudas e crônicas do exercício físico no sistema cardiovascular. Rev Paulista Educação Física. 2004; 18: 21-31.
39. Guyton A, Hall J. Tratado de Fisiologia Médica (11ª ed.). Brasil: Elsevier; 2006.

Funding

This study was support by the Foundation for Research Support of São Paulo State (FAPESP–Proc. 2011/10887-7).

Corresponding Author

Isadora Lessa Moreno
Department of Medicine
Rua Napoleão de Barros, 715, Térreo, São Paulo, SP, Brasil.
Email: moreno.isadoralessa@gmail.com

13

Hypotensive effects of resistance exercise with continuous and intermittent blood flow restriction

Gabriel Rodrigues Neto
Universidade Federal de Paraíba, João Pessoa, Paraíba, Brasil
Universidade Federal do Rio de Janeiro, Rio de Janeiro, RJ, Brasil

Jefferson da Silva Novaes
Universidade Federal do Rio de Janeiro, Rio de Janeiro, RJ, Brasil

Michel Gonçalves
Universidade Federal do Rio de Janeiro, Rio de Janeiro, RJ, Brasil
Instituto de Pesquisa e Capacitação Física do Exército, Rio de Janeiro, RJ, Brasil

Gilmário Ricarte Batista
Rosa Maria Soares Costa de Mendonça
Universidade Federal da Paraíba, João Pessoa, PB, Brasil

Humberto Miranda
Universidade Federal do Rio de Janeiro, Rio de Janeiro, RJ, Brasil

Giovanni da Silva Novaes
Universidade Castelo Branco, Rio de Janeiro, RJ, Brasil
Centro de Investigação em Esporte, Saúde e Desenvolvimento Humano, Vila Real, Portugal

Maria do Socorro Cirilo-Sousa
Universidade Federal da Paraíba, João Pessoa, PB, Brasil

Abstract—The aim of this study was to compare the acute effects of low-intensity (LI) resistance exercise (RE) with continuous blood flow restriction (CBFR) and intermittent blood flow restriction (IBFR) on systolic blood pressure (SBP), diastolic blood pressure (DBP), and mean arterial pressure (MAP). After a one-repetition maximum test, 10 normotensive recreationally trained men performed three experimental protocols. In the three RE protocols, increases in SBP, DBP, and MAP were observed immediately after exercise, but the effect sizes (ESs) were greater for the LI + CBFR and high-intensity protocols. There were hypotensive effects on SBP, DBP, and MAP in all three protocols; however, the effects on MAP lasted longer for the LI + IBFR and LI + CBFR protocols. These long-lasting hypotensive effects on DBP and MAP occurred in all three protocols. Thus, we conclude that the post exercise hypotensive effects on SBP, DBP, and MAP appear to occur in all three RE protocols, with the effect on SBP being longer in the LI + IBFR and LI + CBFR protocols.

Keywords: kaatsu, vascular occlusion, hypotension, resistance training

Introduction

Traditional resistance exercises (REs) have been used to promote post exercise hypotension, which occurs as a result of the reduced vascular resistance observed in these exercise protocols [1-3]. The reduced vascular resistance is caused by an increase in the endothelial substances and by reductions in the sympathetic nervous system activity and cardiac output[4]. In addition, RE enhances the development and maintenance of strength, muscular endurance, power, and muscle hypertrophy[5,6]. However, some individuals cannot be subjected to high-intensity (HI) RE due to several health problems, and therefore, cannot train with heavy loads (>70% one-repetition maximum [1RM]), which are recommended for increasing strength and hypertrophy[5]. Accordingly, low-intensity (LI) RE combined with blood flow restriction (BFR) can be used for these individuals because this method uses low loads (20–30% 1RM) combined with a tourniquet, which reduces the negative effect of heavy loads on the joints[7,8]. The strength and muscle mass gains obtained with this method seem to be as effective as HI training[9,10]; in addition, this method seems to be safe in terms of hemodynamics[11-15].

Few studies have evaluated potential hypotensive effects [systolic blood pressure (SBP), diastolic blood pressure (DBP), and/or the mean arterial pressure (MAP)] after the application of LI RE with continuous blood flow restriction (CBFR)[16,17] and intermittent blood flow restriction (IBFR)[12,18] alone. Among these studies, only three have demonstrated hypotensive responses after LI RE combined with BFR[12,16,17]. However, only Brandner, Kidgell, and Warmington[19] compared the hypotensive effect of CBFR and IBFR RE (unilateral elbow flexion exercise trials). They found no post exercise hypotension and presented some limitations that may have affected the results, such as the amount of exercises used, how they were performed (unilaterally or single-jointed), and the different pressures used for the BFR. In addition, there are few studies showing similar effects when CBFR and IBFR RE were compared in terms of muscle activation, strength, and lean mass[20,21]. While both have benefits for strength and hypertrophy, the best strategy for working with BFR, either in a single exercise or in an exercise session, remains unknown. Thus, it would be interesting to understand the stimuli in blood pressure to verify the degree of change and observe what would be the safest method of BFR (continuous vs. intermittent) in a RE session with BFR. However, it is necessary to conduct studies in healthy populations (e.g., youth and adults) with safe procedures and methods appropriate to later be extrapolated in special populations.

A literature search revealed that no study to date has included analysis of the hypotensive response after a RE session for the upper limbs with CBFR and IBFR. Accordingly, we hypothesized that the hypotensive response observed after HI exercises and after LI RE with CBFR and IBFR would be similar. Therefore, the aim of this study was to compare the acute effects of LI RE with CBFR and IBFR on SBP, DBP, and MAP in normotensive recreationally trained men.

Methods

Subjects

In total, 10 normotensive recreationally trained military men (19 ± 0.8 years old; 78.8 ± 10.8 kg; 174.6 ± 5.4 m; 25.7 ± 2.7 $m^2 \cdot kg^{-1}$) aged 18–21 years performed the three experimental protocols in random order. Those considered recreationally trained had between 1 and 5 years of experience in strength training[22]. The sample was selected by convenience; however, the subjects included should be normotensive men aged between 18 and 30 years. The subjects were randomly divided to undergo the three protocols after selection (crossover design). The exclusion criteria were (1) individuals who responded "yes" to any of the Physical Activity Readiness Questionnaire items[23], (2) individuals who missed one RE session, (3) individuals who had some type of musculoskeletal injury of the upper limbs, and (4) smokers. After being informed of the risks and benefits of the study, the subjects signed an informed consent form prepared in accordance with the principles of the Declaration of Helsinki. The study was approved by the local ethics committee (Protocol 0476/13).

Study Design

Anthropometric parameters and muscle strength were assessed during the first visit to the laboratory. After this visit, the subjects visited the laboratory on three different occasions 72–96 hours apart. During these visits, the subjects completed the three protocols in random order (crossover design): (1) LI RE (20% 1RM) combined with IBFR (LI + IBFR), (2) LI RE (20% 1RM) combined with CBFR (LI + CBFR), and (3) HI RE (80% 1RM). All three protocols were performed at the same time of day to control diurnal blood pressure variation. Blood pressure was measured before (resting); immediately after; and then 15, 30, 45, and 60 min after performing the RE protocols. Subjects were instructed to avoid exhausting exercise, caffeine and chocolate intake, use of nutritional supplements, and intake of alcoholic beverages during and after the effort sessions and were advised to sleep at least 6 hours in the night before the exercise session. In addition, subjects were instructed to maintain the same eating habits during the study period and not to perform the Valsalva maneuver during all RE sessions.

Procedures

Anthropometric Assessment

Height and body mass were measured to the nearest 0.5 cm and 0.1 kg, respectively. A stadiometer and a balance scale (Filizola scale, model 31; Sao Paulo, SP, Brazil) were used in the study.

1RM Test

The exercises were performed bilaterally and included the bench press, lat pulldown, triceps extension, and biceps curl. The subjects performed a warm-up set of 5–10 repetitions at 40–60% of perceived maximum with a 1-min rest interval between the sets. After the 1-min rest interval, the second set was performed with three to five repetitions at 60–80% of the perceived maximum. The strength evaluation started after a 1-min rest interval and measurement within five attempts. The load was adjusted before each new attempt. Rest intervals between the attempts were standardized at 3–5 min, with 20 min elapsed between different exercises. The test was discontinued when the subject failed to properly perform the movement, and the load moved in the last successful attempt was then considered the maximum load. The following strategies were adopted to reduce the margin of error in data collection procedures: (1) all tests were performed at the same time of day in each session; (2) standardized instructions were given before the test so that each subject was aware of the entire data collection routine; (3) the subject was instructed regarding the proper technique to perform the exercise; and (4) all subjects received standardized verbal encouragement during the tests.

Assessment of Blood Pressure

Before and after each RE session, blood pressure was measured using a stethoscope (3M Littmann® Cardiology; 3M, St. Paul, MN, USA) and an aneroid sphygmomanometer (DuraShock™ Tycos®, Model DS-44; Welch Allyn, Skaneateles Falls, NY). The cuff was completely wrapped around the right arm, enclosing at least two-thirds of the upper arm. Blood pressure flow measurements were performed 15 min immediately before (two measures resting); immediately after exercise (post-30–45 s); and approximately 15 min (post-15), 30 min (post-30), 45 min (post-45), 60 min, and more than 60 min (post-60) after each protocol. Immediately after the exercise session, the subject was instructed to sit, then the standard tourniquet was removed and a sphygmomanometer was placed for blood pressure measurement. All measurements were performed by the same expert evaluator according to the guidelines of the American Heart Association[24]. MAP was calculated according to the equation

$$(SBP + 2DBP)/3$$

Determination of BFR

After the assessment of blood pressure using the sphygmomanometer, subjects remained seated and a standard sphygmomanometer was placed in the axillary fold region to measure blood pressure (Riester Komprimeter pneumatic tourniquet for hemostasis in the extremities) in the arm (width of 60 mm and length of 470 mm) to verify blood pressure before starting each protocol of CBFR and IBFR. The total BFR was set at 1.3 times resting SBP[14,19,25]. The cuff was inflated and deflated between sets. The mean pressures used throughout the entire exercise protocols of IBFR and CBFR were 163.8 ± 10.5 mmHg and 160.9 ± 12.9 mmHg, respectively.

Experimental Sessions

Four bilateral REs were performed, including the bench press (with conventional bar and calibrated rings), lat pull-down, triceps extension, and biceps curl (on conventional machines). Subjects performed three protocols in random order: four LI REs (20% 1RM) combined with IBFR (LI + IBFR), four LI REs (20% 1RM) combined with CBFR (LI + CBFR), and four HI RE (80% 1RM). For the LI RE protocols with CBFR and IBFR, the subjects completed 30 repetitions followed by 3 sets of 15 repetitions (20% 1RM), with an interval of 30 s between all sets and a 1-min interval between exercises while wearing a standard sphygmomanometer that was placed on the upper arm (proximal; width 60 mm and length 470 mm) for blood pressure measurement (Riester Komprimeter pneumatic tourniquet for hemostasis in the extremities). The cuff was deflated between sets for the LI + IBFR protocol and maintained inflated between sets for the LI + CBFR protocol. For the HI protocol, subjects completed three sets of eight repetitions (80% 1RM) with 2-min rest intervals between the sets and a 1-min rest interval between exercises. The velocity of the movement was controlled by a metronome set at 3 s (1.5 s for the concentric muscular action and 1.5 s for the eccentric muscular action).

Total Work Exercises

The total work (TW) performed was calculated by multiplying the total load, the sets, and the complete repetitions of the four exercises for each protocol (load × sets × repetitions).

Statistical Analysis

The statistical analysis was initially performed using the Shapiro–Wilk test for normality and Levene's test for homogeneity of variances. The variables were normally distributed and homogeneous ($p > 0.05$). The test of reproducibility was performed between the first and second measurements of blood pressure at rest before starting each protocol (intraclass correlation coefficient [ICC]). A paired *t*-test was used to compare the two BFR pressures used in the LI + IBFR and LI + CBFR protocols, and one-way analysis of variance (ANOVA) with the Bonferroni post hoc test was used to compare TW between protocols. Two-way repeated-measures ANOVA (protocols [LI + IBFR vs. LI + CBFR vs. HI] × time [resting vs. immediately after exercise vs. 15 min vs. 30 min vs. 45 min vs. 60 min]) followed by Bonferroni's post hoc comparisons test was used to analyze the possible differences in SBP, DBP, and MAP. The ES was used to verify the magnitude (trivial <0.35, small 0.35–0.80, moderate 0.80–1.50, and large >1.5) of changes between assessments of the protocols[22], and the percentage change (Δ%) was used to express the possible differences between the significant changes. The level of significance was set at $p \leq 0.05$. All statistical analyses were performed using the IBM SPSS version 20.0 statistical software package (IBM, Armonk, NY).

Results

The blood pressure ICCs calculated by the researcher were as follows: LI + IBFR = 0.975, LI + CBFR = 0.966, and HI = 0.959. All subjects completed the three exercise sessions. The paired *t*-test revealed no significant differences between the two BFR pressures used in the LI + IBFR vs. LI + CBFR protocol ($p = 0.444$). Regarding TW (bench press, lat pulldown, triceps extension, and biceps curl), there was a significant difference between the LI vs. HI RE protocol (LI + IBFR and LI + CBFR [4131.0 ± 608.2] vs. HI [5598.7 ± 836.7], $p < 0.001$); however, there was no significant difference between LI + IBFR and LI + CBFR ($p = 1.000$).

In the comparative analysis of SBP, significant differences were found between LI + CBFR and HI at 15 and 30 min ($p = 0.017$ and $p = 0.050$, respectively). A significant increase in SBP between resting and immediately after the exercises in all protocols was observed (LI + IBFR, $p < 0.001$, Δ% = 24.6%, ES = 3.05; LI + CBFR, $p < 0.001$, Δ% = 35.7%, ES = 5.62; and HI, $p < 0.001$, Δ% = 35.2%, ES = 3.80). Significant reductions were observed between resting and 45 min ($p = 0.021$, Δ% = −6.8%, ES = 0.85) and between resting and 60 min ($p = 0.003$, Δ% = −8.5%, ES = 1.05) in the LI + IBFR protocol. For the LI + CBFR protocol, a significant reduction was observed between resting and 60 min ($p = 0.003$, Δ% = −8.3%, ES = 1.31). In the HI protocol, significant reductions were observed between resting and 15 min ($p = 0.005$, Δ% = −8.1%, ES = 0.88) and between resting and 30 min ($p = 0.022$, Δ% = −7.3%, ES = 0.79) (Table 1). In the LI + CBFR protocol, a significant reduction was observed between resting and 60 min ($p = 0.003$, Δ% = −8.3%, ES = 1.31). For the HI protocol, significant reductions were observed between resting and 15 min ($p = 0.005$, Δ% = −8.1%, ES = 0.88) and between resting and 30 min ($p = 0.022$, Δ% = −7.3%, ES = 0.79) (Table 1).

In the comparative analysis of DBP, significant increases were observed between resting and immediately after exercise in all protocols (LI + IBFR, $p < 0.001$, Δ% = 16.6%, ES = 1.26; LI + CBFR, $p < 0.001$, Δ% = 15.7%, ES = 1.73; and HI $p < 0.001$, Δ% = 22.7%, ES = 2.46). Significant reductions were observed between resting and 60 min in all protocols (LI + IBFR, $p = 0.004$, Δ% = −10.8%, ES = 0.82; LI + CBFR, $p = 0.001$, Δ% = −12.7%, ES = 1.47; and HI, $p = 0.014$, Δ% = −8.8%, ES = 0.95), as shown in Table 2.

In the comparative analysis of MAP, a significant difference was observed between LI + CBFR and AI at 15 min ($p = 0.033$). The analysis of the different times revealed significant increases between resting and immediately after exercise in all protocols (LI + IBFR, $p < 0.001$, Δ% = 20.3%, ES = 2.03; LI + CBFR, $p < 0.001$, Δ% = 24.4%, ES = 3.48; and HI, $p < 0.001$, Δ% = 28.1%, ES = 3.16). Significant reductions were observed between resting and 60 min ($p = 0.001$, Δ% = −9.7%, ES = 0.96) in the LI + IBFR protocol. For the LI + CBFR protocol, there were significant reductions between resting and 60 min ($p < 0.001$, Δ% = −10.7%, ES = 1.52). For the HI protocol, there were significant reductions between resting and 15 min ($p = 0.013$, Δ% = −7.1%, ES = 0.80) and between resting and 60 min ($p = 0.008$, Δ% = −7.1%, ES = 0.80), as shown in Table 3.

Table 1. Comparative analysis of systolic blood pressure in different study protocols.

			Systolic Blood Pressure (mm Hg)			
Protocols	**Resting**	**Immediately after exercise**	**15 minutes**	**30 minutes**	**45 minutes**	**60 minutes**
LI + IBFR	123.5±10.0	154.0±21.7*	120.0±12.4	117.0±12.5	115.0±11.7*	113.0±14.9*
LI + CBFR	126.0±8.0	171.0±17.9*	126.5±11.5†	123.5±12.0†	120.5±8.9	115.5±11.1*
HI	122.0±11.3	165.0±15.8*	112.0±13.9*	113.0±9.4*	117.0±9.4	116.0±9.6

* Significant difference between resting and immediately after exercises, resting and 15 min, resting and 30 min, resting and 45 min, resting and 60 min

† Significant difference between LI + CBFR and HI

LI + IBFR = low-intensity resistance exercises combined with intermittent blood flow restriction; LI + CBFR = low-intensity resistance exercises combined with continuous blood flow restriction; HI = high-intensity resistance exercises

Table 2. Comparative analysis of diastolic blood pressure between the study protocols.

			Diastolic Blood Pressure (mm Hg)			
Protocols	**Resting**	**Immediately after exercise**	**15 minutes**	**30 minutes**	**45 minutes**	**60 minutes**
LI + IBFR	78.0±10.3	91.0±8.7*	75.5±9.5	75.0±10.8	74.5±11.6	69.5±12.1*
LI + CBFR	82.5±7.1	95.5±6.4*	81.0±8.7	79.0±7.3	77.0±9.4	72.0±7.5*
HI	79.0±7.3	97.0±9.4*	74.0±8.4	78.0±8.3	78.0±7.8	72.0±7.8*

*Significant difference between resting and immediately after exercise, resting and 60 min

LI + IBFR = low-intensity resistance exercises combined with intermittent blood flow restriction; LI + CBFR = low-intensity resistance exercises combined with continuous blood flow restriction; HI = high-intensity resistance exercises.

Table 3. Comparative analysis of mean arterial pressure between the study protocols.

			Mean Arterial Pressure (mm Hg)			
Protocols	**Resting**	**Immediately after exercise**	**15 minutes**	**30 minutes**	**45 minutes**	**60 minutes**
LI + IBFR	93.1±9.4	112.0±12.3*	90.3±9.7	89.0±10.3	87.9±11.2	84.0±12.3*
LI + CBFR	96.9±6.8	120.6±9.1*	96.1±8.8†	93.8±7.5	91.4±8.9	86.5±7.7*
HI	93.3±8.3	119.6±9.7*	86.6±9.6*	89.6±6.7	90.9±7.7	86.6±6.8*

* Significant difference between resting and immediately after exercise, resting and 15 min, resting and 60 min

† Significant difference between LI + CBFR and HI

LI + IBFR = low-intensity resistance exercises combined with intermittent blood flow restriction; LI + CBFR = low-intensity resistance exercises combined with continuous blood flow restriction; HI = high-intensity resistance exercises.

Discussion

In this study, we compared the acute effects of RE combined with CBFR and IBFR on SBP, DBP, and MAP in military men. To our knowledge, this study involves the first comparison of the hypotensive responses elicited by upper limb exercises done with CBFR or IBFR. The main findings of this study are (1) the three RE protocols increased SBP, DBP, and MAP immediately after exercises; and (2) hypotensive responses (changes in SBP, DBP, and MAP) were observed in the three protocols without significant differences between them. However, the effects on SBP were longer in the LI+ IBFR and LI + CBFR protocols.

Acute increases in SBP, DBP, and MAP were observed in the three protocols without significant differences between them, but a smaller magnitude was observed in the LI + IBFR protocol than in the other protocols. These increases may have occurred because IBFR promotes lower levels of muscle pain than CBFR[21,] which could cause less tension on the muscles involved. The acute findings of the study conducted by Brandner, Kidgell, Warmington[19] comparing CBFR and IBFR were different from those in the present study. Those authors reported a higher magnitude in the LI + IBFR protocol, a result that may have been due to the pressure used in IBFR (151 mmHg), which was much higher than the pressure used in CBFR (91 mmHg). However, other studies corroborate our findings. Previous studies reported increases in blood pressure immediately after application of LI RE combined with CBFR.[14,15,26] This increase in blood pressure shown in previous studies and in the present study may occur because CBFR potentiates elevations in muscle sympathetic nerve activity, heart rate, and MAP[27]. In contrast, a previous study has found no significant differences in SBP, DBP, and MAP in the IBFR protocol[28]. This finding may have been due to several factors, including the low pressure of the BFR (100 mmHg) used in their protocol, no vascular occlusion (BFR) between sets, and the use of only two single-joint exercises of the lower limbs.

The HI protocol promoted a faster hypotensive response (SBP and MAP) that started 15 min after the end of the exercises. An explanation of this finding is that the TW of the HI protocol was significantly higher than in other protocols. Indeed, it has been stated that TW plays an important role in the hypotensive response[29,30]. These findings are in agreement with previous studies[15-17], that detected hypotensive responses after LI RE combined with CBFR or IBFR. In contrast to other studies[11,18,19] .

Therefore, upon analyzing the methodological procedures according to the body segment used in the exercises and the subjects of the studies, it seems that the greatest magnitude of hypotension occurs in the following scenarios: in individuals who performed RE combined with IBFR in the upper and lower limbs (agonist-antagonist)[12], in hypertensive individuals who performed RE combined with CBFR (lower limbs)[16], and in apparently healthy young individuals who performed RE combined with CBFR at 40% 1RM (upper limbs)[17]. However, it was also observed that the hypotensive response did not occur in apparently healthy young subjects who performed LI RE (≤30% 1RM) with CBFR and IBFR in single body segments[19]. On the other hand, loads ≤30% 1RM are able to promote hypotensive responses after LI RE with CBFR in hypertensive individuals[16].

Additionally, it seems that performing exercises for upper and lower limbs in the same session can promote greater hypotensive effects than the effects after exercises performed with only one segment, which can be associated with the amount of muscle mass involved[31]. Thus, the lower blood pressure observed in the present study (using exercises for upper limbs and trunk) may have occurred due to the larger amount of muscle mass involved leading to increased nitric oxide production via endothelial shear stress, which then plays an important role in protecting vascular tone[32,33].

In the study performed by Brandner, Kidgell, Warmington[19], the first group of investigators who compared the effects of CBFR or IBFR RE (unilateral elbow flexion exercises) on hypotension, no significant hypotensive responses were observed. Some methodological limitations might explain these findings. These authors compared the effects of upper limb RE on hypotensive responses (5, 20, 40, and 60 min post exercise) in four different conditions: HI (80% 1RM, four sets of six to eight repetitions with an interval of 150 s between sets), LI without BFR (20% 1RM, 4 sets, with 30 repetitions in the first set and 15 repetitions in the second, third, and fourth sets; an interval of 30 s between sets), and two LI protocols with application of either CBFR (91 mmHg) or IBFR (151 mmHg) using a cuff with a width of 10.5 cm. The use of only a single-joint exercise (arm flexion) that was performed unilaterally and at different pressures for CBFR (80% resting SBP) and IBFR (130% resting SBP) might explain the lack of hypotensive responses in both BFR protocols. Because of the methodological procedures used, these results are not similar to the results of the present study, where bilateral and multi-joint exercises and not significantly different pressures for CBFR and IBFR were used. Another point worth mentioning is that our training volume was greater than the one used by Brandner, Kidgell, Warmington[19]. In addition, our study has good practical application because four exercises were used, which is similar to a training session.

The faster reduction in SBP observed in the LI + IBFR protocol may have occurred due to the release of the cuff between the sets, which may have promoted reactive hyperemia and shear stress more often than CBFR. These factors, in turn, could increase the production of nitric oxide synthase, the enzyme responsible for the conversion of L-arginine to nitric oxide, a small, electrically neutral molecule capable of promoting positive changes in the endothelium[35], but with less discomfort[21] and lower blood pressure changes, as observed in the present study. This protocol can be an excellent option for hypertensive individuals, as the increase in muscle activation[20] and gains in muscle strength and lean body mass[21] are similar between CBFR and IBFR. In addition, Takano[14] mentioned that the decrease in venous return promoted by the RE performed with BFR causes a reduction in cardiac preload during exercise, which may be an excellent strategy for people with vascular diseases.

Conclusions

The post exercise hypotensive responses occurred in all three protocols (changes in SBP, DBP, and MAP), with longer effects on SBP observed in the LI + IBFR and LI + CBFR protocols, although they were faster in the HI protocol. The LI + IBFR protocol appears to have a smaller effect than the other protocols in increasing SBP, DBP, and MAP immediately after exercise. Therefore, it is important to conduct further experiments in normotensive and hypertensive subjects to address both acute and chronic hypotensive responses, particularly involving different BFR pressures and different cuff sizes.

References

1. Bentes CM, Costa PB, Rodrigues Neto G, Costa e Silva GV, De Salles BF, Miranda HL, Novaes JS. Hypotensive effects and performance responses between different resistance training intensities and exercise orders in apparently health women. Clin Physiol Functional Imaging. 2015; 35:185–190.
2. Matos DG, Aidar FJ, Filho MLM, Silva SR, Oliveira JC, Klain IP, Dantas EHM. Analysis of hemodynamic responses to resistance exercise performed with different intensities and recovery intervals. Health. 2013; 5:159-165.
3. Mohebbi H, Rahmaninia F, Vatani DFH. Post-resistance exercise hypotensive responses at different intensities and volumes. Physical Education Sport. 2009; 7:171-179.
4. Polito MD, Farinatti PTV. Blood pressure behavior after counter-resistance exercises: a systematic review on determining variables and possible mechanisms. Revista Brasileira de Medicina do Esporte. 2006; 12:386-392.
5. ACSM. American College of Sports Medicine. Progression models in resistance training for healthy adults. Medicine Sci Sports Exercise. 2009; 41:687-708.
6. Pollock ML, Franklin BA, Balady GJ, Chaitman BL, Fleg JL, Fletcher B, *et al.* Resistance exercise in individuals with and wihout cardiovascular disease: benefits, rationale, safety, and prescriptionan. An Advisory From the Committee on Exercise, Rehabilitation, and Prevention, Council on Clinical Cardiology, American Heart Association. Circulation. 2000; 101:828-833.
7. Loenneke JP, Wilson JM, Marín PJ, Zourdos MC, Bemben MG. Low intensity blood flow restriction training: a meta-analysis. Eur J Appl Physiol. 2012; 112: 1849-1859.
8. Scott BR, Loenneke JP, Slattery KM, Dascombe BJ. Exercise with blood flow restriction: an updated evidence-based approach for enhanced muscular development. Sports Medicine. 2015; 45:313-325.
9. Laurentino GC, Ugrinowitsch C, Roschel H, Aoki MS, Soares AG, Neves J, *et al.* Strength training with blood flow restriction diminishes myostatin gene expression. Medicine Sci in Sports Exercise. 2012; 44:406-412.
10. Takarada Y, Takazawa H, Sato Y, Takebayashi S, Tanaka Y, Ishii N. Effects of resistance exercise combined with moderate vascular occlusion on muscular function in humans. J Appl Physiol. 2000; 88:2097.
11. Fahs CA, Rossow LM, Seo D, Loenneke JP, Sherk VD, Kim E, *et al.* Effect of different types of resistance exercise on arterial compliance and calf blood flow. European J Appl Physiol. 2011; 111:2969-2975.
12. Neto GR, Sousa MSC, Costa PB, Salles BF, Novaes GS, Novaes JS. Hypotensive effects of resistance exercises with blood flow restriction. J Strength Conditioning Res. 2015; 29:1064-1070.
13. Neto GR, Sousa MSC, Silva GVC, Gil ALS, Salles BF, Novaes JS. Acute resistance exercise with blood flow restriction effects on heart rate, double product, oxygen saturation and perceived exertion. Clin Physiol Functional Imaging. 2016; 36:53-59.
14. Takano H, Morita T, Iida H, Asada K, Kato M, Uno K, *et al.* Hemodynamic and hormonal responses to a short-term low-intensity resistance exercise with the reduction of muscle blood flow. Eur J Appl Physiol. 2005; 95:65-73.
15. Vieira PJC, Chiappa GR, Umpierre D, Stein R, Ribeiro JP. Hemodynamic responses to resistance exercise with restricted blood flow in young and older men. J Strength Conditioning Res. 2013; 27:2288-2294.
16. Araújo JP, Silva ED, Silva JCG, Souza TSP, Lima EO, Guerra I, *et al.* The acute effect of resistance exercise with blood flow restriction with hemodynamic variables on hypertensive subjects. J Human Kinetics. 2014; 43:79-85.
17. Maior AS, Simão R, Rocha MMS, Freitas SB, Willardson JM. Influence of blood flow restriction during low-intensity resistance exercise on the post-exercise hypotensive response. J Strength Conditioning Res. 2015: 29:2894-2899.
18. Rossow LM, Fahs CA, Sherk VD, Seo D, Bemben DA, Bemben MG. The effect of acute blood-flow-restricted resistance exercise on postexercise blood pressure. Clin Physiol Functional Imaging. 2011; 31:429-434.
19. Brandner CR, Kidgell DJ, Warmington SA. Unilateral bicep curl hemodynamics: Low-pressure continuous vs high-pressure intermittent blood flow restriction. Scand J Medicine Sci Sports. 2014.
20. Yasuda T, Loenneke JP, Ogasawara R, Abe T. Influence of continuous or intermittent blood flow restriction on muscle activation during low-intensity multiple sets of resistance exercise. Acta Physiol Hung. 2013; 100:419-426.
21. Fitschen PJ, Kistler BM, Jeong JH, Chung HR, Wu PT, Walsh MJ, *et al.* Perceptual effects and efficacy of intermittent or continuous blood flow restriction resistance training. ClinPhysiol Functional Imaging. 2014; 34:356-363.
22. Rhea MR. Determining the magnitude of treatment effects in strength training research through the use the effect size. J Strength Conditioning Res. 2004; 18: 918-920.
23. Shephard RJ. PAR-Q, Canadian Home Fitness Test and exercise screening alternatives. Sports Medicine. 1988; 5:185-195.
24. Pickering TG, Hall JE, Appel LJ, Falkner BE, Graves J, Hill MN, *et al.* Recommendations for blood pressure measurement in humans and experimental animals part 1: blood pressure measurement in humans: a statement for professionals from the Subcommittee of Professional and Public Education of the American Heart Association Council on High Blood Pressure Research. Circulation. 2005; 111:697-716.
25. Suga T, Okita K, Morita N, Yokota T, Hirabayashi K, Horiuchi M, *et al.* Dose effect on intramuscular metabolic stress during low-intensity resistance exercise with blood flow restriction. J Appl Physiol. 2010; 108:1563-1567.
26. Poton R, Polito MD. Cardiovascular responses during resistance exercise with blood flow restriction. Revista Brasileira de Cardiologia. 2014; 27: 104-110.

27. Victor RG, Seals DR. Reflex stimulation of sympathetic outflow during rhythmic exercise in humans. Am J Physiol. 1989; 257:H2017-H2024.
28. Figueroa A, Vicil F. Post-exercise aortic hemodynamic responses to low-intensity resistance exercise with and without vascular occlusion. Scandinavian J Medicine Sci Sports. 2011; 21:431-436.
29. Mediano MFF, Paravidino V, Simão R, Pontes FL, Polito MD. Subacute behavior of the blood pressure after power training in controlled hypertensive individuals. Revista Brasileira de Medicina do Esporte. 2005; 11: 337-340.
30. Simão R, Fleck SJ, Polito M, Monteiro W, Farinatti P. Effects of resistance training intensity, volume, and session format on the postexercise hypotensive response. J Strength Conditioning Res. 2005; 19:853-858.
31. Lizardo JHF, Simões HG. Effects of different resistance exercise sessions on post-exercise hypotension. Braz J Physical Therapy. 2005; 9:249-255.
32. Loenneke JP, Wilson GJ, Wilson JM. A mechanistic approach to blood flow occlusion. Int J Sports Medicine. 2010; 31: 1-4.
33. Manini TM, Clark BC. Blood flow restricted exercise and skeletal muscle health. Exercise Sport Sci Rev. 2009; 37:78-85.
34. Anderson JE, Wozniak AC. Satellite cell activation on fibers: modeling events in vivo-an invited review. Canadian J Physiol Pharmacol. 2004; 82:300-310.
35. Viaro F, Nobre F, Evora PRB. Expression of nitric oxide synthases in the pathophysiology of diseases cardovasculares. Arquivos Brasileiros de Cardiologia. 2000; 74:365-379.

Corresponding author

Gabriel Rodrigues Neto
Department of Physical Education
Associate Graduate Program in Physical
Education UPE / UFPB
Federal University of Paraíba,
Research Center for Human Movement Sciences
João Pessoa, PB, Brazil.
Email: gabrielrodrigues_1988@hotmail.com

Oxygen uptake in water polo, comparison and agreement in cycle ergometer and eggbeater kick

Ligia Ignêz Engelmann
Giane Veiga Liedtke
Flávio de Souza Castro
Universidade Federal do Rio Grande do Sul, Porto Alegre, RS, Brasil

Abstract—The aim of this study was to compare and verify the agreement of maximal oxygen uptake ($VO_{2\,max}$) values obtained from tests on land and in water. Twelve recreational water polo players (30.5 ± 7.7 years; 79.2 ± 7.2 kg body mass; 179.1 ± 5.9 cm height) were assessed in two phases: (1) in laboratory with maximal test on a cycle ergometer and (2) in a swimming pool with maximal test in eggbeater kick. Maximum values obtained in the two tests (respectively, cycle ergometer, and eggbeater kick: $VO_{2\,max}$ = 40.2 ± 2.7 ml.kg^{-1}.min^{-1} and 38.4 ± 5.7 ml.kg^{-1}.min^{-1}; RER = 1.17 ± 0.08 and 1.19 ± 0.12; HR_{max} = 181.4 ± 11.7 bpm and 179 ± 11.7 bpm; IEP = 20 and 20) did not show significant differences. According to the Bland–Altman analyses, there were acceptable limits of agreement between the two tests (land and water). Therefore, it can be concluded that the eggbeater kick test is a specific and valid protocol to asses $VO_{2\,max}$ in water polo players.

Keywords: water polo, oxygen uptake, assessment

Introduction

Water polo is an invasion sport played with two teams of thirteen players each, consisting of seven fielders and six reserves[1,2]. One common technique used by water polo players include the eggbeater kick, which is a propulsive movement of the lower limbs, also used in synchronized swimming[3]. The skill required in the eggbeater kick in water polo allows the players to (1) remain in the vertical position, (2) receive or execute a pass, (3) shoot for a goal, (4) move in the field, (5) block the opponent, and (6) use the upper body to move upward[4,5]. Specifically, it is a movement of cyclical action performed by the hips, knees, and ankles, with the movements of the right and left lower limbs in opposite directions in the cycle. Hips, knees, and ankles move in an inverse circular direction, i.e., the left leg moves clockwise and the right counter-clockwise[3]. During a match, the players perform the eggbeater kick when in a vertical position. Analyses of water polo matches indicated that the total time spent in the vertical position ranges between 55 and 66.9% of the match[6-8].

In order to perform any type of sport or activity, it is necessary to use energy which comes from different metabolic pathways. Among the assessments of metabolic capabilities, the maximal oxygen uptake ($VO_{2\,max}$) is considered a good indicator of the ability of a person to perform a task. The $VO_{2\,max}$ correct identification is critical in performance analysis for further prescription and for appropriate training[9]. According to Aleksandrovič[10], there is a paucity of information regarding physiological capacity and specific motor skills, such as eggbeater kick, of the players. One possible reason for this may be due to the difficulties imposed by the aquatic environment in obtaining appropriate physiological parameters, such as the $VO_{2\,max}$.

Usually the $VO_{2\,max}$ is identified in tests performed on treadmills, cycle ergometers, or other equipment that allows for control of the load imposed on the subject assessed. In general, several protocols are used to ensure the results are valid, objective, and reproducible[9,11]. However, specific protocols to assess the $VO_{2\,max}$ in water polo players, performing the eggbeater kick, have not being found, except those used in swimming tests[12]. Specifically, Lobenius[13] compared a maximum eggbeater kick test and cycle ergometer test to investigate the validity of a newly developed eggbeater kick test in eight synchronized swimming athletes (20.8 ± 3.4 years; 62.3 ± 6.2 kg; 9.4 ± 5.0 years training). During the eggbeater kick test, the athletes: (a) used both arms for sculling; (b) kept their shoulders above the surface; (c) wore a diving belt where the load increased every 30 seconds; and (d) had their VO_2 measured every 15 seconds. The VO_{2peak} was higher during the eggbeater kick test when compared with the cycle ergometer test and the range of differences between the two tests was large. Furthermore, there was correlation between the tests. It was concluded that the eggbeater kick test could also be a specific test for synchronized swimmers, which enables them technically, physiologically, and psychologically to reach higher values during the test. Nevertheless, there is not information for both tests in reference to load, cadence, and exhaustion time in Lobenius's study[13].

Therefore, the aim of this study is to compare and to verify the agreement between two different maximal protocol tests in water polo players.

Methods

This study included twelve water polo state/recreational level players with a minimum of two years' experience in the sport. The players were training normally two to three times per week for 90 minutes during the test period. All participants were informed about the objectives and protocols of this study through a Term of Consent. This study was approved by the Ethics Committee of the University where the study was conducted (22286613100005347).

The cycle ergometer test was performed in the laboratory (room temperature controlled and maintained at 21°C) and the eggbeater kick test in a 25 m swimming pool (1.90 m deep, heated water temperature of approximately 29°C) during the players' training season. The procedures were divided into two phases:

First Phase

Each player was received in the laboratory where the characteristics of the sample were obtained (wearing shorts and t-shirt): water polo time experience, match position, age, and anthropometric data (skin folds, weight, and height). The physiological variables were measured (VO_2, RER, HR and IEP) at rest, and after standing in an upright position for five minutes. Next, the player warmed-up on a cycle ergometer for five minutes at a cadence of 70–80 RPM and load of 50 W, when HR and IEP were measured. The maximal cycle ergometer test was a progressive protocol with an initial workload of 100 W and increments of 25 W/minute until exhaustion, the cadence was maintained between 70–80 RPM. This test protocol has been used for cyclists and triathletes in many previous studies[14-16]. Exhaustion was identified when the players could not maintain the minimum cadence (70 RPM) or by ending the test voluntarily. In the cycle ergometer test, VO_2, RER, and HR were measured every minute and IEP was measured in the last 15 seconds of every minute.

Second Phase

After a minimum of 48 hours from the completion of the first phase, the second phase was performed in the swimming pool. The player, wearing the usual sport speedo, performed the progressive protocol in eggbeater kick. Initially, the physiological variables (VO_2, RER, HR and IEP) were measured at rest after five minutes in a standing position, and subsequently also at rest by standing upright in the water for five minutes on a pool deep reducer to further investigate the possible effects of immersion on the variables. On the pool deep reducer, the player maintained the water surface between xiphoid process and shoulders. The player then warmed-up for five minutes performing a low-intensity eggbeater kick with both hands in a sculling motion. Following the warm up, the player left the pool to place two adhesive tape marks (approximately 4 cm^2 each) on the acromion process on each shoulder, and to put on the load belt (in the belt there were four pockets, two in front and two in the back for load placement). The second phase test consisted of the player performing the eggbeater kick while maintaining the shoulder marks on the water surface. During the test, the player performed with one arm in sculling and the other held outside of the water. The player could freely choose which arm, but could not change arms during the test.

The maximum eggbeater kick test was a progressive protocol beginning with a 1 kg load and every minute it was increased by 0.5 kg until exhaustion. VO_2, RER, and HR were measured continuously throughout the test. The IEP was collected in the last 15 seconds of every minute. To identify the test cadence, a trained researcher used a manual chronometer (Seiko S140, resolution de 1/100) to control the cycles of eggbeater kick. The cadence was measured in seconds: how long each player performed six complete cycles of eggbeater kick in the last 15 seconds of every minute. Then, the number of cycles (6) was divided by the measured time, and the result was transformed into cycles per minute. The technical criteria suggested by Homma and Homma[4] for the eggbeater kick's performances (keep the highest knees possible and near the surface of the water, keep the heel closest the hip) were controlled. The exhaustion level was identified when the player could not maintain the shoulder marks on the water surface or by voluntarily ending the test.

VO_2 and RER in phases 1 and 2

VO_2 and RER were directly measured using a mixing-box-type portable gas analyzer VO2000® (Portable Metabolic Testing System, Medgraphics, Ann Arbor, USA). Instrument calibration was performed before each assessment according to the manufacturer's specifications. The expired gas concentrations were measured breath by breath and all of the records followed the method of average breathing rate of three respiratory cycles. The data were transferred to a computer via the Aerograph software and exported to Excel for analysis. The neoprene mask was used in both phases to block breathing from the nose. Next, individual curves between load and VO_2 and RER were plotted. RER was calculated from the obtained O_2 and CO_2 data. The O_2 analyzer type was the Galvanic Fuel Cell (range: 0–96%, accuracy: ± 0.1%), and the CO_2 analyzer was Non-Dispersive Infrared (range: 0–10%, accuracy: ± 0.2%). As it was not possible to identify a plateau in VO_2 behavior, in most of the players, VO_2 peak (VO_{2peak}) was used as criteria for VO_{2max}. Therefore, the average was calculated of the two highest VO_{2peak} values identified during the test on the same workload. The associated values of RER of these VO_2 values were also considered maximum values. During the land-resting (phases 1 and 2) and the water-resting (phase 2), the players stood upright for five minutes close to the metabolic gas analyzer. The measurement of metabolic variables began during the last minute in the resting position. The determination of the absolute values of VO_2 ($l.min^{-1}$), and relative to body mass ($ml.kg^{-1}.min^{-1}$) were given after the elimination of dead space, defined as the average of the values collected during the remaining period (1 min).

IEP and HR in Phases 1 and 2

The players performed two familiarization sessions with the scale 6–20 point of the Borg[17] prior to the application of the protocols of this study. Prior to the trial, during training, in order to familiarize the players, the scale was presented to the subjects in exercises at different intensities and distances, and then the subject assigned a numerical value of the corresponding scale of the IEP at the requested time. To measure the HR values at rest (last minute), warm up (pre-test, last minute), during testing (every minute), and post-test in phases 1 and 2, a Polar Electro ® (Finland) Model Polar FT1 heart monitor was used. The maximal heart rate (HR_{max}) of each player was defined as the highest value achieved in both tests. Then, the HR_{max} was considered as: (1) 220 minus age (years) to the test on a cycle ergometer, and (2) 220 minus age and minus the individual value of bradycardia, identified by subtraction between the land-resting heart rate, and the water-resting heart rate for the eggbeater test (phase 2).

Statistical Analysis

The Shapiro-Wilk test was used to verify the normality of the data. Means, standard deviations, and coefficients of variation were calculated. Comparisons between the maximum values of the variables obtained from both tests (land and water) were performed with the Student's t-test for paired data. The comparison between the land rest (phases 1 and 2) and the water rest (phase 2), and the comparison between cadences throughout the test in the water were performed with ANOVA for repeated measures; in this case the sphericity of the data was verified (Mauchly test). When necessary, and indicated by the degrees of freedom in the Fischer test results the Greenhouse—Geisser Epsilon Correction Factor was used. The main effects were tested with Bonferroni post hoc; statistical power was calculated and the effect size was verified with statistical eta^2. The comparison between the eggbeater kick test cadences and the cycle ergometer test fixed cadences was performed with *t* Student simples test (cycle ergometer fixed value cadences were 70–80 RPM). The Intraclass Correlation (ICC) values between both tests outcomes were calculated.

Between the maximum loads reached in the cycle ergometer test (W) and the eggbeater kick test (kg), a Pearson linear correlation test was conducted. In order to verify the agreement between the values obtained from both tests, the Bland–Altmann graphical analysis was performed with the calculation of bias and limits of agreement. The significance level was $\alpha \leq 0.05$ and the SPSS statistical package (15.0) was used for all the analyses.

Results

Twelve state-level, recreational water polo players volunteered to take part in this study; characteristics of the sample are shown in Table 1.

Table 1. General characteristics of the sample, mean ± standard deviation (*SD*); n = 12.

	Age (years)	Body mass (kg)	Height (cm)	∑ cutaneous folds (mm)	Experience time (years)
Mean	30,5	79,2	179,7	179,7	10
SD	7,7	7,2	5,9	5,9	7,7

Resting VO_2, RER, HR, and IEP in three situations: land-resting in phase 1 (pre-test in the cycle ergometer); land-resting in phase 2 (pre-test in the eggbeater kick); and water-resting in phase 2 (pre-test in the eggbeater kick) in means, *SD,* and coefficients of variation are shown in Table 2. In comparison of the resting values (Table 2) in the three situations, effects of immersion were evident only in the resting HR ($F_{2, 22} = 5.11$; $p = 0.015$; $eta^2 = 0.317$, power = 0.766) with lower values in the water-resting (phase 2) compared to land-resting (phase 2). The bradycardia was identified in average of 9.7 ± 5.2 bpm.

Table 2. Means, standard deviation, and coefficients variation of oxygen uptake (VO_2), respiratory exchange ratio (RER), heart rate (HR), the perceived exertion index (IEP) in resting in pre-cycle ergometer test, and pre-eggbeater kick test (land and water); n = 12.

	Cycle ergometer Land-resting	Eggbeater kick Land-resting	Eggbeater kick Water-resting
VO_2 (ml. $kg^{-1}.min^{-1}$)	3.7 ± 1.4 (38.7%)	3.9 ± 0.8 (20.9%)	4.2 ± 1.1 (27.9%)
RER	0.92 ± 0.13 (14.8%)	0.96 ± 0.09 (9.3%)	0.98 ± 0.09 (9.7%)#
HR (bpm)	74.3 ± 14.0 (18.9%)	80 ± 9.2* (11.5%)	70.2 ± 11.8* (16.8%)
IEP (points)	6.25 ± 0.4 (7.2%)	6 ± 0 (0%)	6.08 ± 0.2 (4.7%)

#this case n = 9; *p = 0,019.

Means, *SD,* and coefficients of variation of $VO_{2\,max}$, RER, HR_{max}, IEP_{max}, achieved from load and exhaustion time from the cycle ergometer test and eggbeater kick test are shown in Table 3. There were no differences between the maximum values of the two tests. It is assumed that $VO_{2\,max}$ had been reached in both (in land and water) protocols (although identified by the VO_{2peak}) according to the criteria established by Howley[18]: the percentage of the estimated maximum heart rate reached ≥ 90%; high value for respiratory exchange ratio, and perceived exertion index for the players reported the maximum effort. The cycle ergometer test and eggbeater kick test HR_{max} achieved, respectively, 95.7 ± 5.9% and 99.9 ± 7.7% of the estimated HR_{max}. The Intraclass Correlation Coefficient (ICC) calculated for $VO_{2\,max}$, RER, HR_{max}, and exhaustion time were, respectively, 0.097 (p = 0.43), 0.007 (p = 0.50), 0.948 (p < 0.001), and 0.419 (p = 0.091).

There was no correlation between the maximum loads achieved in both tests. In relation to the eggbeater kick test cadence, considering that there is a need to increase the movement frequency while the load was increased, Figure 1 shows the cadence in cycles per minute for three periods of the test (beginning, middle, and end). There was a significant increase in the movement frequency from the beginning to the end of the test ($F_{1.39;\,14.5} = 32.2$, p <0.001; $eta^2 = 0.746$; power = 1.0). The cycle ergometer test cadence was fixed at 70–80 RPM (permissible cadence range of this test). When comparing the beginning, middle, and end of the eggbeater kick and cycle ergometer test cadence, the eggbeater kick cadence was higher than 70 RPM in all periods (beginning: $t_{11} = 2.4$; $p = 0.035$; middle: $t_{11} = 4.2$; $p = 0.001$; and end: $t_{11} = 7.2$, p <0.001). The eggbeater kick cadence in the beginning and the middle were similar to the cycle ergometer cadence of 80 RPM, while the cadence at the end was higher ($t_{11} = 3.2$; $p = 0.007$).

Table 3. Mean, standard deviation, and coefficients variation of maximum oxygen uptake ($VO_{2\,max}$), maximum respiratory exchange ratio (RER_{max}), maximum heart rate (HR_{max}), maximum perceived exertion index (IEP_{max}), achieved load, and the exhaustion time in cycle ergometer and eggbeater kick tests; n = 12.

	Cycle ergometer test	Eggbeater kick test
$VO_{2\,max}$ (ml.kg^{-1}.min^{-1})	40.2 ± 2.7 (6.9%)	38.4 ± 5.7 (14.1%)
RER_{max}	1.17 ± 0.08 (6.8%)	1.19 ± 0.12 (10.1%)
HR_{max} (bpm)	181.4 ± 11.7 (6.5%)	179 ± 11.7 (5.8%)
IEP_{max} (points)	20 ± 0 (0%)	20 ± 0 (0%)
Achieved load	304.1 ± 29.8 W (9.7%)	4.9 ± 1.03 kg (21.0%)
Exhaustion time (min)	8.7 ± 1.3 (14.9%)	8.1 ± 1.9 (23.4%)

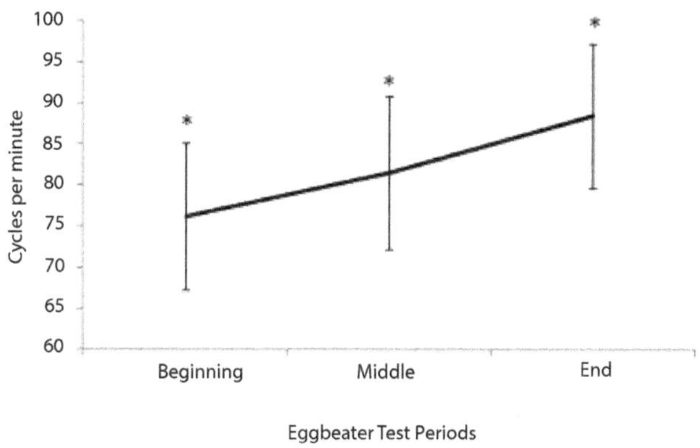

Figure 1. Eggbeater kick test cadence in cycles per minute in three periods (beginning, middle, end); n = 12; * $p < 0.01$ for all comparison

Bland–Altmann graphical analysis, as shown in Figures 2, 3, and 4, illustrate the limits of agreement between the tests. $VO_{2\,max}$ (Bias: 1.74; limits of agreement: –10.40; 13.87), RER (Bias: –0.02; limits of agreement: −0.30; 0.26), and HR_{max} (Bias: 2.41; limits of agreement: −7.31; 12.14). Bland–Altmann analyses indicate acceptable limits of agreement in the three variables. The data obtained from the two tests are considered to be in agreement as they fall within the established limits of agreement.

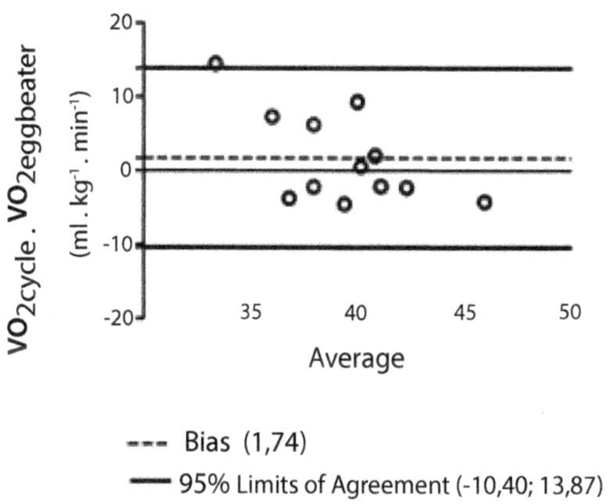

Figure 2. VO_2 values' Bland–Altmann analyses.

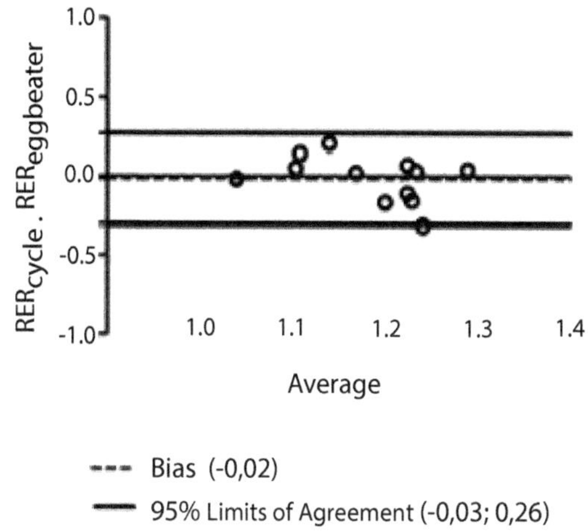

Figure 3. RER's Bland–Altmann analyses.

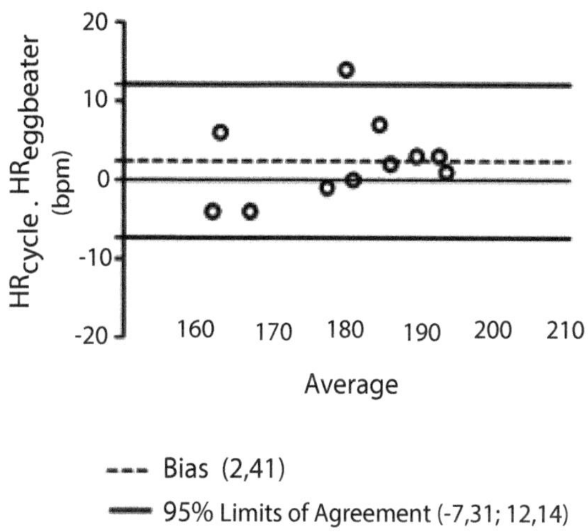

Figure 4: HR's Bland–Altmann analyses.

Discussion

Considering the specifics of water polo, especially the eggbeater kick technique, and its importance for sport performance, this study aimed to compare and to verify the agreement between water polo players' $VO_{2\,max}$ values obtained from two different protocol tests: one test performed on a cycle ergometer (land), and another test in eggbeater kick (water). In general, no differences were evident between the protocols for all analyzed parameters, low values of Intraclass Correlation Coefficient (exception for the HR_{max}), and acceptable agreement results.

The sample characteristics of this study indicate that the participants have lower stature and body mass values than top level players.[8,12,19] These results, in addition to prior knowledge of the assessed players, confirm that the participants of this pilot study are not elite players. Indeed, based on their time spent in training (2–3 times per week for a period of 90 minutes each), and their involvement in regional-level championships, they are considered to be recreational players. These characteristics become relevant for the analyses of $VO_{2\,max}$ values identified in this study.

Possible immersion effects are concern regarding effort tests in an aquatic environment. However, the VO_2 and RER values did not change during the immersion period in this study. Similarly, a previous study compared seven men at rest and during exercise on a cycle ergometer in two situations: land and water[20]. Significant statistical differences were found between the two situations (land VO_2: 3.87 ml.kg^{-1}.min^{-1}; at rest: 35 ml.kg^{-1}.min^{-1}; water VO_2: 3.88 ml.kg^{-1}.min^{-1}; and cycle ergometer: 36 ml.kg^{-1}.min^{-1}). The immersion effect on HR was visible and the results of this study are consistent with the literature regarding immersion bradycardia[21-23]. Specifically, the bradycardia effect averaged 9.7 ± 5.2 bpm. In an aquatic environment, the condition of resting or exercise changes HR, and it is influenced by factors, such as body position, the immersion depth, and the water temperature[24]. The immersion allowed greater hydrostatic pressure which facilitated the venous return that consequently maintains the same cardiac output, reducing HR, and therefore, explains the bradycardia.

The average $VO_{2\,max}$ values in both tests showed lower values when compared with values proposed in the literature[8,25]. Most likely, this fact is due to the sample of this study: recreational-level water polo players. The $VO_{2\,max}$ values described in the literature for elite water polo players with a high-volume and intensity level of training, range between 58 and 63 ml.kg^{-1}.min^{-1}, but these values depend on the study and the type of protocol used. The most frequent protocol found in the literature is swimming tests[8,25]. Among the findings, Tsekouras[12] found VO_{2peak} values of 57.9 ± 7.0 ml.kg^{-1}.min^{-1} in a maximum test of 400 m front crawl for water polo players. These values are similar to those found by Zacca[26] with swimmers using the same distance and the same method (63.5 ± 8.7 ml.kg^{-1}.min^{-1}). Although water polo requires swimming, less than 40% of match time is spent swimming. In fact, most of the matches' time is spent in a vertical position performing the eggbeater kick; therefore, it is more appropriate to test water polo players while performing the eggbeater kick than swimming.

During the cycle ergometer test, the cadence was fixed between 70–80 RPM. In the eggbeater kick test when the load was increased, cadence was increased as well. However, the average cadence in both tests was similar in the majority of periods; the exception was the eggbeater test's end, when the players increased the eggbeater kick cadence more than 80 cycles per minute in order to keep the shoulders above the surface of the water under maximum load. Differences in cadence between the tests could be attributed to a limitation of comparison between them, mostly due to the different strategies of motor unit recruitment under different levels of cadence.

The variability between the results in the eggbeater kick test was higher than in the cycle ergometer test, probably, due to the differences in kinetic and kinematic parameters of the feet in these environments (land and water). Alberton[27] did not find differences in $VO_{2\,max}$ and IEP between treadmill tests (land) when compared to three different water aerobic exercises (water). The $VO_{2\,max}$ data variability of this study could be related to the involved muscle mass during the exercises, rather than the environment in which the individual is exercising. Moreover, as the players are accustomed to training with regard to the eggbeater kick in all sessions, the progressively increased load could lead to increased variability of the task execution, that is, individual strategies of active muscle mass recruitment may be reflected in greater variability in metabolic variables of a water test.

The specific analysis of the results of correlation and agreement, when associated with the comparison results, lead to the first objective of this project:

(1) Correlation was not found between the maximum load of the cycle ergometer test (WATTS) and the maximum load of the eggbeater kick test (kg); this result can be explained by the specifics of both gestures and the responses of the loads;

(2) Low values of ICC indicate poor intraclass correlation, which could be explained by both the level of the athletes and differences between the assessed motor tasks;

(3) the Bland–Altmann analysis indicated agreement, i.e., the cycle ergometer test values (land) agree with the eggbeater kick test values (water), within reasonable agreement limits. The bias values represented, respectively, for the eggbeater kick test data in 4.5% $VO_{2\,max}$; 10% RER, and 1.34% HR_{max}.

Therefore, such findings support the argument that the maximal oxygen uptake can be estimated in a progressive test in the eggbeater kick for water polo players with an error margin of 4.5%. This test is specific to the practiced gesture in water polo matches and respects the particularities of the aquatic environment. The different tests used by coaches and the lack of a specific and valid test makes it difficult to use and provide consistent interpretation of $VO_{2\,max}$ values found for water polo players. Tests using objective physiological measurements, often based on laboratory testing protocols, can be used to form a basis for a valid and reliable specific test for this sport.[8] Therefore, this study was designed for the specific test for water polo, using a laboratory test as a base.

Conclusion

The results of the progressive protocol performed with the water performing eggbeater kick did not differ, and it presented agreement with the results obtained on land on the cycle ergometer, although low ICC values were found. More studies on this topic, beyond this pilot, with larger samples and higher-level water polo players, would aid to further understand the possibility of applying the eggbeater protocol to asses $VO_{2\,max}$.

References

1. Lamas L. Barrera J, Otranto G, Ugrinowitsch C. Invasion team sports: strategy and match modeling. Int J Perform Analysis Sport. 2014; 14 (1):307-29.
2. Snyder P. Water Polo for Players & Teachers of Aquatics. California. LA84 Fondation. USA, 2008. Available from: http://www.la84foundation.org (accessed on January 5 2015).
3. Platanou T. On-water and dryland vertical jump in water polo players. J Sports Med Physical Fitness. 2005; 45: 26-31.

4. Homma M, Homma M. Coaching points for the technique of the eggbeater kick in synchronized swimming based on three-dimensional motion analysis. Sports Biomechanics. 2005; 4 (1):73-88.
5. Sanders R. Strength, flexibility and timing in the eggbeater kick. Available from: http://www.coachesinfo.com (accessed on January 5 2015).
6. Dopsaj M, Aleksandrovic M. Basic anthropomorfological characteristics of elite senior Serbian water polo players according to field position. Int J Fitness. 2009; vol. 5 (2).
7. Dopsaj M, Thanopoulos V. The structure of evaluation indicators of vertical swimming work ability of top water polo players. Rev Port Ciencias Desporto. 2006; 6 (2):124-26.
8. Smith HS. Applied Physiology of water polo. Sports Med. 1998; 26 (5):317-34.
9. Wilmore JH, Costill DL. Fisiologia do Esporte e do Exercício. Editora Manole LTDA, 1° edição brasileira, Barueri/SP, 2001.
10. Aleksandrovic M. Functional abilities as a predictor of specific motor skills of young water polo players. J Human Kinetics. 2011; 29: 123-32.
11. Ferreti G. Maximal oxygen consumption in healthy humans: theories and facts. Eur J Appl Physiol. 2014; 114:2007-2036.
12. Tsekouras YE, Kavouras SA, Campagna A, Kotsis YP, Syntosi SS, Papazoglu K *et al.* The anthropometrical and physiological characteristics of elite water polo players. Eur J Appl Physiol, 2005; 95 (1): 35-41.
13. Lobenius K. Physiological differences during exercise in water and on cycle ergometer for synchronized swimmers. In: Biomechanics and Medicine in Swimming, França. 2002; IX: 539-544.
14. Lucia A, Hoyos J, Perez M, Santalla A, Chicharro JL. Inverse relationship between VO2max and economy/efficiency in world-class cyclist. Med Sci Sports Exerc. 2002; 34(12):2079-84.
15. Bini RR, Senger D, Lanferdini F, Lopes AL. Joint kinematics assessment during cycling incremental test to exhaustion. Isokinetics Exerc Sci. 2012; 20: 99-105.
16. Bini R. Hume PA, Lanferdini FJ, Vaz MA. Effects of body positions on the saddle on pedalling technique for cyclists and triathletes. Eur J Sport Sci. 2014; 14(S1): S413-S420.
17. Borg G. Psychophysical bases of perceived exertion. Med Sci Sports Exerc. 1982; 14 (5):377-81.
18. Howley ET, Basset DR, Welch HG. Criteria for maximal oxygen uptake: review and commentary. Med Sci Sports Exerc. 1995; 27: 1292–1301.
19. Dopsaj M. Pulling force characteristics of 10 s maximal tethered eggbeater kick in elite water polo players: a pilot study. Biomechanics Med Swimming. 2010; XI: 69-71.
20. Nagashima K, Hose H, Yoshida T, Morimoto T. Relationship between atrial natriuretic peptide and plasma volume during graded exercise with water immersion. J Appl Physiol. 1995; 78 (1): 217-24.
21. Hall J, Grant J, Blake D, Taylor G, Garbutt G. Cardiorespiratory responses to aquatic treadmill walking in patients with rheumatoid arthritis. Physiother Res Int. 2004; 9:59-73.
22. Kruel LFM. Peyre-Tartaruga LA,Alberton CL, Muller FG, Petkowizc R. Effects of hydrostatic weight on heart rate during immersion in water. Aquatic Fitness Res J. 2004; 1: 1- 4.
23. Tiggemann CL, Guedes MG, Bgeginski R, Pinto RS, Kruel LFM. Comparação de variáveis cardiorrespiratórias máximas entre a corrida em piscina funda e a corrida em esteira. Motriz. 2007; 13 (4):266-72.
24. Graef FI, Kruel LFM. Frequência cardíaca e percepção subjetiva do esforço no meio aquático: diferenças em relação ao meio terrestre e aplicações na prescrição do exercício – uma revisão. Rev Bras Med Esporte. 2006; 12: nº 4.
25. Platanou T. Physiological demands of water polo goalkeeping. J Sci Med Sport. 2009; 12: 244-50.
26. Zacca R, Teixeira BC, Lopes AL, Matos CC, Engelmann L, Castro FAS. VO_2 assessed by backward extrapolation in 200, 400, 800, and 1500 m front crawl in youth swimmers. In: XII International Symposium on Biomechanics and Medicine in Swimming, 2014, Canberra. Proceedings of the XII International Symposium on Biomechanics and Medicine in Swimming. Canberra: Australian Institute of Sport. 2014; 1: 531-36.
27. Alberton CL, Antunes AH, Beilke DD, Pinto SS, Kanitz AC, Tartaruga MP, Martins Kruel LF. Maximal and ventilatory thresholds of oxygen uptake and rating of perceived exertion responses to water aerobic exercises. J Strength Cond Res. 2013;27(7):1897-903.

Corresponding author

Ligia Ignez Engelmann
Grupo de Pesquisa em Esportes Aquáticos, ESEF, Universidade Federal do Rio Grande do Sul, Rua Felizardo, 750, Bairro Jardim Botânico, Porto Alegre/RS, Brazil.
Email: ligia.engel@gmail.com

15

Electromyographic analysis of riding posture during the bicycling start moment

Johnny Padulo
University e-Campus, Novedrate, Italy
University of Split, Split, Croatia
National Centre of Medicine and Science in Sport, Tunis, Tunisia

Luca Paolo Ardigò
University of Verona, Verona, Italy

Mirjana Milić
University of Split, Split, Croatia

Douglas William Powell
Campbell University, Buies Creek, NC, USA

Abstract — Professional cyclists often adopt a competition-start standing posture, which has been shown to improve performance. The biomechanical basis of this is unclear, and might be due to a greater mechanical advantage or increased key muscle activity. Previous observations in steady state cycling showed greater activation of the *tibialis anterior, erector spinae*, and *biceps brachii* when adopting a standing vs. seated-riding posture. Little is known regarding the effect of riding posture on activation during a standing start. Eleven cyclists performed standing starts in seated and standing-postures using stationary-cycle and on the track. Electromyography of the *gastrocnemius medialis*, tibialis anterior, *erector spinae*, and *biceps brachii* was recorded during first and subsequent pedal strokes. Results showed that the *gastrocnemius medialis* did not modify activity. The tibialis anterior, erector spinae, and *biceps brachii* activity was increased during the standing posture compared to seated, only during the first pedal stroke. These increased activation intensities were accompanied by a corresponding 10% increase in bike speed during the first 5 meters following a standing start in the standing posture compared to the seated one. Adopting a standing posture during a standing start improves performance through greater initial acceleration.

Keywords: sEMG, cycling, performance

Introduction

Many factors are known to affect cycling performance: (i) the geometry of the bike, such as crank length[1] and saddle position[2,3]; (ii) various aerodynamic variables such as proper aero position and (iii) pedaling frequency, which determines maximal power output during cycling[3,4]. Alterations in posture, such as changing from a seated to a standing posture, also result in changes in performance[5,6]. When cycling with a standing posture, a greater production of power output is developed for the same speed, presumably to manage the increased number of degrees of freedom of the lower limbs due to the loss of contact of the buttocks with the saddle[7]. Yet, cycling with a standing posture allows a significant but temporary mechanical power "overboost", which riders can exploit for special situations (e.g., start, attack and sprint at the finish). Such a posture change has therefore a great influence on pedal kinetics[3].

Cyclists predominantly adopt a prolonged standing posture during an all-out standing start (from zero speed as opposed to a flying start) to increase power output compared to a seated posture[3,8,9]. However, the use of a standing posture requires the maintenance of a larger metabolic power and to counterbalance the higher aerodynamic drag due to an increased drag area associated with the overall postural change[9,10]. Therefore, a standing posture seems to be advantageous and metabolically sustainable only for short duration, high-acceleration, and high-torque periods, such as an all-out standing start. For these periods, skilled cyclists prefer to adopt a standing posture.

The specific motor control of the lower extremities during standing *vs.* seated cycling postures has been previously described using surface electromyography (sEMG)[11-14]. The findings of these investigations have suggested that a standing posture is associated with greater force applied to the pedals and that this increased for application is likely due to the pedals supporting the mass of the cyclist. Conversely, in a seated posture, the cyclist's mass is mostly supported by the saddle[15]. The findings of this study are supported by individual power profiles and demonstrate that instantaneous power is strongly correlated to pedal normal force[16]. However, the same study has also shown that the overall maximum power is highly correlated to the cyclist's muscle mass. Although previous research has demonstrated that a standing posture is associated with greater pedal force and overall powers applied to the pedals, few differences have been observed in lower extremity joint kinetics between standing and seated cycling postures[3]. It has been suggested that when cycling with a standing posture, forces produced by the upper extremity enhance overall power production[17]. Limited research has investigated the contributions of the upper extremity musculature to cycling performance, and changes in muscle activation of the upper extremity have not been previously investigated in standing *vs.* seated cycling postures.

An understanding of the changing contributions of upper and lower extremity musculature to the observed differences in standing start performance using a standing compared to seated cycling posture, would enhance individually optimized training programs. In addition to improving performance, individualized training programs may also reduce the incidence and prevalence of training-related injuries in cyclists. Therefore, the purpose of this study was to quantify changes in muscle activation of ankle, trunk, and elbow musculature in standing compared to seated cycling postures during a maximal standing start. It was hypothesized that the standing posture would be associated with significantly greater muscle activation intensities compared to seated postures.

Methods

Participants

Eleven male amateur cyclists participated in this study (age: 31 ± 3 years [range 27 ÷ 36], mass: 69.0 ± 4.1 kg, height: 1.76 ± 0.04 meters, BMI: 22.1 ± 1.5 kg/m^2; data reported as mean ± SD; with no history of major lower extremities injuries). All participants were highly skilled cyclists with more than six years of sport-specific training, had a cycling-specific training volume of more than 400 km *per* week and were ranked regionally or nationally within their category. This study was conducted in accordance with the Declaration of Helsinki. The experimental protocol was approved by the University e-Campus research ethics board, and each participant gave signed informed consent prior to participation in this study.

Laboratory measures and procedures

The participants were asked to pedal on a commercial and commonly available cycle ergometer (Schwinn, Johnny G Pro Spin Bike; crank length: 17 cm; resistance mob: halfway), wearing their competition cycling shoes and pedals with toe clips. Seat height was adjusted for each participant according to his preferred seated cycling posture on a road bike, such that his knee was nearly fully extended and the sole of the foot was perpendicular to the shank when the crank was at the bottom-dead-center. Crank position was considered to be at 0° when the crank was aligned with the positive Y-axis and the clockwise (anterior) rotation (facing rider's right side) was considered positive (Figure 1B). The handlebars were positioned according to each individual participant's preferred seated cycling posture on a road bike.

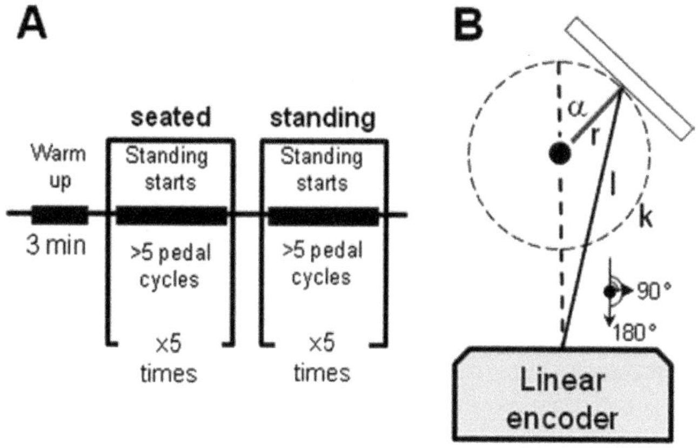

Figure 1. (A) Schematic description of the experimental procedure. (B) Schematic description of the measurement of the crank angle using a linear encoder attached to the pedal (see text for details). k = distance of the linear encoder from crank center; l = distance pedal-linear encoder (measured by the linear encoder); α = crank angle; r = crank length.

Participants completed the whole experimental procedure during one single visit. Experimental procedure laboratory temperature was comfortable (i.e., ~ 20°C) and participants were allowed to drink water *ad libitum* to keep their hydration *status* adequate. Participants were first required to perform a 3-min warm up consisting of low-resistance pedaling (Figure 1A). All participants started pedaling with their right (dominant) limb. The dominant limb was defined as the limb the athlete would use to kick a ball, and was the only limb evaluated for each participant. Participants performed five maximal effort trials with hands positioned on the bottom of the handlebar and a 70° starting crank angle for a minimum of five consecutive pedaling cycles (maximum of ten consecutive pedaling cycles; average trial duration 5 s[18]. Between trials, participants were asked to stop completely and rest for 4 min (Figure 1A). A minimum of 25 pedaling strokes was collected from each participant. Participants completed this protocol for each experimental condition (seated and standing cycling postures). The sequence of riding posture conditions (seated *vs.* standing) was randomized across participants. To standardize the exercise in the seated compared to standing posture, participants were required to accelerate as quickly as possible from a standing start (zero speed) and then to pedal at same (seated) warm up cadence.

The crankshaft pedal was connected to a customized linear encoder (sEMG system with encoder included, MuscleLab™ 4020e, Bosco System, Ergotest Technology, Langensund, Norway), which recorded the vertical displacement of the pedal to synchronize with sEMG signals (Fig. 1B) as previously described[19-22]. The linear encoder had a spatial resolution of 0.1 mm (range 3.5 m, max speed 24 m/s) and a sampling frequency of 100 Hz. The vertical displacement of the pedal was then converted into the angular position of the pedal according to the following equation (Figure 1B): $\alpha = \cos^{-1}(k^2 + r^2 - l^2) / (2\ k\ r)$

where α = crank angle; k = distance of the linear encoder from crank center; l = distance pedal-linear encoder; r = crank length. The angular resolution was determined to be 0.03°. Surface EMG of the *gastrocnemius medialis* (GAS), *tibialis anterior* (TA), *erector spinae* (at L3 level; ES), and *biceps brachii* (BB) were recorded at 1500 Hz using pre-amplified bipolar silver–silver chloride (Ag/AgCl) sEMG electrodes. Previous studies have shown that the selected muscles play a major contribution to the production of power during sprint cycling exercises[6,11,18]. The disc electrodes had a diameter of 1 cm and inter-electrode distance of 2 cm. The input impedance was 2GΩ, common mode rejection rate 100 dB, band-pass filter 6–1,500 Hz, and gain ×600. The electrodes were positioned longitudinally with respect to the orientation of muscle fibers and located according to the recommendations of SENIAM[23]. To reduce electrical impedance, the participant's skin was shaved and cleansed using an alcohol pad prior to electrode placement. To prevent movement artifacts due to movement of electrode cables, the cables were secured using elastic bands (Vetrap™). The raw EMG signal was band-pass filtered (8–1,200 Hz) and converted to root mean square (RMS) with a 20-ms smoothing window as previously reported in the literature. Maximal voluntary isometric contractions (MVIC) for each muscle of interest were systematically determined by averaging the integrated sEMG (iEMG) signal during a 3-s period of sustained maximal force output after the initial peak in the force curve during a maximal contraction of each muscle as previously described[24,25]. Normalized iEMG values were calculated as the quotients of the recorded iEMG values from dynamic trials divided by the iEMG values recorded during the MVIC trials and were represented as percentages of MVIC[26].

To ensure correct riding posture and to investigate cycling kinematics, sagittal plane kinematic data were recorded (210 Hz, 480×360 resolution, Exilim EX-FH20, Casio, Tokyo, Japan). The high-speed digital camera was placed perpendicular to the sagittal plane of the participant's right side at a distance of 5 meters with the camera height at the vertical height of each participant's estimated center of mass[27,28]. Markers were positioned on main body joints (Figure 2A).

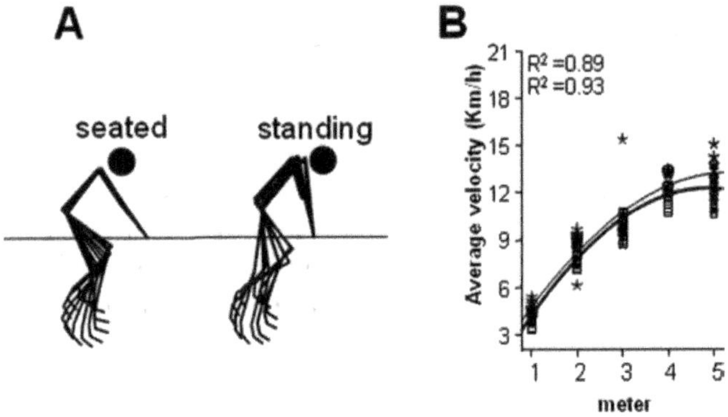

Figure 2. (A) Stick figure of body angles during a standing start in seated and standing positions. (B) Effect of riding position on average speed following a standing start at different distances from the start.

To investigate changes in muscle activation patterns associated with seated compared to standing cycling posture, sEMG, and kinematic data were recorded in a laboratory setting. However, to verify the effect of the two riding postures on instantaneous cycling speed in a real cycling environment, participants were also required to perform a similar experimental protocol on a race bicycle on a sport-specific oval track. This protocol has been used previously to assess cycling performance[19].

Track measures and procedures

To verify the effects of riding posture on instantaneous speed during a standing start, participants repeated the testing protocol using a race bicycle (FP1, Pinarello, Italy; crank length 17 cm). The participant's hand position was similar to the stationary cycling task (bottom of the handle bar) and the gear selected was consistent with the stationary cycling task[19]. The same bicycle was used to test all participants. The participants wore standard cycling shoes and pedals with toe clips. The seat height was adjusted for each participant according to his preferred cycling posture on a road bike, such that his knee was fully extended and the sole of the foot was perpendicular to the shank when the crank was at bottom-dead-center. The handlebars were positioned according to each participant's preferred posture on a road bike. After a 3-min pedaling warm up, participants were asked to pedal as fast as possible starting in each experimental posture (seated and standing) again with a 70° starting crank angle[18]. Participants were given 4 min rest between trials. The first 5 meters of each standing start trial were recorded with a high-speed digital camera (210 Hz, 480×360 resolution, Exilim EX-FH20, Casio, Tokyo, Japan). The camera was placed on a tripod, perpendicular to the sagittal plane of the participant's right side at a distance of 5 meters from the 5-meter run with the camera placed at the vertical height of each participant's estimated center of mass. To calculate the instantaneous speed of the bicycle the center of the anterior wheel was tracked using Dartfish 5.0 Pro (Dartifish, Fribourg, Switzerland).

Statistical analysis

The RMS signal of each muscle for each experimental condition was averaged over 36 × 10° intervals constituting the entire crank cycle. Previous research has suggested that 10° intervals are most efficacious in the analysis of muscle activation patterns during cycling[29]. For each trial, custom software was used to calculate the average sEMG amplitude across each 10° pedal angle interval (MatLab 2013, MathWorks, Inc., Natick, MA, USA). Average data were then analyzed using a univariate analysis of variance (ANOVA) to identify significant differences in sEMG activity due to riding posture (seated *vs.* standing) and crank angle (36 intervals). All data were provided as mean ± standard deviation. The Shapiro-Wilk test was used to ensure normal distribution of the data.

A two-way repeated measures ANOVA was used to assess the influence of riding posture (seated *vs.* standing) and crank angle (36 intervals) on the average instantaneous speed during the first 5 m of the standing start performance with repeated measures for cycling posture and crank angle factors. In the presence of a significant main effect of posture or posture by crank angle interaction, *post-hoc t*-tests were used to determine the source of the significant findings. Statistical analyses were performed using Excel 2003 and SPSS 15 software. The statistical significance level was set at $P < 0.05$.

Results

Quantitative sEMG elicited during the first and subsequent pedal strokes (i.e., as steady state was achieved), in the seated and standing cycling postures are presented in Figure 3. Peak sEMG amplitudes are showed in normalized data, a finding that is consistent with previously published data[11,30,31].

The univariate ANOVA with pedaling intervals (i.e., 10° pedal intervals) and riding posture as factors revealed no significant changes in iEMG among the different conditions. The time of occurrence and the intensity of the peak activity were not significantly different between the two riding postures (Figure 3, $P > 0.05$) in contrast with the finding by Hug, Turpin, Couturier, Dorel[5]. Similar to the first stroke, there were no significant changes in iEMG during the subsequent pedal strokes. The univariate ANOVA with pedaling order (i.e., first pedal stroke *vs.* subsequent pedal strokes) and riding posture as factors revealed significant differences for both pedaling order ($P < 0.05$) and riding posture ($P < 0.01$) as well as a significant pedaling posture interaction ($P < 0.05$). The standing compared to seated cycling posture was associated with significantly greater iEMG amplitude (Figure 3).

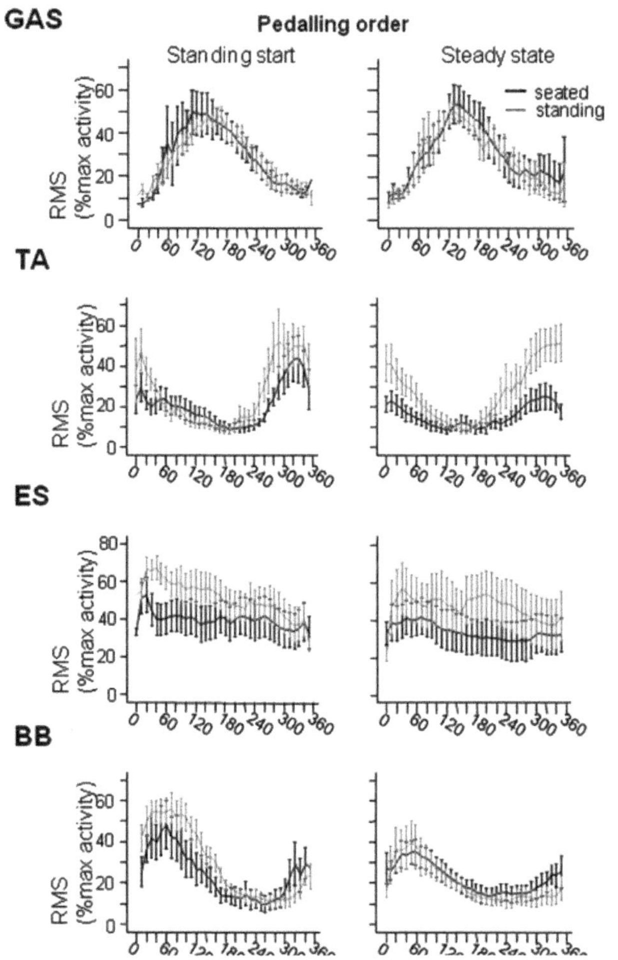

Figure 3. Average sEMG RMSs (% max activity) of the *gastrocnemius medialis* (GAS), *tibialis anterior* (TA), *erector spinae* (ES), and *biceps brachii* (BB) while pedaling the cycle in seated and standing positions are shown for standing start (left panels) and for following cycling ("Steady state", right panels). Values are shown as mean ± SEM.

The analysis of the peak activity of TA muscle revealed no change in peak activity between the two riding postures ($P < 0.05$). Similarly there was no difference between the first pedal stroke compared to subsequent pedal strokes. However, the intensity of the iEMG signal was significantly greater during the first pedal stroke ($P < 0.01$) and during the standing posture compared to the seated one ($P < 0.001$). Unsurprisingly, univariate ANOVA showed significant effect for riding posture on sEMG, but not for pedaling cycle phase, without interaction effect.

Riding posture did not significantly affect BB sEMG. However, univariate ANOVA with riding posture and pedaling order as factors showed that pedaling order (e.g., first *vs.* subsequent pedal strokes) had a significant effect on iEMG data. iEMG was higher during the first pedal stroke. Therefore, as a preliminary key message, we may suggest specific TA strengthening to improve all-out standing start performance.

The basic kinematic analysis of the riding posture during the pedaling cycle phase showed that with standing posture there was little vertical displacement of the hip (Figure 2A). Analysis of the instantaneous speed during on-track standing starts showed that with standing posture the mean acceleration during the first 5 meters was 10% greater than with seated posture (Figure 2B). A *t*-test showed significant differences in the acceleration ($P < 0.05$) between the two postures. The acceleration was 1.32 ± 0.22 and 1.59 ± 0.24 m/s^2 (mean ± SD) for the seated and standing posture, respectively.

Discussion

The purpose of this study was to investigate the effects of seated *vs.* standing posture on muscle activation intensity in muscles of the lower extremities, trunk, and upper extremities in two cycling conditions including a standing start (zero speed) and steady state cycling. The major findings of this study demonstrate that during a standing start (zero speed), muscle activation intensities of the TA and ES are significantly greater in the standing *vs.* seated posture. Additionally, during steady state cycling, greater muscle activation intensities were observed in the TA and BB in the standing compared to seated cycling posture. These data demonstrate that cycling posture significantly alters muscle activation of the lower extremities, trunk, and upper extremities.

In competitive cycling and cycling-inclusive sports such as triathlon, it is not uncommon for races to be decided by small differences in time. Therefore, optimizing performance during training and competition are of the utmost importance to maximize athlete performance. To our knowledge, this is the first study to provide data pertaining to changes in muscle activation intensity associated with a standing compared to seated posture during a standing start and steady state cycling.

The standing start (zero speed) is commonly used in time trials and cycling-inclusive sports to begin the cycling portion of the competition. Successful sprint cyclists produce greater accelerations from a standing start resulting in greater speeds earlier in the race. This is achieved by generating greater crank torques and powers. The results of the current study indicate that the standing start was associated with significantly greater TA and BB muscle activation intensity compared to steady state cycling. It is theorized that these alterations in muscle activation would result in greater lower extremity power output to be transferred to the crank during the standing start[3,8,9]. Specifically, the increased amplitude of the BB activation would produce greater elbow flexion torques to the cycle handles and aid in reducing unwanted vertical displacement of the center of mass, allowing greater downward force to be applied to the pedals in the standing start condition [11-14]. This increased transfer of lower extremity power would generate greater accelerations for the standing start. Therefore, increased BB activation intensity may result in improved efficiency of lower extremity kinetics by maintaining a stable platform from which the lower extremity can apply torques to the cycle. Similarly, greater TA activation may be present to functionally stiffen the ankle joint through antagonist co-activation in response to greater loading from the lower extremity[32]. By increasing ankle joint stiffness, the joint torques and powers produced by large anti-gravity muscles of the lower extremities are more optimally applied to the cycle pedals. Although TA-GAS co-activation was not empirically calculated in the current study, no differences were observed in GAS activation while TA activation was significantly increased. Further, previous research has supported our hypothesis by suggesting that TA function in cycling is associated with enhanced power transmission to the crank[22,33]. These findings would strongly suggest that an increase in TA co-activation is associated with improved cycling performance. While the postulated mechanics offer plausible explanations for the observed changes in muscle activation of the lower extremities, no quantitative data was included in the present study to support these proposed mechanisms of function including handle forces or joint stiffness data.

Conversely, previous data has been published pertaining to differences in lower extremities muscle activation during steady state cycling in a standing compared to seated posture. Specifically, previous research data has shown that cycling in a standing posture is associated with significantly greater muscle activation intensities of the *vastus lateralis* and *gluteus maximum* compared to a seated posture[11-14]. The observed increases in hip and knee extensor muscle activation may serve to increase hip and knee joint torques and powers to improve cycling performance when cycling with a standing compared to seated postures. Conversely, greater hip and knee extensor muscle activation may be due to the requisite need to increase hip and knee extensor forces to support the greater load associated with a standing posture.

During steady state cycling, no significant differences in GAS and BB muscle activation intensities were observed in the standing compared to seated cycling posture. These findings contrast with previously published data[11,12]. Specifically, it has been shown that cycling with a standing posture is associated with significantly greater lower extremity muscle activation intensities compared to a seated posture[11,12]. Further, it was also noted that uniarticular muscles exhibited larger increases in muscle activation intensity compared to biarticular muscles[12]. It is possible that the methodological differences between each of these studies underlie these conflicting findings.

While the current study presents unique findings pertaining to differences in the intensity of muscle activation when cycling with a standing compared to seated posture, the authors acknowledge several limitations of the current study. First, the sample size was relatively small. Although several statistically significant differences were observed, it is possible that the study was underpowered to detect all significant differences. Second, the low number of muscles recorded during testing. Previous studies investigating cycling performance with changing postures have collected data from a greater number of muscles[11,12]. It is possible that by collecting from a greater number of muscles, this study could have captured other differences in neuromuscular strategy that exist in a standing compared to seated cycling posture. Third, there was a lack of joint and crank kinetic data (i.e., crank torque and power output). The presence of kinetic data would provide greater insight into the biomechanical efficacy of the observed neuromuscular changes associated with a standing *vs.* seated posture. Fourth, lateral sway of the cycles used in field testing were not recorded. It is possible that energy was expended in the frontal plane, which was not accounted for in our analysis of cycling performance.

Conclusions

The findings of this study demonstrate that the enhanced performance during a standing start (zero speed) when adopting a standing cycling posture, is associated with increased muscle activation of the *biceps brachii* and *tibialis anterior* muscles. Although these muscle activations do not drive the pedal stroke, they may indirectly benefit cycling performance by providing a more stable platform and more efficient lever to improve power transfer to the crank. A straight practical indication provided by this study is that the standing posture allows a bike standing start speed 10% increase with respect to the seated posture. Therefore, this finding may potentially be useful for specific training protocols for cyclists to improve the technique for a standing start. Further research is required to more fully understand the biomechanical effects of altering cycling posture during both steady state cycling and a standing start.

References

1. Martin JC, Malina RM, Spirduso WW. Effects of crank length on maximal cycling power and optimal pedaling rate of boys aged 8-11 years. Eur J Appl Physiol. 2002; 86:215–217.
2. Bini RR, Hume PA, Kilding AE. Saddle height effects on pedal forces, joint mechanical work and kinematics of cyclists and triathletes. Eur J Sport Sci. 2014; 14:44–52.
3. Martin JC, Davidson CJ, Pardyjak ER. Understanding sprint-cycling performance: the integration of muscle power, resistance, and modeling. Int J Sports Physiol Perform. 2007; 2:5–21.
4. Gardner AS, Martin JC, Martin DT, Barras M, Jenkins DG. Maximal torque- and power-pedaling rate relationships for elite sprint cyclists in laboratory and field tests. Eur J Appl Physiol. 2007; 101:287–292.

5. Hug F, Turpin NA, Couturier A, Dorel S. Consistency of muscle synergies during pedaling across different mechanical constraints. J Neurophysiol. 2011; 106:91–103.
6. Padulo J, Laffaye G, Bertucci W, Chaouachi A, Viggiano D. Optimisation of starting conditions in track cycling. Sport Sci Health. 2014; 10:189–198.
7. Millet GP, Tronche C, Fuster N, Candau R. Level ground and uphill cycling efficiency in seated and standing positions. Med Sci Sports Exerc. 2002; 34:1645–1652.
8. Martin JC, Gardner AS, Barras M, Martin DT. Modeling sprint cycling using field-derived parameters and forward integration. Med Sci Sports Exerc. 2006; 38:592–597.
9. Hansen EA, Waldeland H. Seated versus standing position for maximization of performance during intense uphill cycling. J Sport Sci. 2008; 26:977–984.
10. Harnish C, King D, Swensen T. Effect of cycling position on oxygen uptake and preferred cadence in trained cyclists during hill climbing at various power outputs. Eur J Appl Physiol. 2007; 99:387–391.
11. Duc S, Bertucci W, Pernin JN, Grappe F. Muscular activity during uphill cycling: effect of slope, posture, hand grip position and constrained bicycle lateral sways. J Electromyogr Kinesiol. 2008; 18:116–127.
12. Li L, Caldwell GE. Muscle coordination in cycling: effect of surface incline and posture. J Appl Physiol. 1998; 85:927–934.
13. Sakamoto M, Endoh T, Nakajima T, Tazoe T, Shiozawa S, KomiyamaT. Modulations of interlimb and intralimb cutaneous reflexes during simultaneous arm and leg cycling in humans. Clin Neurophysiol. 2006; 117:1301–1311.
14. Usabiaga J, Crespo R, Iza I, Aramendi J, Terrados N, Poza JJ. Adaptation of the lumbar spine to different positions in bicycle racing. Spine, 1997; 22:1965–1969.
15. Minetti AE, Pinkerton J, Zamparo P. From bipedalism to bicyclism: evolution in energetics and biomechanics of historic bicycles. Proc Biol Sci. 2001; 268:1351–1360.
16. Bolourchi F, Hull ML. Measurement of rider induced loads during simulated bicycling. Int J Sport Biomechan. 1985; 1:308–329.
17. Davidson CJ, Horscroft RD, McDaniel J, Tomas A, Hunter EL, Grisham JD et al. The biomechanics of producing standing and seated maximal cycling power. Med Sci Sports Exerc. 2005; 37, S393.
18. Padulo J, Powell DW, Ardigò LP, Viggiano D. Modifications in activation of lower limb muscles as a function of initial foot position in cycling. J Electromyogr Kinesiol. 2015; 25:648–652.
19. Padulo J, Di Capua R, Viggiano D. Pedaling time variability is increased in dropped riding position. Eur J Appl Physiol. 2012; 112:3161–3165.
20. Padulo J, Annino G, Tihanyi J, Calcagno G, Vando S, Smith L, et al. Uphill racewalking at iso-efficiency speed. J Strength Cond Res. 2013; 27:1964–1973.
21. Padulo J, Mignogna P, Mignardi S, Tonni F, D'Ottavio S. Effect of different pushing speeds on bench press. Int J Sports Med. 2012; 33:376–380.
22. Padulo J, Tiloca A, Powell D, Granatelli G, Bianco A, Paoli A. EMG amplitude of the biceps femoris during jumping compared to landing movements. Springerplus. 2013; 9:520.
23. Hermens HJ, Freriks B, Disselhorst-Klug C, Rau G. Development of recommendations for SEMG sensors and sensor placement procedures. J Electromyogr Kinesiol, 2000; 10:361–374.
24. Cormie P, McGuigan MR, Newton RU. Changes in the eccentric phase contribute to improved stretch-shorten cycle performance after training. Med Sci. Sports Exerc. 2010; 42:1731–1744.
25. Padulo J, Laffaye G, Ardigò LP, Chamari K. Concentric and eccentric: muscle contraction or exercise? J Human Kinetics. 2013; 37:5–6.
26. Burden A. How should we normalize electromyograms obtained from healthy participants? What we have learned from over 25 years of research. J Electromyogr Kinesiol. 2010; 20:1023–1035.
27. Padulo J, Chamari K, Ardigò LP. Walking and running on treadmill: the standard criteria for kinematics studies. Muscles Ligaments Tendons J. 2014; 4:159–162.
28. Padulo J, D'Ottavio S, Pizzolato F, Smith L, Annino G. Kinematic analysis of soccer players in shuttle running. Int J Sports Med. 2012; 33:459–462.
29. Ting LH, Kautz SA, Brown DA, Zajac FE. Phase reversal of biomechanical functions and muscle activity in backward pedaling. J Neurophysiol. 1999; 81:544–551.
30. Hug F, Dorel S. Electromyographic analysis of pedaling: a review. J Electromyogr Kinesiol. 2009; 19:182–198.
31. Caldwell GE, Li L, McCole SD, Hagberg JM. Pedal and crank kinetics in uphill cycling. J Appl Biomech. 1988; 14:245–259.
32. Hortobágyi T, DeVita P. Muscle pre- and coactivity during downward stepping are associated with leg stiffness in aging. J Electromyogr Kinesiol. 2000; 10: 117–126.
33. Ryan MM, Gregor RJ. EMG profiles of lower extremity muscles during cycling at constant workload and cadence. J Electromyogr Kinesiol. 1992; 2:69–80.

Acknowledgements

The authors thank Davide Viggiano for his useful suggestions.

Corresponding author

Luca Paolo Ardigò
School of Exercise and Sport Science, Department of Neurosciences, Biomedicine and Movement Sciences, University of Verona, Via Felice Casorati, 43
37131 Verona, Italy
Email: luca.ardigo@univr.it

Anthropometric analysis and performance characteristics to predict selection in young male and female handball players

Juan J. Fernández-Romero
University of A Coruña, Corunã, Spain

Helena Vila Suárez
Jose Mª Cancela
Universidade de Vigo, Vigo, Spain

Abstract — The aim of this study was two-fold. The first aim was to determine if there were any anthropometric and physical performance differences (controlling for maturation) between male and female handball players selected in training categories as well as the relation of these differences with the performance level achieved. The second aim was to identify the discriminatory variables between the performance levels achieved. A total of 216 young handball players (125 men and 91 women) participated in the study. The data were classified by selection level (regional n=154; national n=62), gender (men; women) and age category (under-15; under-17). The use of MANCOVA analyses, controlling for maturation, identified how gender could determine variables related to handball players' future competitive levels. The results revealed that anthropometric variables such as height, arm span, trochanter height, thigh girth, and leg girth were more influential in men than in women. In addition, the physical performance tests of vertical jump (squat jump and counter movement jump with/without arm) and 10x5 m shuttle run were determinants in both gender. Discriminatory analysis predicted that a combination of five variables (counter movement jump with arm, body mass, 10x5 m shuttle run, dominant hand length and trochanter height) would successfully distinguish between regional and national players, with a predictive accuracy of 81.9% for all players.

Key words: talent, maturity, performance, VO_2 max, explosive strength

Introduction

The process of a steady increase in professional sport has led to an interest in identifying prospective top players as soon as possible. For this reason, clubs spend increasing amounts of time and resources on the process of identifying and selecting young talent. This article expands on the existing relation between anthropometric characteristics, physical performance and identification of talent[1,2] in young male and female handball players.

The concept of 'talent' is still very complex to pinpoint, although it has been suggested that it consists of trying to identify, right from the earliest developmental stages, which players could become elite[3]. In team sports, this prediction about the player's potential performance is more complex than in individual sports because of the involvement of genetic, physiological, morphological, psychological, and environmental factors[4,5].Therefore, the model of talent identification, largely influenced by the particular design of individual sports, is currently being reviewed. These models make it difficult to forecast the best possible performance levels in a number of sports from a very young age and with reasonable probability levels. Over the last few years, a new focus on the study of talent identification in team sports seems to have gained pre-eminence[2,6,7]. Various player characteristics are quantified with the aim of uncovering a series of key factors that might facilitate early talent identification. Previous studies have assessed how anthropometric and physical performance characteristics are important to achieve outstanding levels of performance in team sports such as basketball[8], soccer[9,10], rugby[11] and handball[2,12-14]. According to these authors, anthropometric, and physical performance characteristics are considered fundamental for talent identification. The present study expanded on these ideas and tried to determine which anthropometric and physical performance variables, by means of discriminatory analysis, were most significant at the time of selecting male and female handball players; this follows the trend of research established by other academics and practitioners[7,15,16].

The aim of this study was two-fold. The first aim was to determine if there were any anthropometric and physical performance differences (controlling for maturation) between male and female handball players selected in accordance with training categories, in relation to the competitive levels achieved (either regionally or nationally). The second aim was to identify which of the variables could discriminate between the performance levels achieved.

Methods

Participants

A total of 216 young handball players (125 men and 91 women) who belonged to the Galician Handball Federation (Galicia, Spain) took part in the study. This particular federation has one of the highest numbers of teams and player licenses in the country; this provided the research team with a large enough resource pool to carry out a compelling statistical analysis.

A committee of experts consisting of five members of the technical section of the handball federation selected groups of participants between the ages of 12 and 17 from a total of 1,568 young players. No member of the research team was involved in this selection. The participants were assessed longitudinally during the 1998/1999 season and performance level tracking was followed up until March 2013 to try to determine the performance level they had achieved.

The data were classified according to selection level (regional n=154; national n=62), gender (men; women) and age category (under-15; under-17). The average age of the sample was 15.1±1.6 years (men: 15.7±1.3 years; women: 14.4±1.5 years). The male national level players had played in the highest category of the Spanish Handball Federation (ASOBAL) for a minimum of the duration of a season. The female national level players fulfilled the same condition in the B Honor Division. All the other participants were classified under the label "regional level," which comprised the rest of the leagues and divisions.

All the players took part in an anthropometric and fitness assessment. All the protocols received the institutional approval of two ethics committees: the Ethics Committee of the Galician Handball Federation, and the Ethical Principles for Medical Research involving Human Objects (Declaration of Helsinki). Parental or guardian consent was also obtained.

Procedures

The players performed a battery of fitness tests at the beginning of the competitive season before their pre-season training period and as a part of their respective training programs. All the assessments were carried out by the Sport Science Department of the University of A Coruña. Standard anthropometry, maturation, and physical performance data were compiled for each participant who competed at the regional level and all the tests were completed on the same day.

Anthropometry: Anthropometric measurements were conducted, following standardized procedures by ISAK (International Society for the Advancement of Kinanthropometry), a society of certified anthropometrists[17]. The measurements included height, sitting height, weight, arm span, trochanter height, arm length, dominant hand length, four skinfold measurements (triceps, subscapular, supraspinal and abdominal), two breadths (biacromial and biepicondylar), and two girths (thigh and leg). The sum of the four skinfolds was used as the main adiposity index. Height and sitting height were measured using a Seca Alpha stand (Barcelona, Spain) to the nearest 0.1 cm. Weight was measured using calibrated Seca alpha scales (model 770) to the nearest 0.01 kg. Skinfolds were measured with a Harpenden skinfold caliper (British Indicators Ltd., Luton), with 10 $g \cdot mm^{-2}$ constant pressure. Girths were measured using a Lufkin Metal Tape (Lufkin Executive Thinline, W606PM, USA). Breadths and lengths were measured using an anthropometer (GPM, Siber Hegner Zurich, Switzerland) with an accuracy of 0.01 cm.

Maturation (age at PHV): The players' maturity status was determined using Mirwald, Baxter-Jones, Bailey and Beunen's[18]prediction equation. This technique is a non-invasive method that predicts years from peak height velocity (PHV) as a measure of maturity, offset using anthropometric variables. Years from PHV was calculated by subtracting age at PHV from the player's chronological age.

Physical Performance: The EUROFIT test battery[19] was used to assess general physical fitness and was applied using the official protocols and materials in the following order: 1) Shuttle run test assessed aerobic endurance; 2) Flamingo balance assessed general balance; 3) Plate tapping assessed segment velocity of the upper limbs; 4) Sit and reach assessed flexibility of the trunk and lower limbs; 5) Standing long jump assessed explosive strength of the lower limbs; 6) Hand dynamometry assessed grip; 7) Sit-ups for 30 seconds assessed trunk power; 8) Flexed arm hang assessed muscular resistance of the arms and shoulders, and; 9) Shuttle run test of 10x5 m assessed agility and speed. Additional tests were also performed by each player to calculate explosive strength.

Each participant performed three kinds of maximal jumps (Squat Jump [SJ], Countermovement Jump [CMJ] and Avalakov Jump) on a jump mat (Ergo Jump Bosco System Byomedics, SCP, Barcelona, Spain). The participants completed three trials of each type of jump, and the best one was used for the subsequent statistical analysis. Between jumps, the participants were allowed to recover for three minutes to avoid fatigue. Jump height was calculated using flight time. The SJ showed an ICC of 0.94 and a CV of 24.2%, and the CMJ showed an ICC of 0.97 and a CV of 22.1%. Aerobic capacity was expressed as estimated maximal oxygen uptake (VO_2 max) using a 20 m shuttle run test and predicted by a regression equation according to age and running speed at the last completed stage[20]. A 15 minute warm-up was performed before the physical testing.

Statistical analysis

Mean and Standard Deviation (SD) scores were calculated for all dependent variables with selection level acting as the independent variable. None of the data violated the normality assumption necessary to conduct parametric statistical tests (Kolmogorov-Smirnov; $p>0.05$). A multivariate analysis of covariance test (MANCOVA) was applied with selection level (regional vs. national) as the fixed factor. Maturity (years from PHV) was used as a covariate to adjust for variations in maturation status. Partial eta squared effect sizes (η^2) were also calculated. To identify discriminating variables between regional and national players, a stepwise discriminant analysis was applied with selection level being used as the discrete outcome variable. SPSS version 15.0 was employed for all analyses with the significance set at $p<0.05$.

Results

The anthropometric characteristics and physical performance parameters of the mean and standard deviation, and taking into account the selection level (i.e., regional and national) are shown in Table 1. The results indicate that maturation age influenced players' performance level independently of sex. MANCOVA analyses between selection levels for all players revealed that national players outperformed regional players significantly for height, arm span, trochanter height, body mass, sum of skinfolds, thigh circumference, leg circumference, vertical jump (SJ, CMJ, and CMJ with arm Avalakov), standing broad jump, flamingo balance, plate tapping, sit and reach, sit-ups, ups, 10x5 m shuttle rum, 20 m shuttle run and VO_2 max in male players.

Table 1. Selection level characteristics (national vs. regional) of male and female handball players

		Men (n=125)					Women (n=91)				
				Covariate					Covariate		
		Regional (n=93)	National (n=32)	Years PHV	MAN-COVA	η^2	Regional (n=61)	National (n=30)	Years PHV	MAN-COVA	η^2
Age (years)		15.5±1.1	15.2±0.9	-	-	-	14.6±1.5	14.3±1.5	-	-	-
Age at PHV (years)		14.6±0.9	14.3±0.6*	-	-	-	12.4±0.8	12.1±0.8*	-	-	-
Years from PHV (years)		0.8±1.5	0.9±0.9	-	-	-	2.1±1.1	2.2±0.9	-	-	-
Anthropometry											
Height (cm)		171.8±8.9	176.4±8.3	0.001	0.001	0.135	162.5±6.8	166.1±4.8	0.001	0.207	
Arm span (cm)		176.5±11.6	180.6±10.7	0.001	0.040	0.049	165.5±7.3	169.6±6.5	0.001	0.232	
Height trochanter (cm)		89.1±6.4	93.1±4.7	0.679	0.002	0.112	81.3±8.9	84.4±7.6	0.659	0.109	
Arm length (cm)		32.9±4.3	33.5±4.8	0.001	0.541		36.9±17.2	40.8±15.1	0.004	0.560	
Body mass (kg)		61.8±10.6	70.9±12.2	0.001	0.001	0.222	58.1±14.5	60.2±10.3	0.001	0.004	0.094
Sum of skinfolds (mm)		49.8±21.4	28.7±6.5	0.878	0.001	0.249	60.1±25.9	44.6±21.9	0.004	0.001	0.192
Dominant hand length (cm)		22.9±1.4	23.1±2.1	0.002	0.142		19.8±1.3	20.1±1.1	0.001	0.903	
Biacromial breadths (cm)		38.7±3.2	38.5±2.4	0.003	0.401		36.4±2.1	36.8±1.7	0.001	0.959	
Biepicondylar breadths (cm)		6.8±0.5	6.7±0.4	0.001	0.503		4.5±0.3	4.7±0.2	0.036	0.899	
Thigh girth (cm)		49.9±5.5	52.9±4.6	0.001	0.001	0.130	50.7±3.3	50.8±5.5	0.001	0.136	
Leg girth (cm)		37.2±2.9	34.8±2.8	0.002	0.001	0.173	34.5±4.7	34.9±3.1	0.001	0.068	
Physical performance											
Squat Jump (cm)		22.8±3.9	27.6±6.5	0.005	0.001	0.179	20.6±6.4	23.3±3.6	0.149	0.002	0.106
Counter Movement Jump (cm)		28.8±5.1	33.5±6.0	0.021	0.001	0.218	23.9±6.9	27.3±3.9	0.902	0.002	0.105
Counter Movement Jump with arm (cm)		34.2±6.0	40.3±7.0	0.019	0.001	0.231	28.1±5.4	32.3±3.5	0.460	0.001	0.139
Eurofit Test	Flamingo balance (rep)	16.9±5.7	12.7±6.6	0.867	0.006	0.100	14.7±6.3	12.3±3.7	0.267	0.063	
	Plate tapping (s)	116.1±13.6	108.9±9.8	0.034	0.015	0.081	116.1±10.7	115.8±11.5	0.272	0.812	
	Sit and reach (cm)	18.3±7.0	22.1±7.4	0.012	0.011	0.055	24.5±6.6	25.1±6.7	0.009	0.319	
	Standing broad jump (cm)	187.8±22.9	203.1±25.3	0.025	0.001	0.137	152.1±42.7	158.7±32.1	0.076	0.926	
	Handgrip strength (kg)	40.7±11.7	42.5±8.8	0.001	0.313		29.4±6.3	30.7±5.3	0.004	0.691	
	Sit – ups (rep)	24.3±3.3	26.9±3.5	0.339	0.001	0.166	23.1±2.7	23.5±3.1	0.090	0.860	
	Flexed arm hang (s)	302.2±157.2	348.9±202.5	0.543	0.341		98.5±88.7	131.3±86.2	0.486	0.089	
	10 x 5 m shuttle run (s)	196.9±12.6	183.7±11.1	0.003	0.001	0.457	228.8±16.7	213.5±15.4	0.097	0.001	0.141
	20 m shuttle run (rep)	9.6±1.5	8.5±1.6	0.022	0.001	0.141	6.2±1.2	6.7±1.7	0.027	0.045	0.046
	VO_2 max (ml kg–1 min–1)	46.1±4.7	49.5±3.8	0.022	0.001	0.141	39.1±4.2	40.7±2.9	0.027	0.045	0.046

Table 2 presents the means and standard deviations of the anthropometric characteristics and physical performance of the selection level by age category (under-15 and under-17). Maturity status (PHV) did not condition players' performance levels; there were other parameters that determined these differences. The parameters that had a significant influence on players' performance level (globally and regardless of gender and age category) were the following: body mass, sum of skinfolds, explosive strength (SJ, CMJ, Avalakov jump, 10x5 m shuttle run) and VO_2 max.

Table 2. Mean and standard deviation of the anthropometric and conditional characteristics of male and female handball players by category and performance level

		Men (n=125)				**Women (n=91)**			
		under-15 (n=62)		under-17 (n=63)		under-15 (n=48)		under-17 (n=43)	
		Regional n=44	National n=18	Regional n=49	National n=14	Regional n=33	National n=16	Regional n=28	National n=14
	Age (years)	14.6±0.4	14.6±0.6	16.4±0.8	16.5±0.8	13.2±0.6	13.3±0.8	15.8±0.8	15.9±0.9
	Age at PHV (years)	14.2±0.7	14.6±0.5	14.5±0.9	14.6±0.8	11.5±0.4	11.9±0.6	12.8±0.5	13.1±0.7
	Years from PHV (years)	0.4±0.7	0.1±0.1	1.8±1.2	1.8±1.2	1.7±0.6	1.4±0.9	3.0±0.6	2.7±1.8
	Anthropometry								
	Height (cm)	169.1±9.0	173.6±7.3	175.3±7.2	181.4±8.6*	161.6±6.1	163.9±10.1	163.0.±5.7	168.5±5.2*
	Arm span (cm)	176.9±9.1	173.4±12.9	180.5±11.6	187.7±7.5*	164.5±80.6	167.3±11.2	166.8±5.7	172.1±2.6*
	Height trochanter (cm)	89.2±5.4	91.5±4.3	89.1±7.3	95.8±2.9*	76.6±6.5	83.5±9.2*	85.8±4.8	86.4±22.6
	Arm length (cm)	31.8±2.8	32.5±5.1	34.8±2.9	34.8±4.6	36.5±2.8	36.8±5.1	37.4±26.6	37.5±17.3
	Body mass (kg)	66.6±11.0	57.6±10.5*	78.5±11.6	67.3±17.7**	57.2±10.4	56.3±12.9*	64.1±9.7	60.0±4.5*
	Sum of skinfolds (mm)	49.9±19.7	29.3±7.1**	48.4±16.0	28.1±5.8**	54.4±24.1	43.1±9.2*	67.4±21.3	46.2±9.5*
	Dominant hand length (cm)	22.5±1.4	22.3±2.1	22.8±1.4	24.2±1.8*	20.0±1.1	20.0±1.3	20.1±1.3	20.5±1.0
	Biacromial breadths (cm)	37.2±2.4	37.7±2.3	39.1±2.5	39.9±2.1	36.0±2.9	36.7±2.3	36.8±1.6	36.9±1.7
	Biepicondylar breadths (cm)	6.7±0.3	6.7±0.5	7.0±0.4	6.8±0.3	4.1±0.3	4.3±0.3	4.9±0.2	5.1±0.2
	Thigh girth (cm)	48.8±4.7	51.7±4.4*	51.3±5.8	55.1±4.4*	49.6±4.5	50.3±4.9	51.1±4.4	52.4±8.6
	Leg girth (cm)	33.9±3.0	36.4±2.9*	36.0±3.5	38.6±2.9*	34.1±4.3	34.5±3.3	34.5±2.6	36.1±5.6*
	Physical performance measures								
	Squat Jump (cm)	22.4±5.9	26.2±4.1*	23.5±7.6	29.6±2.8*	20.4±4.1	23.2±7.6*	20.8±3.2	23.4±1.8*
	Counter Movement Jump (cm)	28.3±4.9	31.5±4.7*	29.7±6.9	36.0±2.4*	23.1±8.2	27.2±4.1*	25.2±2.9	27.3±3.6*
	Counter Movement Jump with arm (cm)	33.3±5.9	37.5±5.8*	35.8±8.1	43.8±5.6*	27.1±9.7	32.2±4.4*	29.5±2.6	32.5±3.9*
Eurofit Test	Flamingo balance (rep)	17.1±7.1	12.6±5.6*	16.5±6.3	12.8±3.1	15.3±6.4	13.4±3.8	14.1±6.1	11.0±3.9
	Plate tapping (s)	119.2±12.6	111.5±11.1	110.4±8.4	105.3±13.1	118.2±10.6	118.5±9.8	112.6±10.1	113.4±19.0
	Sit and reach (cm)	17.1±7.5	21.8±4.6*	20.6±7.4	22.3±6.1	20.4±5.6	23.7±6.6	26.9±9.7	28.9±5.7
	Standing broad jump (cm)	181.8±21.8	196.4±19.5*	199.6±25.2	211.5±18.3	143.4±38.7	144.8±50.3	162.9±10.8	174.2±17.5
	Handgrip strength (kg)	38.1±6.9	38.4±9.7	45.1±8.7	48.2±10.8	27.8±5.8	29.0±7.2	31.4±3.6	32.4±4.5
	Sit ups (rep)	23.6±3.6	26.4±3.5*	25.7±2.9	27.7±2.9	22.3±2.9	23.5±3.6	24.0±2.9	24.2±2.1
	Flexed arm hang (s)	295.6±215.7	368.3±140.1	315.0±196.9	324.3±201.6	93.6±90.4	127.9±76.7	104.9±88.2	136.0±112.0
	10 x 5 m shuttle run (s)	198.9±9.2	186.3±12.4*	193.2±9.9	180.3±11.5*	235.8±19.1	216.4±17.2*	220.9±10.5	210.2±8.1*
	20 m shuttle run (rep)	8.3±1.7	9.6±1.8*	8.8±1.2	9.6±1.6*	6.1±1.4	6.6±1.4*	6.3±1.0	6.8±2.5*
	VO_2 max (ml kg−1 min−1)	45.5±5.3	49.4±4.3*	47.2±3.5	49.6±3.4*	38.8±4.3	40.3±3.7*	39.6±4.1	41.2±1.7*

APHV = age at peak height velocity; *0.005;**0.001

Within the under-15 male category, we identified more parameters that condition performance in a significant way. These parameters were thigh and leg girth, flamingo balance, sit and reach, standing broad jump and sit-ups. In the case of female players, the only parameter incorporated was trochanter height. Regarding the under-17 male category, the following parameters were identified as determining factors of performance: height, arm span, trochanter height, dominant hand length, and thigh and leg girth. Regarding the under-17 female category, the parameters were height, arm span and leg girth.

The stepwise discriminatory analysis predicted that a combination of five variables would successfully discriminate between regional and national players: CMJ with arm (0.826), body mass (0.759), 10x5 m shuttle run (0.701), dominant hand length (0.630), and trochanter height (0.599). The average squared canonical correlation was 0.634, showing that these five variables accounted for 63.4% of the overall variance in the data set. Cross-validation results were calculated to identify the correct classification of regional and national players based on the discriminatory analysis. The discriminatory analysis corresponded to an overall predictive accuracy of 81.9% for all players with an accuracy of 78.9% and 87.7% for regional and national players respectively.

Discussion

The first aim of the present study was to determine if there were any anthropometric and physical performance differences (controlling for maturation) in male and female handball players selected in training categories, with relation to the competitive level achieved (regional and national). The second purpose of this study was to identify which variables could be taken into account at the time of selecting handball players to reach maximum performance levels.

When the results are analyzed in terms of physical performance and anthropometric characteristics in the training period and ages of the players, it must be taken into consideration that performance data need to include maturation[2, 13,21, 22]. As stated earlier, maturation is a variable that influences male and female handball players when they try to achieve their maximum performance level (national). Anthropometric characteristics, explosive strength, agility-velocity, and aerobic capacity discriminate male and female players with regard to their performance level.

In accordance with previous studies where maturation was statistically controlled[7, 15], we found that PHV (maturation status) influences the performance level of male and female handball players. National level handball players (male and female) show better values in both anthropometric parameters and physical performance when compared to regional level players. These differences are highly significant in the case of anthropometric parameters (height, arm span, body mass, biacromial breadth, and hand length), even though other authors have also referred to these differences as key to performance levels[2, 23, 24, 25].

Taking into consideration the players' gender, differences in physical performance are connected with the explosive strength of the lower limbs and with the maximum isometric strength of the forearm for male players. However, for female players the differences are found in the maximum isometric strength of the forearm and aerobic power. These results are in accordance with a study conducted by Malina, Cumming, Morano, Barron and Miller[21] on the maturation of young football players.

A limited number of studies have assessed some anthropometric parameters, physical performance and maturity status in handball[1, 13, 26].Mohamed, Vaeyens, Matthys, Multael, Lefevre, Lenoir and Philippaerts[2] carried out a cross-sectional study with players (elite vs. non-elite) between the ages of 12 and 16, and concluded that maturation had influenced anthropometric parameters and not physical performance, except in the case of hand-grip. However, a study carried out by Matthys, Vaeyens, Vandendriessche, Vandorpe, Pion, Coutts, Lenoir and Philippaerts[13] with players between the ages of 12 and 17 concluded that maturation was a determining factor in anthropometric and physical performance parameters, which coincides with the results reported in the present study. Other soccer-related studies [15,22,27] have reported results that are also in line with the results obtained in the present study. Nevertheless, given the clear methodological divergences observed in these studies, such conclusions should be reflected upon carefully. Very little information is available on young female players, which renders comparisons quite challenging.

When the maturity status is statistically controlled, results show how the group with the maximum level of performance (national) presents fewer differences with regard to the regional level group, which reinforces the importance of maturity as a key factor in executing talent selection[2, 13, 21, 22], with both males and females.

Once the effect of player maturity is neutralized, it is observed how anthropometric parameters (sum of skinfolds, body mass, leg girth, height, thigh girth, trochanter height and arm span) and physical performance parameters (vertical jump SJ, CMJ, Avalakov jump, standing broad jump, flamingo balance, plate tapping, sit and reach, sit-ups, 10x5 m shuttle run, 20 m shuttle run and VO_2 max) are responsible for the difference in performance levels. This behavior is not shown when female players are analyzed; therefore, maturity is a fundamental factor that strongly determines performance level. The only anthropometrical variables that are not affected by maturity are weight and body fat; the latter variable is inversely correlated to performance[23, 28]. This behavior would need to be taken into consideration in future research. Regarding physical performance parameters, the data analysis suggests that explosive strength, sprinting for short distances and aerobic capacity can discriminate across levels for female players.

The results of the study carried out by Vaeyens, Malina, Janssens., Van Renterghem, Bourgois, Vrijens and Philippaerts[22] are in accordance with the results of the present study. They confirmed that anthropometric parameters, once maturity is controlled, are conditioned by the analyzed category, so the anthropometric data show differences between performance levels in 50% of the analyzed categories (under-14 and under-15). Taking gender into consideration, maturity is a key factor for females and it determines 80% of the variables under study; in the case of male maturity, it is only 55.5%. The results shown by Matthys, Vaeyens, Vandendriessche, Vandorpe, Pion, Coutts, Lenoir and Philippaerts[13], which are directly linked to physical performance parameters, revealed that maturation is not the only variable responsible for the differences between handball players of different performance levels in parameters such as explosive strength, speed and agility; these parameters are also conditioned by the category that is analyzed, which also seems to be the case for females when the parameters of explosive strength, speed and aerobic resistance are considered.

The analysis carried out within each age (under-15 and under-17) and the gender group revealed that the maturity parameter does not determine performance level within each age category; the selection process carried out by the group of experts could have influenced this. These results confirm the findings presented by Till, Cobley, O'Hara, Chapman and Cooke[11]. A more detailed study of each age group (under-15 and under-17) showed how the behavior of anthropometric and physical performance variables for the under-15 category is not conditioned by gender. In fact, the parameters that best identify maximum performance are linked to physical performance (explosive strength, speed, aerobic resistance). These results coincide with those reported in Vaeyens, Malina, Janssens, Van Renterghem, Bourgois, Vrijens and Philippaerts[22] for male soccer players, as well as with the study conducted by Till, Cobley, O'Hara, Chapman and Cooke[11] for male rugby players. If we analyze the under-17 group, anthropometrical variables (height, arm span, body mass, sum of skinfolds, leg girth) become more predictive of handball players' performance levels, while physical performance variables remain stable in both age groups and they reassert the importance of explosive strength, speed-agility and aerobic power in handball[2, 23]. These results are also in accordance with the research carried out by Matthys, Vaeyens, Vandendriessche, Vandorpe, Pion, Coutts, Lenoir and Philippaerts[13], which reflected that category (age group) influences the stage at which distinguishing anthropometric variables of players' performance levels are identified.

A discriminatory analysis indicated that five variables could help distinguish between regional and national players. This model combines tests that assess explosive strength (CMJ) and speed (10x5 m) with anthropometric variables (body mass, hand length and trochanter height), accounting for 81.9% of the overall variance. The parameters highlighted by the discriminatory analysis correspond to anthropometric characteristics and physical performance demands, viewed as essential in senior handball players[2, 23, 29]. Three of the five variables were associated with PHV. It must be noted, however, that variation of maturity status did not feature as a variable in the model. Nevertheless, our model fails to account for 18% of the variance. This could be explained by the complexity of handball, and the fact that certain tactical and technical aspects have not been dealt with in this study. Lidor et al.[30] indicated that assessments of technical skills would need to be found in light of the difficulty involved in deciding which systematic approach, among those presented in recent studies, would be better suited for the purpose. With this study it has been advanced that physical performance and anthropometric characteristics may be used to distinguish players that will potentially achieve high performance levels playing handball.

Main findings and conclusion

This study analyzed the evolution of the sporting performance of young handball players for 13 years; 28.7% of the participants assessed in the 1998/1999 season reached elite levels.

As regards the first objective specified above and taking into account the results derived from the data analysis, we conclude that gender conditions performance-related variables and even more so in the case of anthropometric variables (height, arm span, trochanter height, thigh girth and leg girth) with a greater impact on males than on females. The physical performance tests of vertical jump (SJ and CMJ with/without arm) and the 10x5 m shuttle run were the most influential for both gender.

As regards the second objective, it should be noted that the selection of young talent in handball requires the combination of five variables (CMJ with arm, body mass, 10x5 m shuttle run, dominant hand length and trochanter height), which would contribute to distinguish between regional and national players successfully, with a predictive accuracy of 81.9% for all players.

References

1. Matthys SP, Fransen J, Vaeyens R, Lenoir M, Philippaerts R. Differences in Biological Maturation, Anthropometry and Physical Performance between Playing Positions in Youth Team Handball. J Sports Sci. 2013; 1-9.
2. Mohamed H, Vaeyens R, Matthys S, Multael M, Lefevre J, Lenoir M, Philippaerts R. Anthropometric and Performance Measures for the Development of a Talent Detection and Identification Model in Youth Handball. J Sports Sci. 2009; 27: 257-266.
3. Abbott A, Collins D. Eliminating the Dichotomy between Theory and Practice in Talent Identification and Development: Considering the Role of Psychology. J Sports Sci. 2004; 22: 395-408.
4. Pearson D, Naughton G, Torode M. Predictability of Physiological Testing and the Role of Maturation in Talent Identification for Adolescent Team Sports. J Sci Med Sport. 2006; 9: 277-287.
5. Williams AM. Perceptual Skill in Soccer: Implications for Talent Identification and Development. J Sports Sci. 2000; 18: 737-750.
6. Elferink-Gemser MT, Visscher C, Lemmink KA, Mulder T. Multidimensional Performance Characteristics and Standard of Performance in Talented Youth Field Hockey Players: A Longitudinal Study. J Sports Sci. 2007; 25: 481-489.
7. Till K, Cobley S, O'Hara J, Brightmore A, Cooke C, Chapman C. Using Anthropometric and Performance Characteristics to Predict Selection in Junior UK Rugby League Players. J Sci Med Sports. 2011; 14: 264-269.
8. Karalejic M, Jakovljevic S, Macura M. Anthropometric Characteristics and Technical Skills of 12 and 14 Year Old Basketball Players. J Sports Med Phys Fitness. 2011; 51: 103-110.
9. Buchheit M, Mendez-Villanueva A. Reliability and Stability of Anthropometric and Performance Measures in Highly-Trained Young Soccer Players: Effect of Age and Maturation. J Sports Sci. 2013; 1-12.
10. Huijgen BC, Elferink-Gemser MT, Lemmink KA, Visscher C. Multidimensional Performance Characteristics in Selected and Deselected Talented Soccer Players. Eur J Sports Sci. 2012; 1-9.
11. Till K, Cobley S, O'Hara J, Chapman C, Cooke C. A Longitudinal Evaluation of Anthropometric and Fitness Characteristics in Junior Rugby League Players Considering Playing Position and Selection Level. J Sci Med Sports. 2012.
12. Ingebrigtsen J, Jeffreys I, Rodahl S. Physical Characteristics and Abilities of Junior Elite Male and Female Handball Players. J Strength Cond Res. 2013; 27: 302-309.
13. Matthys SP, Vaeyens R, Vandendriessche J, Vandorpe B, Pion J, Coutts AJ, Lenoir M, Philippaerts RM. A Multidisciplinary Identification Model for Youth Handball. Eur J Sports Sci. 2011; 11: 355-363.
14. Visnapuu M, Jürimäe T. Relations of anthropometric parameters with scores on basic and specific motor tasks in young handball players. Percept Mot Skills. 2009; 108: 670-676.
15. le Gall F, Carling C, Williams M, Reilly T. Anthropometric and Fitness Characteristics of International, Professional and Amateur Male Graduate Soccer Players from an Elite Youth Academy. J Sci Med Sports. 2010; 13: 90-95.
16. Zibung M, Conzelmann A. The Role of Specialisation in the Promotion of Young Football Talents: A Person-Oriented Study. Eur J Sports Sci. 2012; 1-9.
17. Ross WD, Marfell-Jones MJ. Kinanthropometry. Physiological testing of elite athlete. London. Human Kinetics. 1991; 223-308.
18. Mirwald RL, Baxter-Jones AD, Bailey DA, Beunen GP. An Assessment of Maturity from Anthropometric Measurements. Med Sci Sports Exerc. 2002; 34: 689-694.
19. Adam C, Klissouras V, Ravazzolo M, Renson R, Tuxworth W. EUROFIT: European Test of Physical Fitness. Rome, Italy: Council of Europe, Committee for Development of Sport 1988.

20. Leger L, Mercier D, Gadoury C, Lambert J. The Multistage 20 Metre Shuttle Run Test for Aerobic Fitness. J Sports Sci. 1988; 6: 93-101.
21. Malina RM, Cumming SP, Morano PJ, Barron M, Miller SJ. Maturity Status of Youth Football Players: A Noninvasive Estimate. Med Sci Sports Exerc. 2005; 37: 1044-1052.
22. Vaeyens R, Malina RM, Janssens M, Van Renterghem B, Bourgois J, Vrijens J, and Philippaerts RM. A Multidisciplinary Selection Model for Youth Soccer: The Ghent Youth Soccer Project. Br J Sports Med. 2006; 40: 928-934.
23. Gorostiaga E, Granados C, Ibanez J, Izquierdo M. Differences in Physical Fitness and Throwing Velocity among Elite and Amateur Male Handball Players. Int J Sports Med. 2005; 26: 225-232.
24. Skoufas D, Kotzamanidis C, Hatzikotoylas K, Bebetsos G, Patikas D. The Relationship between the Anthropometric Variables and the Throwing Performance in Handball. J Hum Mov Stud. 2003; 45: 469-484.
25. Zapartidis I, Vareltzis I, Gouvali M, Kororos P. Physical Fitness and Anthropometric Characteristics in Different Levels of Young Team Handball Players. TOSSJ. 2009; 2: 22-28.
26. Hasan A, Reilly T, Cable N, Ramadan J. Anthropometric Profiles of Elite Asian Female Handball Players. J Sports Med Phys Fitness. 2007; 47: 197-202.
27. Roescher C, Elferink-Gemser M, Huijgen B, Visscher C. Soccer Endurance Development in Professionals. Int J Sports Med. 2010; 31: 174-179.
28. Milanese C, Piscitelli F, Lampis C, Zancanaro C. Anthropometry and Body Composition of Female Handball Players According to Competitive Level Or the Playing Position. J Sports Sci. 2011; 29: 1301-1309.
29. Vila H, Manchado C, Rodriguez N, Abraldes JA, Alcaraz PE, Ferragut C. Anthropometric Profile, Vertical Jump, and Throwing Velocity in Elite Female Handball Players by Playing Positions. J Strength Cond Res. 2012; 26: 2146-2155.
30. Lidor R, Falk B, Arnon M, Cohen Y, Segal G, Lander Y. Measurement of talent in team handball: the questionable use of motor and physical tests. J Strength Cond Res. 2005; 19(2): 318-325.

Acknowledgments

The authors would like to thank the Galician Handball Federation (Galicia, Spain) and all the coaches involved in this study for their collaboration and unconditional support. No financial assistance was obtained for this project.

Corresponding author

Jose Mª Cancela
Faculty of Education and Sport Sciences. University of Vigo. Spain.
Faculty of Education and Sport Sciences. C. A Xunqueira, s/n, 36005. Pontevedra, Spain
Email: chemacc@uvigo.es

17

The influence of rules manipulation on offensive patterns during small-sided and conditioned games in football

João Cláudio Machado
Chellsea Alcântara
Carlos Palheta
João Otacílio Libardoni dos Santos
Universidade Federal do Amazonas, Manaus, AM, Brasil

Daniel Barreira
Universidade do Porto, Porto, Portugal

Alcides José Scaglia
Universidade Estadual de Campinas, Limeira, SP, Brasil

Abstract— This study analyzed the influence of rules manipulation on offensive patterns in different Small-Sided and Conditioned Games (SSCGs). Fourteen young soccer players (13.82 ± 1.94 years) performed two different SSCG formats (6v6+Gk): Maintenance of Ball Possession Game (MPG) and Progression to the Target Game (PTG). Both games were played on a field 52 m long by 32 m wide. We used the Offensive Sequences Characterization System (OSCS) and SoccerEye software to analyze offensive sequences. For statistical analysis, we used the Mann-Whitney test to compare variables that compose the OSCS between the two SSCGs, while the SDIS-GSEQ software allowed us to detect offensive patterns. We concluded that the rule manipulation of SSCGs influenced changes in teams' offensive patterns, in which they self-organized according to manipulation of key task constraints.

Keywords: football, constraints-led approach, tactical behavior

Introduction

A football match can be understood as a complex and dynamic system because multiple sources of information influence many decisions, actions, and interactions among the system's components[1,2]. Despite performance based in a complex inter-relation among physical, technical, tactical, and psychological aspects, due to the game's high variability and contextual complexity, tactical, perceptual, and decision-making components are highlighted as essential to players and teams' performance.

According to Costa, Guilherme Oliveira, and Garganta[3], tactics in football can be understood by how players and teams manage game space through constant movements and their positioning, according to different match contexts. Teams and players' behavior depends on their interpretation of a large amount of relevant information that emerges from the match context. This information originates from interaction of four classes of constraints (Organismic, Team, Environment, and Tasks), providing players' perception of opportunities for action (affordances)[4,5]. Thus, as interpersonal coordination occurs, players must share their perceptions of affordances, with players coordinating action possibilities that one player provides to another, thus establishing interpersonal synergies[6].

Thus, when handling a task constraint, the coach leads players to perceive different sources of contextual information, providing the team with self-organization toward new possibilities for action, that is, new tactical behaviors emerging from formation of new interpersonal synergies[6,7]. In this sense, task constraints are important tools for enhancing players' decisions and actions in the game environment, as well as for shaping players and teams' tactical behavior[8].

Therefore, Small-Sided and Conditioned Games (SSCGs) are an excellent example of task constraints manipulation that enable coaches to shape specific tactical behaviors through modifications and adaptations of the competitive context[9,10]. SSCGs allow coaches to manipulate several constraints, for example, field dimension, the player's number, game rules, and others, to stimulate different self-organization processes in which players must adapt according to new action possibilities generated from perception of new information sources[10,11]. In addition, SSCGs provide players maintenance of an environment similar to regular competition, in contrast to traditional teaching and training methodology[12,13].

However, to reach efficiency in the teaching and training process, the coach must have some knowledge that allows him to manipulate key task constraints, thus influencing emergence of specific tactical behaviors aligned with training aims and the game model he has defined[11,14]. In recent years, due to technological and methodological developments that allow investigation of emerging coordinative patterns in team sports, particularly in football, research has attempted to analyze the influence of key task constraint manipulations, such as field dimension and number of players[15-17].

As for SSCG rules manipulation, Dellal, Chamari, Owen, Wong, Lago-Peñas, and Hill-Haas[18] found that reducing the amount of ball touches allowed each professional player in different SSCGs tended to decrease the number of successful passes and to increase the amount of lost ball possessions. Thus, the authors[18] emphasized that manipulating this specific rule makes it possible to prepare players better to deal with more complex situations in football matches.

Almeida, Ferreira, and Volossovitch[19] investigated the influence of rules manipulation on teams' offensive performance in different SSCGs (3v3+Gk); they found that "two touches" rule would condition players to perceive information and make decisions quickly, while "four passes" rules would induce longer offensive sequences, favoring occurrences of an attack method that prioritized maintenance of ball possession. Studying SSCGs, Lizana, Reverdito, Brenzikofer, Macedo, Misuta, and Scaglia[20] also found that the manipulation of different game rules influenced teams' technical-tactical performance.

However, not enough information yet exists about rule manipulation's influence on offensive patterns performed by teams during different SSCGs. Therefore, this study analyzes the influence of rules manipulation on teams' offensive patterns in different SSCGs. Thus, SSCG manipulations are intended to assist coaches in developing more specific exercises, thereby increasing the probability of transferring certain tactical behaviors to competitive games.

Methods

Study Design:

This research employed observational methodology because it allows observation and recording of team and players' behavior in natural match contexts[21]. This study's design, according to a specific taxonomy[22], is nomothetic (two teams observed in each SSCG), has follow-up (registration is continuous during the SSCG), and is multidimensional (the observation tool comprises seven field criteria combining field formats with systems of categories).

Subjects:

Fourteen young soccer players (13.82 ± 1.94 years) on a team in the city of Manaus-AM participated in this study. The team and players were informed of the experimental study protocol as they signed the free and informed consent form (ICF), approved by the Ethics Committee in Research of the Federal University of Amazonas (CAE: 31081614.6.0000.5020).

Procedures:

Two different formats of SSCG were used—Maintenance of Ball Possession Game (MPG); Progression to the Target Game (PTG)—by Lizana, Reverdito, Brenzikofer, Macedo, Misuta, and Scaglia[20]. Each of the SSCGs lasted 30 minutes and was performed in a field dimension of 52 m long and 32 m wide (Figure 1); teams were composed of six players and a goalkeeper (6v6+Gk). All SSCGs were played between 09:00 and 10:00 a.m., at 48-hour intervals. For each SSCG, two familiarization games (i.e., a period during which players became accustomed to the proposed rules) and two experimental games were played, with a 48-hour interval between them. Games were preceded by a standardized warm-up of 15 minutes, with 5 minutes each of acyclic low-intensity movements and coordinative running, of dynamic stretching, and of intermittent high-intensity activities. During data collection of these games, 173 offensive sequences were recorded from the MPG and 196 from the PTG.

Table 1 contains the different rules included in the two SSCG formats used in this investigation.

The rules used in the MPG and PTG emphasized operational principles of maintaining ball possession and progression to the target, respectively[23]. Importantly, with the exception of the rule that determines the minimum number of passes needed to perform a goal shot in the MPG, breaking the game's rules did not interrupt game dynamics, but some minimum points were given to the opposing team.

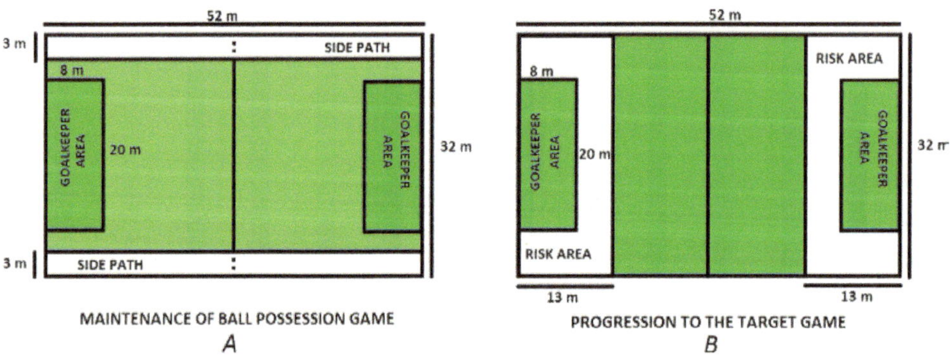

Figure 1. Field dimensions used at the different SSCG.

Table 1. Rules included in the different SSCGs used in this study.

Small-Sides and Conditioned Games	Rules	Definition
Maintenance of Ball Possession Game (MPG)	First Rule	Each player could do a maximum of two touches on the ball, where extra points to the opposing team were registered for each extra touch on the ball given by the same player.
	Second Rule	The players of the team who were with the ball possession should make constant switches of lines/ zones, which were pre-determined in the field with cones of different colors, and were registered an extra point to the team that could circulate the ball from one side path to the other.
	Third Rule	Each time that the team that was with the ball possession could make five passes without returning the ball to the player who had just made the pass, the team obtained two points.
	Fourth Rule	The goal could only be scored after five passes, thus earning eight points.
Progression to the Target Game (PTG)	First Rule	The passes made by the players could only be carried out towards the opposing goal, in which each time the player disrespected this rule it would result in an extra point given to the opposing team, being allowed the performance of backwards passes only on two occasions, in the recovery of the ball possession and in an assistance
	Second Rule	Every goal scored made through a backwards pass would worth five points, while the goal scored in an offensive sequence in which the last pass were performed just towards the opposing goal it would worth ten points
	Third Rule	Whenever the team could break into a pre-defined area by the cones (risk area) would obtain three points.

Observation Instrument:

In this study, two observational instruments were used to characterize and detect offensive patterns by teams in each SSCG: the Offensive Sequences Characterization System (OSCS) and SoccerEye. Those instruments have been properly validated and tested in different studies published elsewhere[19,24-26].

The OSCS is composed of simple indicators previously used in other investigations: Duration of Ball Possession[27], number of Players involved[28], number of Ball Touches[28], number of Passes[29], and number of Shots[27]. A simple ratio established between performance indicators makes it possible to access more accurate information about characteristics of teams' offensive sequences[19]. The OSCS has the following composite indicators: Players involved/Duration of ball possession, Ball Touches/ Duration of ball possession, Passes/Duration of ball possession, Ball Touches/Players involved, Passes/Players involved, Passes/ Ball Touches, and Goal/Shots.

To detect teams' offensive patterns, we also used the SoccerEye observation instrument (Table 2)[25], consisting of 80 unique, mutually exclusive categories, distributed according to seven criteria that combine field formats with systems of categories: (1) Start of the offensive phase/ball recovery (BR); (2) Development of defense/attack transition-state (DT); (3) Progress of ball possession (DP); (4) End of the offensive phase (F); (5) Patterns of pitch space position; (6) Centre of the game (CJ); and (7) Spatial patterns of teams' interaction (CEI).

The first four criteria relate to behaviors of the observed team's players, while the fifth is a structural criterion dividing the pitch into 12 zones or categories. The sixth and seventh criteria characterize interaction contexts on micro and macro scales, respectively, taking into account relations of opposition and cooperation between teams and players.

Table 2: SoccerEye Observation Instrument[25].

Criteria	Sub-criteria	N° categories	Categories
Start of the offensive phase/ball recovery (BR)	1.1 Direct/ Dynamic ball recovery	4	BRi: Interception; BRt: Tackle; BRgk: Intervention of the goalkeeper in the defensive phase; BRp: Defensive behavior followed by a pass;
	1.2 Indirect/ Static ball recovery	6	BRst: Start/restart of the offensive phase; BRv: Opponent's violation of the laws of the game; BRc: Corner kick; BRgki: Goal kick; BRdb: Dropped ball; BRti: Throw-in
Development of defense/ attack transition-state (DT)		14	DTpsp: Positive short passing; DTnsp: Negative short passing; DTplp: Positive long passing; DTnlp: Negative Long Passing; DTpcr: Positive Crossing; DTncr: Negative Crossing; DTrb: Running with the ball; DTd: Dribbling (1x1); DTbc: Ball control; DTdu: Duel; DTs: Shooting; DTns: Opponent's intervention with no Success; DTogk: Intervention of the goalkeeper in the offensive phase; DTdgk: Intervention of the goalkeeper in the defensive phase

Progress of Ball Possession (DP)		19	DPpsp: Positive Short passing; DPnsp: Negative short passing; DPplp: Positive Long Passing; DPnlp: Negative Long Passing; DPpcr: Positive Crossing; DPncr: Negative Crossing; DPrb: Running with the ball; DPd: Dribbling (1x1); DPd: Ball control: DPdu: Duel; DPs: Shooting; DPns: Opponent's intervention with no success; DPogk: Intervention of the goalkeeper in the offensive phase; DPdgk: Intervention of the goalkeeper in the defensive phase; DPi: Violation of the laws of the game; DPc: Corner kick; DPgki: Goal kick; DPdb: Dropped Ball; DPti: Throw-in
End of the Offensive Phase (F)	4.1 With Efficacy	4	Fws: Wide shot; Fst: Shot on target; Fso: Shot stopped, with no continuation of ball possession; Fgl: Goal
	4.2 With no Efficacy	4	Fled: Loss of ball possession by error of the ball carrier/defender's intervention; Fgk: Loss of ball possession by intervention of the opponent's goalkeeper; Fo: Throwing the ball out of the pitch; Fi: Violation of the laws of the game
Patterns of pitch space position		12	Zones 1 to 12 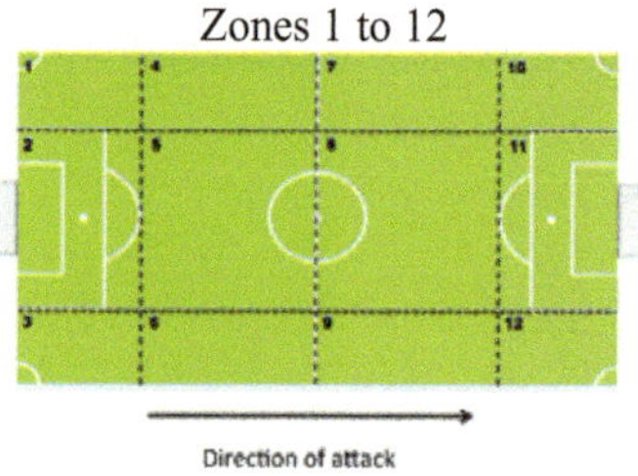
Centre of the Game (CJ)	6.1 With Pressure (P)	3	Pr: Relative numerical inferiority; Pa: Absolute numerical inferiority; Pe: Pressure in numerical equality
	6.2 With no Pressure (NP)	3	NPe: No pressure in numerical equality; NPr: Relative numerical superiority; NPa: Absolute numerical superiority
Spatial patterns of teams interaction (CEI)		11	EF: Ball in the empty zone (goalkeeper) versus offensive line; BF: Back line versus offensive line; BM: Back line versus mid line; BE: Back line versus exterior zone; MF: Mid line versus offensive line; MM: Mid line versus mid line; MB: Mid line versus back line; FM: Offensive line versus mid line; FB: Offensive line versus back line; EB: Exterior zone versus back line; FE: Offensive line versus empty zone (goalkeeper)

Recording Instrument:

To record offensive sequences, we used an adaptation of SoccerEye recording software (v 3.2, October 2012)[30]. The software simultaneously enables visualization and recording of players' actions; it is a versatile and adaptable tool, including contextual variables such as "match status" and "duration of the offensive sequence." SoccerEye's user manual contains definitions and guidelines for its use, helping the viewer perform more affordable, reliable data collection.

Before recording behaviors, field areas, and contexts of players/team's interactions, the observer recorded match status, duration of the attack sequence, and two OSCS variables[19,24] were also included — the "number of players involved" and the "number of touches on the ball" (Figure 2).

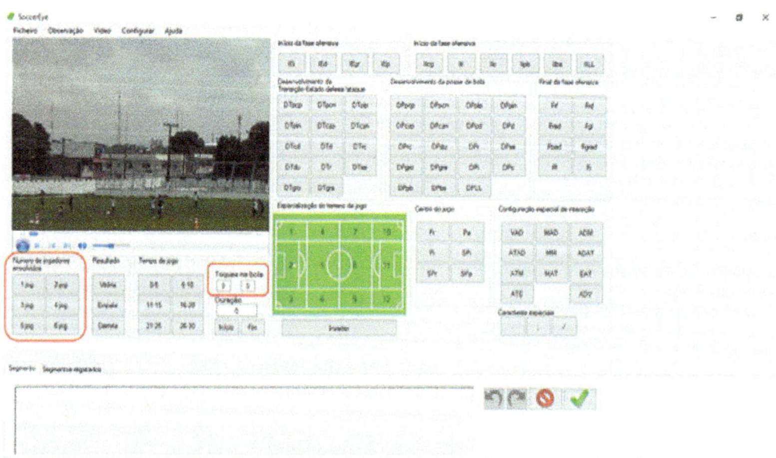

Figure 2. Adaptation of SoccerEye recording instrument[30].

Data quality:

SDIS-GSEQ software (version 5.0.77)[31] was used to determine inter- and intra-observer reliability through the value of Kappa de Cohen (k)[21]. Observers twice (with an interval of 15 days) analyzed the first 45 minutes of a football game. Values for inter-observer reliability ranged from 0.79 to 0.99, while values for intra-observer reliability ranged from 0.91 to 0.96. Therefore, according to Bakeman, Gottman, Portal, Anguera, and Villaseñor[32], the study data shows good reliability.

Statistical Analysis

Shapiro-Wilk and Levene tests were performed to verify the normality and homogeneity of variances, respectively, of data related to variables belonging to the OSCS. Once the data did not show normal distribution, a descriptive statistic (median and range) and the Mann-Whitney test were employed to characterize and compare simple and composite indicators of the OSCS (dependent variables) between the two SSCGs (MPG and PTG as independent variables). The significance level of 5% ($p < 0.05$) was adopted. Statistical analysis was performed with the SPSS 20.0 program.

Using SDIS-GSEQ software (v5.0.77, 2010)[31], we conducted a Lag Sequential Analysis, which enables identification of teams' offensive patterns during SSCGs. Lag Sequential Analysis allows identification of behavioral patterns more likely to occur than those dependent on chance, assuming that behaviors are probably repeated in a football match with some frequency and that their sequences are visible in the match[33].

Therefore, a retrospective analysis of the ten behaviors previous to the attack's end, assuming indicator categories of offensive efficacy (criterion 4) in SoccerEye as conduct criteria. Through selection of respective conduct criteria, analysts counted the times that a certain conduct, considered an object conduct, succeeds that conduct retrospectively, setting the standard conduct (max-lag). The z-score value ($z \geq 1.96, p \leq 0.05$) determines the significance level between those conducts, thus detecting teams' offensive patterns during different SSCGs. Sackett[34] conventional rules, used to determine maximum delay, were not applied.

Results

Characterization of offensive sequences

Table 3 shows results of simple and composite indicators of performances belonging to the OSCS. All performance indicators showed statistically significant differences, with the exception of composite indicators "Players involved/Duration" ($p = 0.301$) and "Ball Touches/Duration" ($p = 0.055$).

Regarding simple performance indicators, the MPG had longer offensive sequences ($p = 0.005$), with more players involved in attacks ($p < 0.001$), besides a larger amount of ball touches ($p = 0.011$) and passes performed ($p < 0.001$). The PTG had a greater amount of shots on the opponent's goal ($p < 0.001$).

As for composite indicators, the MPG obtained a larger number of passes per time ($p < 0.001$), passes performed by players involved ($p < 0.001$), and by ball touches ($p < 0.001$). In the PTG, there occurred a greater number of ball touches by players involved in offensive sequences ($p = 0.003$) and a greater number of goals scored by shots performed ($p < 0.001$).

Table 3: Indicators of performance that characterize the offensive sequences in different Small-Sided and Conditioned Games.

Performance Indicators	Maintaining Ball Possession Game			Progression to the Target Game		
	Median	Min.	Max.	Median	Min.	Max.
Duration of Ball Possession (s)	15,00*	2	94	11,00*	2	86
Players Involved	4,00*	1,0	7,0	3,00*	1,0	6,0
Ball Touches	8,00*	1,0	32,0	6,00*	1,0	22,0
Passes	4,00*	0,00	21	2,00*	0,00	9
Shots	0,00*	0,00	2,0	0,00*	0,00	2,0
Players Involved/ Duration	0,27	0,06	1,00	0,25	0,04	0,67
Ball Touches/ Duration	0,51	0,17	1,25	0,58	0,06	2,00
Passes/Duration	0,25*	0,00	0,67	0,18*	0,00	0,43
Ball Touches/ Players Involved	2,00*	1,00	5,33	2,25*	1,00	13,00
Passes/Players Involved	1,00*	0,00	3,50	0,66*	0,00	2,00
Passes/Ball Touches	0,50*	0,00	0,80	0,33*	0,00	0,80
Goal/Shots	0,00*	0,00	1,0	0,00*	0,00	1,00
Offensive Sequences (Total)	173			196		

* Statistically significant difference between the Maintenance of Ball Possession Game and the Progression to the Target Game ($p < 0,05$).

Analysis of offensive patterns

Figure 3 displays offensive patterns that resulted in wide shots (Figure 3A) and in goals scored (Figure 3B) in the MPG. Shots in the MPG tended to occur in the central path of the offensive sector (Fws: $z = 2.85$; Fgl: $z = 3.75$) or in the left path of the offensive sector (Fws: $z = 2.05$). Wide shots tended to be preceded by a positive short pass ($z = 3:58$) or a positive crossing ($z = 4.99$), both during progress of ball possession (Figure 3A). Goals scored strongly tended to occur before a positive short pass ($z = 2.89$), which was in turn preceded by a positive crossing ($z = 5.17$), also in progress of ball possession (Figure 3B).

Figure 4 displays offensive patterns that resulted in wide shots (Figure 4A), in shots on target (Figure 4B), and in goals scored (Figure 4C) in the PTG. For offensive sequences that resulted in wide shots (Fws) in the PTG, it was possible to identify offensive patterns with behaviors in progress of ball possession; these tended to occur after an opponent's

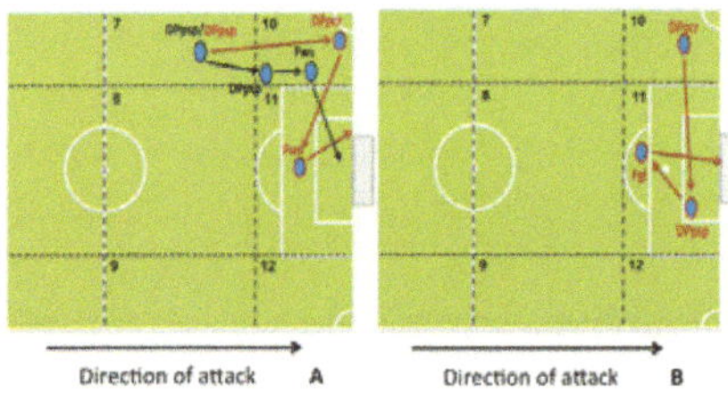

Figure 3. Illustration of the offensive patterns that resulted in a wide shot (A) and in goals scored (B) in the Maintenance of Ball Possession Game. See Table 1.

intervention with no success (z = 3.16), preceded by a negative short pass (z = 3.08). Wide shots were preceded by a goalkeeper intervention (DPdgk; z = 2.44) after a shot (DPs; z = 2.36), when these behaviors were preceded by a positive long pass (z = 2.81) (Figure 4A).

As for offensive sequences ending in shots on target (Fst), these tended to be preceded by a positive long pass (z = 3.16) after running with the ball (z = 2.44), both in development of defense/attack transition-state. Shots preceded by dribbling (z = 3.76) and by running with the ball (DPrb; z = 2.19) in progress of ball possession could also be detected. Another offensive pattern indicated shots preceded by a positive short pass (z = 4:41) after the goalkeeper's intervention in the defensive phase (z = 3.48) (Figure 4B). Shots on target were preceded by a defensive behavior followed by a pass (BRp; z = 3.32), demonstrating shorter offensive sequences.

Goals scored in the PTG tended to occur from an unsuccessful opponent's intervention (z = 2.87), preceded by a shot (z = 2.02) or a negative short pass (z = 2.02) in development of defense/attack transition-state (Figure 4C); another pattern showed that the shot also tends to occur after a goalkeeper's intervention (z = 2.66), from a shot in development of ball possession (z = 2.59) (Figure 4C). Detected also were goals scored after a recovery of ball possession by tackle (BRt; z = 2.07) or a positive crossing in Development of defense/attack transition-state (z = 3.34).

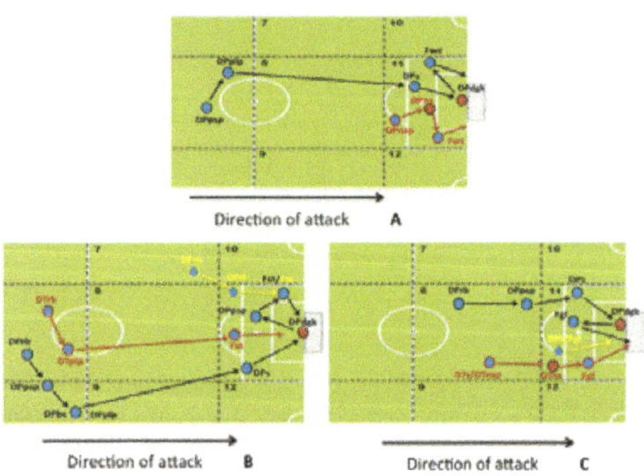

Figure 4. Illustration of offensive patterns that resulted in wide shot (A), in shot on target (B) and in goal scored (C) in Progression to the Target Game. See Table 1.

Discussion

This study analyzed the influence of rules manipulation on teams' offensive patterns in different SSCGs. These results showed that MPG rules influenced the emergence of offensive sequences of long duration, with a large number of players involved and with a great amount of touches on the ball and passes made. One possible explanation for this occurrence is the manipulated rule attributing extra points to the team that could replace five passes without returning the ball to the player who had just made the pass (Rule 3), and especially the rule that limited the minimum amount of passes required for shooting (Rule 4). Corroborating this study, Almeida, Ferreira, and Volossovitch[19] found that manipulation of a rule that defines a minimum number of passes required for a shot tends to condition teams to self-organize so that they opt to attack by prioritizing maintenance of ball possession and circulation of the ball over the pitch, requiring collective construction of offensive actions.

Regarding performance's composite indicators, observers could see that MPG teams had a higher rate of ball transmission among players (Passes/Duration) and a greater contribution by players of ball circulation (Passes/Players involved). Through variable Passes/Ball touches in the MPG, teams used a play style that prioritized exchange of passes among players, adopting a method of positional attack[35]. The rule that assigns a number of points to a team if they circulate the ball from one side path to the other encourages them to do so constantly, to create an advantageous situation for scoring or advancing through offensive game space.

Results from the detection of offensive patterns assist in confirming that teams seek to choose a method of attack that prioritizes maintenance of ball possession. Offensive patterns detected in the MPG consisted largely of behaviors to develop ball possession, prioritizing positional attack by using side paths. MPG rules eventually inhibited the emergence of individual behaviors, enabling a collective attack with more players' participation.

These results corroborate findings by Lizana, Reverdito, Brenzikofer, Macedo, Misuta, and Scaglia[20], who found that in maintenance possession games, players create favorable situations to score a goal only after ball circulation, in search of a clear space to shoot. Use of side bands in the MPG game field probably facilitated ball circulation, since, when occupying these side paths, players successfully increased the width of effective play-space, thus conducting tactical principles that favor maintenance of ball possession as a spatial principle[36].

Regarding the PTG, manipulated rules influenced the emergence of faster offensive sequences, in which teams seek faster progression, attempting to take advantage of the opposing team's defensive unbalance, thus making more shots. Almeida, Ferreira, and Volossovitch[19] observed that rules limiting the amount of ball touches (two) per player influence fast advance, enabling a greater number of shots. However, in this study, offensive sequences' shorter duration seemed to be influenced by manipulation of the rule that constrains the direction of passes toward the opposing goal (Rule 1), but not by the rule that limits the minimum amount of ball touches per player, as used by the authors.

In these games, players sought to intervene more with the ball (Ball touches/Players involved), most likely because of a nonexistent rule that limits the amount of ball touches per player. In addition, shots tended to be more effective (Goal/Shots), probably because faster progression through the field seems to help the team take advantage of the opposing team's possible defensive unbalance. However, Almeida, Ferreira, and Volossovitch[19] found that a rule that conditions performance of an attack with greater player participation, like the rule that limits the number of passes required to perform a shot, tended to influence shots' greater effectiveness. One possible explanation for this divergence is that the MPG, in this study, had a rule that determined the minimum number of passes needed to shoot and a rule that limited the amount of touches on the ball per player, difficult in both performance of shots as well as their effectiveness.

Offensive patterns in the PTG tended largely to occur in the development of defense/attack transition-state from faster attacks, in which teams look for ball progression through direct connections by a long pass, or through individual behaviors such as a running with the ball and dribbling.

Detection of shots made immediately after a direct ball recovery showed how rules of the game tended to encourage emergence of fast attacks. One possible explanation for emergence of shots on target after a direct ball recovery is that teams can have greater difficulty making passes only toward the opposing goal (rule manipulated in SSCG), thus increasing the probability of losing ball possession in areas close to their own goal. Dellal, Chamari, Owen, Wong, D. Lago-Peñas, and Hill-Haas[18] observed that manipulation of a rule that conditions the increase of games' dynamics and intensity might influence the effectiveness of passes and loss of ball possession.

With this study's results, we found that manipulated rules in both SSCGs (MPG and PTG) influenced the emergence of opposite play conditions. MPG rules constrained teams to maintain ball possession and circulate it to unbalance the opposing team's defensive organization. The PTG influenced the emergence of faster attacks, when the teams tended to advance quickly through the field to take advantage of the opponent's momentary defensive unbalance. Almeida, Ferreira, and Volossovitch[19] found that the manipulated rules in their investigation, rules of "two touches" and "four passes," also caused different self-organizing processes in teams, corroborating our findings.

Importantly, however, we highlight that this research sought to use two rules: one that limits each player's ball touches and another that limits the number of passes required to shoot to the opponent's goal, all in the same SSCG (MPG). These two rules were used in MPG in order to condition the teams to adopt a play style prioritizing ball possession through quick passes, promoting highly dynamic offensive sequences. As we know, match dynamics are increasingly faster in today's football, with a higher rate of passes[37]; thus, teams tend to have greater difficulty creating finalization situations, possibly due to choosing more defensive play strategies, which require greater collective work[38-40]. Therefore, when choosing an offensive method that prioritizes maintenance of possession, players and teams need to unbalance the opposing team's defensive organization through faster ball circulation, with greater player participation in sustained attacks.

Therefore, we found that the manipulation of games rules caused distinct self-organizing processes in teams. Coaches may choose to use both games in training, since offensive effectiveness will occur in terms of how teams can switch methods and play styles, imposing their plays in different match contexts[26].

Conclusion

With this investigation, we concluded that players and teams tend to self-organize according to games rules used in SSCGs. The MPG rules tended to influence the emergence of offensive patterns in the progress of ball possession, inducing positional attacks, with more players participating and using, preferably, side paths. The PTG rules tended to influence the emergence of faster offensive sequences through long passes and individual behaviors.

The amount of players and teams analyzed can be a limitation of the present study. Therefore, future studies should investigate whether players and teams in different categories (U-13 and U-15, for example) seek to self-organize in different ways, depending on rules manipulation. However, this study provides important information for coaches, since the knowledge about the influence of key tasks constraints manipulation may help them in shaping their teams' specific tactical behaviors.

References

1. Duarte R, Araújo, D Correia V, Davids, K. Sports Teams as Superorganisms. Sports Med. 2012; 42(8): 633-642.
2. Davids K, Araújo D,Shuttleworth R. (2005). Applications of dynamical system theory to Football. In T. Reilly, J. Cabri and D. Araújo (Eds.), Science and Football V (pp. 556-569). Oxon: Routledge.
3. Costa IT, Guilherme Oliveira J, Garganta J. Para um futebol jogado com ideias: Concepção, treinamento e avaliação do desempenho tático de jogadores e equipes. Curitiba: Appris; 2015.
4. Davids K, Araújo D. A abordagem baseada nos constrangimentos para o treino desportivo. In D. Araújo (Ed.), O contexto da decisão–A acção táctica no desporto (pp. 37-60). Lisboa: Visão e Contextos; 2005.
5. Gibson JJ. The ecological approach to visual perception. Hillsdale: Lawrence Erlbaum Associates: 1979.
6. Silva P, Garganta J, Araújo D, Davids K, Aguiar P. Shared knowledge or shared affordances? Insights from an ecological dynamics approach to team coordination in sports. Sports Med. 2013; 43(9): 765-772.
7. Riley MA, Richardson MJ, Shockley K, Ramenzoni VC. Interpersonal synergies. Front Psychol. 2011; 2.
8. Passos P, Araújo D, Davids K, Shuttleworth R. Manipulating constraints to train decision making in rugby union. Int J Sports Sci Coach. 2008; 3(1): 125-140.

9. Davids K, Araújo D, Correia V, Vilar L. How small-sided and conditioned games enhance acquisition of movement and decision-making skills. Exerc Sport Sci Rev. 2013; 41(3): 154-161.
10. Hill-Haas SV, Dawson B, Impellizzeri FM, Coutts AJ. Physiology of small-sided games training in football. Sports Med. 2011; 41(3): 199-220.
11. Clemente F, Couceiro M, Martins FM, Mendes R. The usefulness of small-sided games on soccer training. JPES. 2012; 12(1): 93-102.
12. Castelo J. (2003). Futebol: Guia prático de exercícios de treino. Lisboa: Edição Visão e Contextos.
13. Reverdito RS, Scaglia AJ, Paes RR. Pedagogia do esporte: panorama e análise conceitual das principais abordagens. Motriz: J. Phys. Ed. 2009; 15(3): 600-610.
14. Júlio L, Araújo D. Abordagem dinâmica da acção táctica no jogo de futebol. In D. Araújo (Ed.), O Contexto da Decisão: A Acção Táctica no Desporto. Lisboa: Visão e Contextos; 2005 p. 157-178.
15. Folgado H, Lemmink KA, Frencken W, Sampaio J. Length, width and centroid distance as measures of teams tactical performance in youth football. Eur J Sport Sci. 2014; 14(supl): S487-S492.
16. Silva P, Duarte R, Sampaio J, Aguiar P, Davids K, Araújo D, Garganta J. Field dimension and skill level constrain team tactical behaviors in small-sided and conditioned games in football. J Sport Sci. 2014; 32(20): 1888-1896.
17. Silva P, Esteves P, Correia V, Davids K, Araújo D, Garganta J. Effects of manipulations of player numbers vs. field dimensions on inter-individual coordination during small-sided games in youth football. Int J Perform Anal Sport. 2015; 15(2): 641-659.
18. Dellal A, Chamari K, Owen AL, Wong DP, Lago-Peñas C, Hill-Haas S. Influence of technical instructions on the physiological and physical demands of small-sided soccer games. Eur J Sport Sci. 2011; 11(5): 341-346.
19. Almeida CH, Ferreira AP, Volossovitch A. Manipulating task constraints in small-sided soccer games: Performance analysis and practical implications. The Open Sports Sciences Journal. 2012; 5: 174-180.
20. Lizana CJR, Reverdito RS, Brenzikofer R, Macedo DV, Misuta MS, Scaglia AJ. Technical and tactical soccer players' performance in conceptual small-sided games. Motriz: J. Phys. Ed. 2015; 21(3): 312-320.
21. Sánchez-Algarra P, Anguera MT. Qualitative/quantitative integration in the inductive observational study of interactive behavior: impact of recording and coding among predominating perspectives. Qual Quant. 2013; 47(2): 1237-1257.
22. Anguera MT, Villaseñor AB, Mendo AH, López JLL. Diseños observacionales: ajuste y aplicación en psicología del deporte. Cuadernos de psicología del deporte. 2011; 11(2): 63-76.
23. Bayer C. O ensino dos jogos desportivos colectivos. Paris: Vigot; 1994.
24. Almeida CH, Ferreira AP, Volossovitch A. Offensive sequences in youth soccer: effects of experience and small-sided games. J Hum Kinet. 2013; 36(1): 97-106.
25. Barreira D, Garganta J, Prudente J, Anguera MT. Desenvolvimento e validação de um sistema de observação aplicado à fase ofensiva em Futebol: SoccerEye. Rev Port Cien Desp. 2012; 12(3).
26. Machado JC, Barreira D, Garganta J. Eficácia ofensiva e variabilidade de padrões de jogo em futebol. Rev Bras Educ Fís Esporte. 2013; 27(4): 667-677.
27. Hughes M, Churchill S. Attacking profiles of successful and unsuccessful teams in Copa America 2001. In T. Reilly, J. Cabri and D. Araújo (Eds.), Science and football V: The Proceedings of the Fifth World Congress on Science and Football; 2005. p. 222-228.
28. Garganta JM, Marques A, Maia J. Modelação táctica do jogo de futebol: Estudo da organização da fase ofensiva em equipas de alto rendimento. In J. Garganta (Ed.), A investigaçao em futebol: estudos ibéricos; 2002. p. 51-66. Universidade do Porto: Faculdade de Ciências do Desporto e de Educaçao Física.
29. Hughes M, Franks I. Analysis of passing sequences, shots and goals in soccer. J Sport Sci. 2005; 23(5): 509-514.
30. Barreira D, Garganta J, Castellano J, Anguera MT. SoccerEye: A software solution to observe and record behaviors in sport settings. The Open Sports Sciences Journal. 2013; (6): 47-55.
31. Bakeman R, Quera V. Analyzing interaction: Sequential analysis with SDIS and GSEQ: Cambridge University Press; 1995.
32. Bakeman R, Gottman JM, Portal MDG, Anguera MT, Villaseñor AB. Observación de la interacción: introducción al análisis secuencial: Morata; 1989.
33. Anguera MT. Metodología de la Observación en las ciencias Humanas. Madrid: Cátedra; 1992.
34. Sackett GP. The lag sequential analysis of contingency and cyclicity in behavioral interaction research. In J. Osofsky (Ed.), Handbook of infant development. New York: Wiley; 1979. p. 623-649.
35. Castelo J. Futebol–A organização do jogo. Lisboa: Edição do autor; 1996.
36. Costa IT, Garganta J, Greco PJ, Mesquita I. Princípios Táticos do Jogo de Futebol: conceitos e aplicação. Motriz: J. Phys. Ed. 2009; 15(3): 657-668.
37. Wallace JL, Norton KI. Evolution of World Cup soccer final games 1966–2010: Game structure, speed and play patterns. J Sci Med Sport. 2014; 17(2): 223-228.
38. Barreira D Garganta J, Castellano J, Prudente J, Anguera MT. Evolución del ataque del ataque en el fútbol de élite entre 1982 y 2010: aplicación del análisis secuencial de retardos. Rev Psicol Deporte. 2014; 23(1): 139-146.
39. Barreira D, Garganta J, Castellano J, Machado J, Anguera MT. How elite-level soccer dynamics has evolved over the last three decades? Input from generalizability theory. Cuadernos de Psicología del Deporte. 2015; 15(1): 51-62.
40. Bloomfield J, Jonsson G, Polman R, Houlahan K, O'Donoghue P. Temporal Pattern Analysis and its Applicability in Soccer. In L. Anolli, S. D. Jr, M. S. Magnusson and G. Riva (Eds.), The Hidden Structure of Interaction: From Neurons to Culture Patterns Amsterdam: IOS Press; 2005. p. 238-251.

Acknowledgments

We gratefully acknowledgment the support of Fundação de Ampara à Pesquisa do Estado do Amazonas (FAPEAM).
We gratefully acknowledge the support of two Spanish government projects (Ministerio de Economía y Competitividad): (1) La actividad física y el deporte como potenciadores del estilo de vida saludable: Evaluación del comportamiento de-

portivo desde metodologías no intrusivas [Grant number DEP2015-66069-P]; (2) Avances metodológicos y tecnológicos en el estudio observacional del comportamiento deportivo [PSI2015-71947-REDP]; and the support of the Generalitat de Catalunya Research Group, GRUP DE RECERCA I INNOVACIÓ EN DISSENYS (GRID). Tecnología i aplicació multimedia i digital als dissenys observacionals [Grant number 2014 SGR 971].

Corresponding author

João Cláudio Machado.
Federal University of Amazonas, Faculty of Physical Education
and Physiotherapy, Brazil; Av, General Rodrigo Octávio, 3000; Campus
Universitário; Manaus/AM
Email: joaoclaudiomachado@gmail.com

Specific warm-up exercise is the best for vertical countermovement jump in young volleyball players

Fernando Nazário de Rezende
Universidade Federal do Triângulo Mineiro, Uberaba, MG, Brasil
Universidade Presidente Antônio Carlos, Uberlândia, MG, Brasil

Gustavo Ribeiro da Mota
Universidade Federal do Triângulo Mineiro, Uberaba, MG, Brasil

Charles Ricardo Lopes
Universidade Metodista de Piracicaba, Piracicaba, SP, Brasil
Faculdade Adventista de Hortolândia, Hortolândia, SP, Brasil

Bruno Victor C. da Silva
Centro Universitário de Belo Horizonte, Belo Horizonte, MG, Brasil

Mário A. M. Simim
Universidade Federal de Belo Horizonte, Belo Horizonte, MG, Brasil

Moacir Marocolo
Universidade Federal de Juiz de Fora, Juiz de Fora, MG, Brasil

Abstract — We evaluated the effect of performing various distinct warm-up exercises on vertical countermovement jump (VCMJ) performance. Eight volleyball players (age 15.4 ± 0.5 yrs) performed five different warm-up activities (in a counterbalanced, randomized crossover study) over five days, at 24-h intervals: stretching (4 × 30 s, 30 s between sets), cycloergometer (5 min at 50 W + 5 min at 100 W), resistance exercise (leg press 45°, 3 × 5 repetitions maximum, 3-min pause between sets), specific vertical jumping (4 × 10 VCMJ, 2-min pause between sets), and no warm-up at all (control condition). Beginning 3 min after their warm-up, the players performed 3 attempts (at intervals of 3 min) of VCMJ (on a contact carpet), and each player's best jump was considered in the analysis. All warm-up activities presented higher VCMJ performance ($p < 0.05$) than the control condition, with the exception of stretching. Vertical jumping revealed a large effect size (0.8) than other interventions. We conclude that in practical terms, vertical jumps are the best warm-up exercise (when applied by itself) to acutely improve VCMJ performance in volleyball players, but that other exercises can make a complementary contribution.

Keywords: performance, jumping technique, team sport, potentiation, athletes

Introduction

Vertical countermovement jumps (VCMJs) are considered essential to success in volleyball, as they are used in both defensive (blocking) and offensive (attacking, passing, and serving) motions[1,2] VCMJs are performed frequently by volleyball players during training and competitions, and several studies have focused on how athletes can enable themselves to jump most effectively[3,4] Volleyball players must jump frequently in matches, making good jumping technique crucial. An analysis of two matches showed that the average player executed about 45 jumps and subsequent landings, and that the players' overall performance depended heavily on these actions[5].

The importance of VCMJs in volleyball makes understanding the factors that influence jumping ability essential. Limiting factors such as flexibility in the joints involved in jumping movements, the strength and muscle power of athletes (e.g., maximal force, maximal velocity, and stretch-shortening cycle utilization), and specific techniques seem to be reasonable variables to consider.

Sports scientists and coaches are constantly seeking the best ways to maximize players' performance. Examining the phenomenon known as post-activation potentiation is one pathway associated with this purpose, at least acutely[6]. Most studies about post-activation potentiation have used VCMJs because studying this movement can detect variations in lower limb performance (i.e., muscle power, strength) and because these jumps are important in several sports such as volleyball[7].

Although particular exercises are commonly performed during warm-up before practices and matches, aiming at a better transition from a resting state to high-intensity activity, little is known about the effect of this activities (e.g., stretching, resistance exercise, jumps, jogging) on VCMJ performance by volleyball players. Thus, the aim of this study was to evaluate the acute effect of each of four distinct warm-up activities (performed as the subjects normally completed them, not influenced by researchers) on VCMJ performance in young volleyball players. We hypothesized that a more specific warm-up (e.g. jumps) would induce greater improvement than other activities.

Methods

Subjects and ethical concerns

Eight female volleyball players who participated in a Brazilian state championship competition (age 15.4 ± 0.5 years; 4.3 ± 1.2 years of training; 5 training sessions/week; 90 min/session) participated voluntarily, having been recruited through by convenience sampling. They had experience in strength training (1 repetition maximum [RM] for leg press 45° = about 335.8 ± 16.5 kg). This study was conducted according to the Declaration of Helsinki, and the protocol was fully approved by the ethics committee of the local university before we began conducting our assessments. All participants were informed that they could withdraw from the study at any time without penalty, and their parents (or guardians) signed an informed consent form.

Inclusion and exclusion criteria

We sought participants with no history of lower limb musculoskeletal injury diseases that could affect the results. All participants had to meet the following inclusion criteria: (1) having at least two years of experience playing volleyball; (2) having participated in the state championship competition; (3) not consuming nutritional supplements or potential ergogenic aids of any kind (exogenous anabolic androgenic steroids); (4) non-smoker; (5) normal blood pressure; (6) not diabetic; and (7) familiar with the exercises used in the evaluation.

General design of the experiment

To address the question of whether any exercises usually used in warm-ups could influence VCMJ performance by themselves (i.e., if performed alone without any other exercise), we performed a counterbalanced, randomized crossover study. In the course of five days (at 24-h intervals), participants performed the control activity (no warm-up) and four distinct warm-up protocols, following the same general procedures carried out in training or before matches, and then had their VCMJ performance measured. We did not influence the content (i.e., type, duration, and intensity) of each warm-up and simply asked the players to perform each warm-up activity by itself. The four warm-ups selected were as follows.

Resistance exercise: This exercise (leg press 45°) consisted of 3 sets of 5 repetitions maximum (RM) with a 3-min pause between sets. The intensity (5 RM) was determined by the team's fitness coach, because he already had information on the players' abilities. The velocity of the movement was observed (without influence) by a pacer alarm (SEIKO DM50, Tokyo, Japan), and the average for all players was about 4 s for each repetition (2-s concentric and 2-s eccentric phases).

Static stretching: Four sets (30 s stretching and 20 s pause) for the following muscles: lateral/medial and adductors/abductors of hip, flexor/extensor of hip, and knee and ankle plantar flexors. The players' fitness controlled the intensity of the stretching by using the visual analog pain scale, from 0 ("no pain") to 10 ("maximum pain"). Players were instructed to keep their intensity level between 3 and 4 ("annoying, uncomfortable, troublesome pain")(8), as they normally did during daily warm-up activities.

Stationary cycloergometer (bicycle): The players spent 10 min riding a cycloergometer (Maxx-Pro standard Monark®, Varberg, Sweden). The initial load was 5 min at 50 W (1 kp, 50 RPM), followed by an additional 5 min at 100 W (2 kp, 50 RPM).

Vertical jump: This warm-up consisted of 4 sets of 10 jumps, simulating VCMJs, with a 2-min pause between sets. The fitness coach asked the players to jump vertically as high as they were capable of doing during the sets.

The order of the warm-up protocols was counterbalanced to avoid potential bias associated with the warm-up protocol sequence. The sequence of the warm-up protocols for each participant was determined by lot. The only changes was that players performed each warm-up exercise by itself, whereas they would usually combine two or more exercises (e.g., stretching, bicycling, and vertical jumps) in their typical warm-up rather than performing only one. Since the warm-up exercises used in this study were already part of the players' daily routine, they were fully familiar with how to execute each activity.

The study was carried out at the beginning of the volleyball season, and the players were instructed to arrive at the gym in a rested and fully hydrated state, at least 2 h postprandial, and to avoid strenuous exercise in the previous 24 h. Each subject was tested at the same time of day (10:00–12:00 h), at a temperature of 25 ± 2° C, and strong verbal encouragement was given to all players to motivate them to perform each test action. Additionally, the players wore exactly the same uniforms for all protocols. The experimental protocol design is displayed in Figure 1, and the sequence in which each participant performed the warm-ups is shown in Table 1.

VCMJ test

To measure the jumping height, a contact platform measuring 100 x 60 x 8 cm, sensitive to small changes in pressure and coupled with Jump Test® software (CEFISE, Jump System Pro, Nova Odessa, Brazil; interface connection cable, 25-pin, parallel USB port; sampling frequency 1Mhz, mean error ± 3 ms) was used. The VCMJ performance test consisted of a bilateral

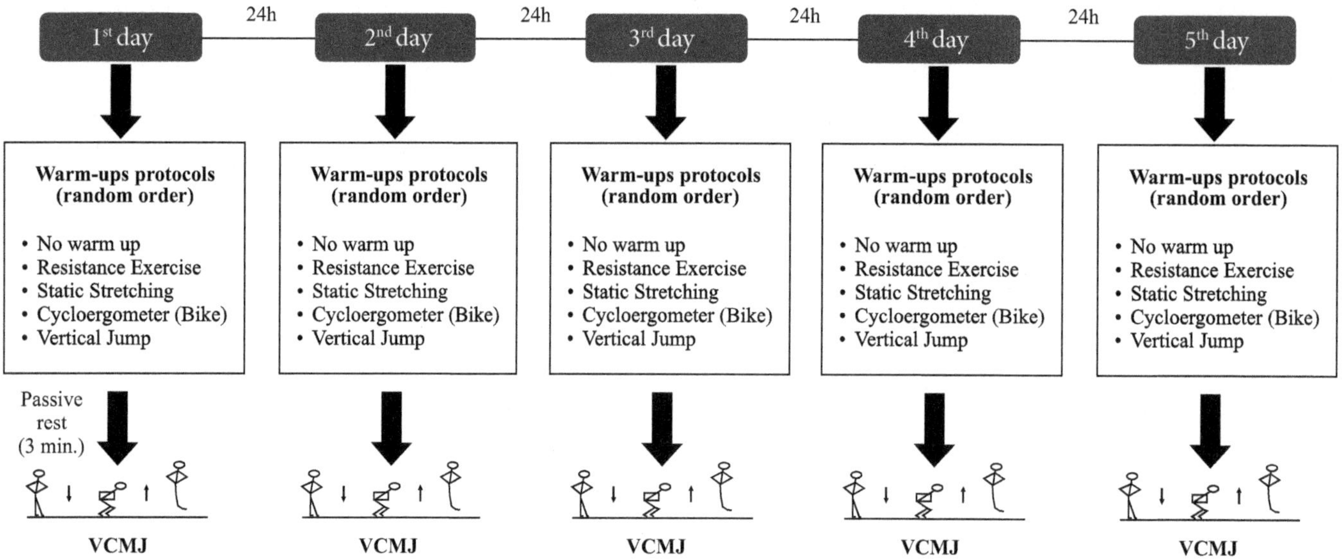

Notes: No warm up (control) / Resistance Exercise (Leg Press 45°, 3x5 repetitions, 3 min. pause between sets) Static Stretching (4x30s, 30s between sets) / Cycloergometer = Bike: (5 min. 50W + 5 min. 100W) Vertical Jump (4x10 VCMJ, 2 min. pause between sets)

Figure 1. Experimental design of the study (n = 8)

Table 1. Sequence in which each participant performed the warm-up protocols. The interventions are coded as follows: 1 = control; 2 = resistance exercise; 3 = bicycling; 4 = vertical jumps; 5 = stretching.

Participants	1st day	2nd day	3rd day	4th day	5th day
1	3	5	2	4	1
2	1	2	4	5	3
3	2	1	3	4	5
4	5	2	3	1	4
5	4	3	1	2	5
6	1	5	3	2	4
7	4	1	2	3	5
8	5	3	2	1	4

vertical jump from an orthostatic position with hands on the hip (no arm swing allowed), in the suprailiac region. Leg-thigh flexion relation occurred until about 90°. The participants then did a fast leg and hip extension, trying to push the body upward and vertically without previous movement of any other body part. The trunk was held upright vertically without excessive advance. Another important technical detail is that the knees remained extended during the flight. All technical evaluations were performed beginning 3 min after the warm-up. Each participant performed three trials with 3 min of recovery between trials, and we used only the best performance in our analysis. The test was invalidated if the players violated any of these conditions: (1) did not start or complete the jump with both feet inside the platform; (2) used upper body movement during the jump; or (3) adopted a sort of "group" (i.e. flexion of the hip, approaching the thighs of the trunk) at the time of landing (which increases the time of flight).

Statistical Analysis

All data were checked for normality using the Shapiro-Wilk test. Data were presented as means ± standard deviations, delta (Δ%) compared to the control group, and effect sizes. The effect sizes were interpreted using the scale of magnitudes proposed by Cohen(9). Repeated measures ANOVAs were used to examine the main effects between the warm-up protocols. Mauchly's Test of Sphericity was conducted initially, followed by ANOVAs, with Greenhouse-Geisser correction where appropriate. Alpha was set at $p < 0.05$.

Results

All warm-up protocols presented higher VCMJ performance ($F_{(3,20)} = 14{,}8$; $p < 0.01$; $\eta^2 = 0.679$) than the control condition, except for static stretching (Table 2). Vertical jump warm-up led to the highest VCMJ performance (12% greater than control, $p < 0.01$, effect size 0.8), followed by bicycling (7% greater, $p = 0.049$, effect size 0.5) and resistance exercise (6% greater, $p = 0.031$, effect size 0.4).

Discussion

The main finding of this study was that a skill-specific warm-up (vertical jumping) was the best exercise (largest effect size) to improve VCMJ performance when applied by itself. Thus, the use of jumping exercises in warm-up appears to be effective prior to training and matches, but other methods can also be applied as complementary warm-up activities.

The exact mechanisms supporting the potentiation effect elicited by plyometric exercise (vertical jump) as preload are still unclear[2]. Although electromyography was not performed in the present study,

Table 2. VCMJ performance changes following warm-up protocols (n = 8)

Warm-up protocols	Mean ± SD	CI 95%	In relation control condition	
Control	28.2±3.5	25.2 - 31.1	Δ%	Effect size
Stretching	28.4±3.4	25.5 - 31.3	1%	0,06
Bicycling	30.1±4.0*[a]	26.7 - 33.4	7%	0,5
Resistance exercise	29.8±3.7*	26.7 - 32.9	6%	0,4
Vertical jumps	31.5±4.4*[a]	27.9 - 35.2	12%	0,8

CI: confidence interval; *significant differences ($p < 0.05$) between warm-ups protocol and control; [a]significant differences from stretching. Effect sizes of < 0.09, 0.10–0.49, 0.50–0.79, and > 0.80 were considered trivial, small, moderate, and large, respectively (Cohen, 1988). Data represent mean ± standard deviation.

we can suggest that post-activation potentiation effects could be attributed to such neural mechanisms as increased motor neuron excitability, enhanced motor unit recruitment patterns, or increased activation of synergists (or all of these)[2,10].

Bicycling showed better results than control and stretching, but not better than resistance exercises and vertical jumping. This result relative to the latter two exercises is not surprising, because to obtain the benefits from post-activation potentiation, type II (fast twitch) fibers must be recruited during conditioning activities (size principle). Because the bicycling warm-up was performed at a low intensity, it was probably unable to activate type II muscle fiber and generate post-activation potentiation. Nevertheless, it has been found that exercise with low loads also can create an optimal environment for power production[11]. This improvement in neuromuscular function can occur through the increase of body temperature and the acceleration of metabolism[12]. In this way, although through different mechanisms, the bicycle warm-up at low intensity was also somewhat effective in improving VCMJ.

In the present study, VCMJ performance increased after resistance exercise, similar to the results of other investigations that demonstrated a positive change in jumping performance after high-intensity squat exercises[13,15]. Although the leg press is a multi-joint exercise (similar to jumping), biomechanically the two have some differences (e.g., the ballistic nature of jumping, and the different body positions) that could influence the post-activation potentiation response[16]. Despite this, warming up with high-intensity leg presses improved VCMJ performance, probably due to the increase of phosphorylation of myosin regulatory light chains and the recruitment of higher-order motor units[17]. There is also evidence to suggest that acute changes in the pennation angle may contribute to post-activation potentiation. All these mechanisms result in greater cross-bridge attachments and higher muscle power[17].

The stretching protocol was the only exercise that did not improve VCMJ relative to the control condition (i.e., no warm-up at all) in the present study. Also, we did not observe a negative influence of the stretching protocol on VCMJ, in agreement with some previous studies[18,19]. However, other studies have shown negative effects on vertical jump performance after static stretching[20,23]. The differences among studies could be due to the volume and/or intensity level of the stretching protocol. The fact that our protocol applied a relatively high volume (4 sets of 30 s) but low intensity of exercise could be related to the lack of negative impact on jumping performance. In addition, the participants performed a similar stretching protocol to their normal training routine, and this fact could also help to explain the maintenance of VCMJ capacity.

Another interesting finding in our study was that resting for 3 min was sufficient to avoid negative impact on VCMJ performance in all protocols. Generally, the rest interval needed to obtain post-activation potentiation effects has ranged between 5 and 18.5 min. [24]. Although several factors can interfere with post-activation potentiation, including the rest interval[17,24-26], our data showed that the interval used (3 min) did not decrease VCMJ performance.

Once we carried out a crossover randomized assignment to avoid any influence of treatments, our findings were robust, reinforcing our initial hypothesis that a more specific warm-up (i.e., vertical jumping) would be better than others when applied in an isolated way to acutely improve VCMJ.

Finally, the current data should be interpreted with caution, because we analyzed isolated warm-up protocols. This method was suited to our purpose, as it enabled us to compare the impact of four distinct warm-up exercises, but single-exercise warm-ups rarely if ever happen in the real world of high-level sports. Thus, future research could elucidate the impact of combined warm-up protocols and other possibilities.

Conclusion

In practical terms, vertical jumping is the best warm-up exercise to acutely improve VCMJ performance in volleyball players, when compared to other exercises and when each one is applied by itself. The results suggest that acute-response, high-intensity resistance exercises and low-intensity bicycling on an ergometer can improve VCMJ performance to a lesser degree, whereas static stretching exercises do not.

References

1. Nikolaidis PT, Ziv G, Arnon M, Lidor R. Physical characteristics and physiological attributes of female volleyball players - The need for individual data. J Strength Cond Res. 2012; 26(9): 2547–2557.
2. Ziv G, Lidor R. Vertical jump in female and male volleyball players: a review of observational and experimental studies. Scand J Med Sci Sports. 2010; 20(4): 556-567.
3. Ebben WP, Simenz C, Jensen RL. Evaluation of plyometric intensity using electromyography. J Strength Cond Res. 2008; 22(3): 861-868.
4. Pereira G, Freitas PB, Barela JA, Ugrinowitsch C, Rodacki ALF, Kokubun E, Fowler NE. Vertical jump fatigue does not affect intersegmental coordination and segmental contribution. Motriz: J. Phys. Ed. 2014; 20(3): 303-309.
5. Tillman MD, Hass CJ, Brunt D, Bennett GR. Jumping and Landing Techniques in Elite Women's Volleyball. J Sports Sci Med. 2004; 3(1): 30-36.

6. Seitz LB, Haff GG. Factors Modulating Post-Activation Potentiation of Jump, Sprint, Throw, and Upper-Body Ballistic Performances: A Systematic Review with Meta-Analysis. Sport Med. 2016; 46(2): 231-240.
7. McCann MR, Flanagan SP. The effects of exercise selection and rest interval on postactivation potentiation of vertical jump performance. J Strength Cond Res. 2010; 24(5): 1285-1291.
8. Turner AP, Bellhouse S, Kilduff LP, Russell M. Postactivation potentiation of sprint acceleration performance using plyometric exercise. J Strength Cond Res. 2015; 29(2): 343-350.
9. Cohen J. Statistical power analysis for the behavioral sciences. New Jersey: Lawrence Erlbaum; 1988.
10. Masamoto N, Larson R, Gates T, Faigenbaum A. Acute effects of plyometric exercise on maximum squat performance in male athletes. J Strength Cond Res. 2003; 17(1): 68-71.
11. Crow JF, Buttifant D, Kearny SG, Hrysomallis C. Low load exercises targeting the gluteal muscle group acutely enhance explosive power output in elite athletes. J Strength Cond Res. 2012; 26(2): 438-442.
12. Pagaduan JC, Pojskić H, Užičanin E, Babajić F. Effect of various warm-up protocols on jump performance in college football players. J Hum Kinet. 2012; 35(1): 127-132.
13. Esformes JI, Cameron N, Bampouras TM. Postactivation potentiation following different modes of exercise. J Strength Cond Res. 2010; 24(7): 1911-1916.
14. McBride JM, Nimphius S, Erickson TM. The acute effects of heavy-load squats and loaded countermovement jumps on sprint performance. J Strength Cond Res. 2005; 19(4): 893-897.
15. Weber KR, Brown LE, Coburn JW, Zinder SM. Acute effects of heavy-load squats on consecutive squat jump performance. J Strength Cond Res. 2008; 22(3): 726-730.
16. Robbins DW. Postactivation potentiation and its practical applicability. J Strength Cond Res. 2005; 19(2): 453-458.
17. Tillin MNA, Bishop D. Factors modulating post-activation potentiation and its effect on performance of subsequent explosive activities. Sport Med. 2009; 39(2): 147-166.
18. Power K, Behm D, Cahill F, Carroll M,Young W. An acute bout of static stretching: effects on force and jumping performance. Med Sci Sports Exerc. 2004; 36: 1389-1396.
19. Unick J, Kieffer HS, Cheesman W, Feeney A. The acute effects of static and ballistic stretching on vertical jump performance in trained women. J Strength Cond Res. 2005; 19(1): 206-212.
20. Behm DG, Kibele A. Effects of differing intensities of static stretching on jump performance. Eur J Appl Physiol. 2007; 101(5): 587-594.
21. Bradley PS, Olsen PD, Portas MD. The effect of static, ballistic, and proprioceptive neuromuscular facilitation stretching on vertical jump performance. J Strength Cond Res. 2007; 21(1): 223-226.
22. Cornwell A, Nelson AG, Sidaway B. Acute effects of stretching on the neuromechanical properties of the triceps surae muscle complex. Eur J Appl Physiol. 2002; 86(5): 428-434.
23. Young W, Behm D. Effects of running, static stretching and practice jumps on explosive force production and jumping performance. J Sports Med Phys Fitness. 2003; 43(1): 21-27.
24. Wilson JM, Duncan NM, Marin PJ, Brown LE, Loenneke JP, Wilson SM, et al. Meta-analysis of postactivation potentiation and power: effects of conditioning activity, volume, gender, rest periods, and training status. J Strength Cond Res. 2013; 27(3): 854-859.
25. Rixon KP, Lamont HS, Bemben MG. Influence of type of muscle contraction, gender, and lifting experience on postactivation potentiation performance. J Strength Cond Res. 2007; 21(2): 500-505.
26. Seitz LB, de Villarreal ES, Haff GG. The Temporal Profile of Postactivation Potentiation Is Related to Strength Level. J Strength Cond Res. 2014; 28(3): 706-715.

Acknowledgments

The authors would like to thank the players and coaches that contributed in this study.

Corresponding author

Gustavo Ribeiro da Mota, PhD.
Federal University of Triangulo Mineiro, UFTM, Department of Sport Sciences, Av. Frei Paulino, 30, Uberaba, MG, Brazil.
Email: grmotta@gmail.com

Applicability of an Indirect VO2max Test: Its Association with the 400 Meters Freestyle Performance

Adalberto Veronese da Costa
Universidade do Estado do Rio Grande do Norte, Rio Grande do Norte, RN. Brasil
Universidade de Trás-os-Montes e Alto Douro, Vila Real. Portugal

Manoel da Cunha Costa
Jorge Luiz de Brito Gomes
Fernando José de Sá Pereira Guimarães
Universidade de Pernambuco, Recife, PE, Brasil

Tiago Manuel Barbosa
National Institute of Education, Nanyang Technological University, Singapore

Abstract – The aim of this study was to evaluate the VO2max using a previously validated indirect test for non-expert adult swimmers and to verify its connection with the 400 meters freestyle test. A total of 17 non-expert male swimmers (21.5 ± 3.12 years) were evaluated. Body composition measurements included body weight (74 ± 9.41 kg), height (172.9 ± 5.21 cm) and body fat percentage (15.2 ± 4.15 %). Two tests were conducted on different days; the 400 meters freestyle (400 MF) and the Progressive Swim Test (PSwT), respectively. The participant's heart rate frequency before and after the test (BHR and AHR) was analyzed, as well as the subjective perception of effort (RPE), the number of laps covered (NLP), and the time of test execution measured in minutes. Significant differences were identified in all variables ($p < 0.05$) with the exception of BHR. An inverse correlation ($r > -0.60$) was found between AHR and execution time ($r > -0.70$), as well as between the VO2max estimated by the PSwT and the 400 MF performance test ($r > -0.70$). The Bland-Altman Plot showed that the values discovered were within the established concordance limits of 95% (±1.96 SD). A negative correlation between a swimming test and a test that estimates the VO2max occurred, and the PSwT showed results of greater approximation of the aerobic power of non-expert swimmers. In conclusion, the PSwT is applicable for non-expert adult swimmers.

Keywords: swimming, VO2max, health, training program, performance

Introduction

Physical evaluation has been of great use for swimmers as the results contribute to guiding intensity, duration, and objectives to be achieved during physical exercise, whether for competition or health purposes[1,2,3]. In this sense, there is a trend to conduct research in order to evaluate the swimmers' cardiorespiratory fitness, and it is imperative that the choice of test is the closest possible to their sport reality. Thus, the design or adaptation of swimming tests require caution to meet the criteria of scientific authenticity, providing greater precision through their consistency (reproducibility), authenticity (validity), and association to real-life situations (applicability)[4,5].

There is a solid set of evidence that the 400 meters freestyle swimming test is closely related to the VO2max (ml/kg.min^{-1}) of high-performance swimmers when evaluated in a laboratory setting[6]. Specifically, Ribeiro evaluated the ability of different metabolic indexes to predict the swimming performance in the 400 meters freestyle, noting 85% of the VO2max (ml/kg.min^{-1}) and the concentration of 4 mmol/l blood lactate are significant predictors for mid-distance events[7]. Another study measured the time to exhaustion at the minimum speed that matches the VO2max of high-performance swimmers (in swimming conditions through direct oximetry) and showed the average time with values of 260.20 ± 60.73 s, demonstrating the relationship of VO2max (ml/kg.min^{-1}) and mid-distance tests[8]. Further, when investigating the anthropometric and physiological characteristics of young competitive swimmers in relation with their swimming performance, Oliver Hue, selected the 400 meters freestyle test as a reference[9].

Recently, the previous test proposed by Léger and Boucher was adapted[10], developed, and validated for the aquatic environment, and was coined the *Progressive Swim Test* (PSwT), which has the purpose of determining the VO2max (ml/kg.min^{-1}) based upon the greater number of laps in a 25-meter swimming pool, with phased intensity established by sound signals at each 50 meters[11]. Through the reproducibility obtained in the test, it was possible to see that the number of laps swum during the test (NLP) may determine the physical conditioning of non-expert swimmers, due to the distances with pre-determined time (r and ICC > 0.90, $p < 0.01$)[11].

In addition, a prediction equation was created from its validation, which could estimate the VO2max of non-expert swimmers where the mean value was within the 45 ml.kg^{-1}min^{-1}. These results are in accordance with other studies that evaluated the VO2max at the end of the 400 meters freestyle in maximum speed by elite swimmers, which showed results between 45 and 62 ml.kg–1min^{-1} [12]. Following the adaptation, design reproducibility, and validity stages of PSwT [11,12], the next step should be its application in order to verify its sensibility and its use as a source of information regarding the cardiorespiratory aptitude of swimmers.

Since there is a strong connection between the performance in the 400 meters freestyle test and VO2max, there is a good chance to verify whether or not the VO2max estimated with the PSwT is also related to this test. Therefore, the study hypothesis contends there is a significant connection between the estimated VO2max and the performance in the 400 meters freestyle test. Thus, the purpose of this study was to evaluate VO2max through a previously validated indirect test for non-expert adult swimmers and to establish its connection with the 400 meters freestyle test.

Methods

Participants

The size of the sample in relation to the local swimming schools was estimated using the GPower 3.0.10. software[13]. Thus, in a pilot study conducted under the same conditions of the validation experiment, we attempted to verify the extent of the effect size (ES) of preliminary analysis. Therefore, while examining the high correlation that exists between VO2max and the distance swum, an ES of 0.75 was observed. Accordingly, taking into account the great power of analysis from 0.8 and a corresponding alpha error of 0.05, we reached a minimum sample of 11 swimmers for this investigation. However, 17 non-expert male swimmers with ages between 18 and 30 years participated in the study (age: 21.5 ± 3.12 years; body mass: 74 ± 9.41 kg; height: 172.9 ± 5.21 cm and body fat percentage: 15.2 ± 4.15 %), submitting to two tests on different days. On the first day, the 400 meters freestyle (400 MF) was simulated and on the following day (24 hours later), the Progressive Swim Test (PSwT) was performed.

The criteria for participation in this study were as follows: a) swimmers with accurate technique for crawl style; b) taking swimming lessons three times a week with a duration of one hour per session; c) the ability to swim 800 meters uninterrupted; d) swimmers who have eaten three hours before the test; e) who have not taken any type of food supplements; f) who have not ingested any alcohol, carbonated drinks or caffeine, and who have not smoked or taken drugs; g) have not performed any type of moderate to vigorous physical activity 24 hours prior to testing. Excluded from this study were: a) elite swimmers, affiliated with the National Swimming Federation or athletes who have been affiliated in the three years prior to the survey; b) non-expert swimmers that have responded negatively to one of the questions in the Physical Activity Readiness Questionnaire – PAR-Q[14]; c) who performed the test in less than four minutes (1,15,16); d) visibly presenting any kind of infection that would compromise their musculoskeletal condition.

All procedures followed the guidelines of the Declaration of Helsinki, which deals with the ethics of experiments involving human beings. This study was approved by the ethics committee of the University of Pernambuco / PROPEGE / UPE, Brazil – Protocol 035/2012. Prior to beginning the test, all participants signed a Statement of Informed Consent.

Procedures

The body composition of the subjects was assessed by weight (Finizola Weighing-machine, São Paulo, Brasil – accuracy 100 g), stadiometer (Sanny, São Paulo, Brasil – accuracy 1 mm) and to determine the percentage of fat, the Jackson e Pollock protocol of tree skin fold (adipometer Lange Skinfold Caliper, Beta Technology, California, United States of America – accuracy 1 mm) was employed[17,18].

In order to the perform tests (400 MF and PSwT) under the same conditions, both were conducted in a 25-meter swimming pool, with a mean water temperature of 27 ±1 °C, without jumping from the block, leaning against the side with one foot placed on the wall, and executed at the same hour. A chronometer (Casio HS3, São Paulo, Brasil–accuracy in hundredths of seconds) was used to verify the execution time of the 400 MF. A heart rate monitor (Model Polar FT1, Polar Electro Oy, Kempele, Finland) was used before each test to identify the condition of the swimmer when at rest (BHR), using values below 90 bpm for starting criteria. The heart rate after the test (AHR) was also measured to verify the maximum reached, as well as the rate of perceived exertion (RPE) through the Borg's Category Ratio-Scale – CR-10 was applied at the end of the test[19,20]. Also tested were the number of laps performed (NLP) and the duration of the performance in each of the tests, measured in minutes. During the simulated 400 MF test, swimmers were asked to execute it in the least amount of time possible.

In the PSwT protocol, swimmers used an underwater MP3 which was attached to the their glasses (SwiMP3 V2, Finis Inc., Livermore, CA) and the evaluators used a 50/60 Hz (18W) Micro System, to ensure that all subjects could hear the audio sounds recorded during the test. The PSwT was applied according to the protocol of Veronese da Costa[12], which corresponds to an increase of swimming intensity of one second for every two laps (meaning every 50 meters). The test ends when the swimmer cannot arrive at the distance which marks the first or last five meters of the swimming pool twice in a row. From the application of the PSwT[12], it was possible to estimate the VO2max of non-expert adult swimmers through the following equation:

$$VO2max\ (ml.kg^{-1}.min^{-1}) = 14.085 + 1.858[NLP] - 0.192[BM(kg)] + 0.111[AHR]$$

Note: NLP–Number Laps Performed, BM–Body Mass, AHR–After Heart Rate

Analysis

The Shapiro-Wilk and Levene tests were conducted to test the normality and homogeneity of the data and whether the presuppositions of parametric statistics were met. The results are presented in mean and standard deviation. To compare the variables, the paired t-test was selected. To verify the association between the tests, the Pearson linear correlation (r) was computed between the variables BHR–Before Heart Rate; AHR – After Heart Rate; RPE – Rate of Perceived Exertion (Scale from 1 to 10); NLP – Number Laps Performed; bpm – beats per minute; min–time in minutes, as well as between the equation which uses time in minutes to estimate the VO2max of the PSwT and 400 MF. The coefficient of variation (CV = standard deviation / mean x 100) was assessed in each individual between the two tests so the CV general mean and the Standard Error of Measurement (SEM) could be calculated. Thus, it was considered that the greater the R and smaller the CV and SEM percentages, the greater the test applicability levels would be[11]. The limits of agreement and bias of the variables between the two tests were analyzed using the Bland-Altman Plot, and taking as satisfactory that 80% of the plots are within a confidence interval of 95% (± 1.96 SD)[21,22]. The data was analyzed using the SPSS for Windows statistical package (v 17.0, SPSS, Inc., Chicago, IL) and MedCalc for Windows (v 12.2.1.0, Mariakerke, Belgium). In all analyses, the significance level was 5%.

Results

Table 1 presents the descriptive data between the simulated 400 MF test and the PSwT. It was observed that all swimmers began the tests with their BHR at less than 90 bpm, the AHR displayed larger values in the PSwT than 400 MF, the RPE was classified as very strong, and the NLP mean in the PSwT was inferior to the 400 MF in terms of time and distance (difference of 140 meters).

Table 1. Descriptive data between the distance of the 400 meters freestyle and Progressive Swim Test

Variables	Test	Mean	Standard Deviation
BHR (bpm)	400MF	82.8	16.8
	PSwT	76.8	8.7
AHR (bpm)	400MF	155.2	18.8
	PSwT	176.9	4.0
RPE	400MF	8.0	0.8
	PSwT	8.4	0.5
NLP	400MF	16	–
	PSwT	10.4	2.9
Time (min)	400MF	7.29	0.82
	PSwT	4.67	1.52

Abbreviation: BHR – Before Heart Rate; AHR – After Heart Rate; RPE – Rate of Perceived Exertion (Scale from 1 to 10); NLP – Number Laps Performed; bpm – beats per minute; min–time in minutes (Test Duration).

Table 2 shows an inverted correlation in AHR and in the execution times between the simulated 400 MF test and the PSwT. We also observed significant differences in the paired t-test, a coefficient of variation, and a standard error of measurement smaller than 10% in most variables.

Table 2. Statistical analyses between the 400 meters freestyle and Progressive Swim Test

Variables	r	t-test	SEM	CV (%)
BHR (bpm)	0.50	0.16	3.87	14%
AHR (bpm)	-0.67*	<0.01**	3.99	9%
RPE	0.32	0.05**	0.20	6%
NLP	–	<0.01**	0.76	12%
Time (min)	-0.79*	<0.01**	0.54	8%

Note: * Significant correlation ($p \leq 0.05$); ** Significant difference in t-test ($p \leq 0.05$).
Abbreviation: r – Pearson linear correlation; SEM – Standard Error of Measurement; CV (%)–Coefficient of Variation; BHR – Before Heart Rate; AHR – After Heart Rate; RPE – Rate of Perceived Exertion (Scale from 1 to 10); NLP – Number Laps Performed; bpm – beats per minute; min–time in minutes (Test Duration).

Figure 1 shows the limits of agreement between the 400 MF and PSwT. It was observed that most plots were above the 80% considered to be satisfactory and within the IC limits of 95%.

Figure 2 presents the relation between the VO2max estimated by the PSwT and the simulated 400 MF test, highlighting an inverse correlation between the variables.

Discussion

The aim of this study was to verify the existence of an association between the estimated VO2max for non-expert swimmers test (PSwT) and the swimming performance in the simulated 400 meters freestyle test. It was observed, in fact, a connection occurred between the two tests, and we can state that the PSwT is a test with applicability for non-expert adult swimmers.

The BHR, AHR, RPE, and NLP variables (adding the time for conducting the tests) were necessary to the standardization with previous studies regarding the PSwT, since these presented security and consistency in the reproducibility and validity verification[11,12]. These variables were essential to determine the physical condition of these swimmers, and especially HR and RPE, were important in the verification of the state of the swimmers immediately before and after the tests[5,19], in the verification of the longest distance incrementally swum by the swimmer in the PSwT[11], and in the least amount of time in the simulated 400 MF test[1,23].

In the NLP and time needed to perform the test, significant differences were observed, as well as the inverse correlation between the two tests (Table 2), taking into account the fact that the mean time for the 400 MF test was larger than that of the PSwT, and the distance that the swimmers swum to reach VO2max in the PSwT had smaller mean values than those of the 400 MF. This is evidence demonstrating that for non-expert swimmers, a phased test can be better employed than the simulation of a swimming test which references the lesser time swum

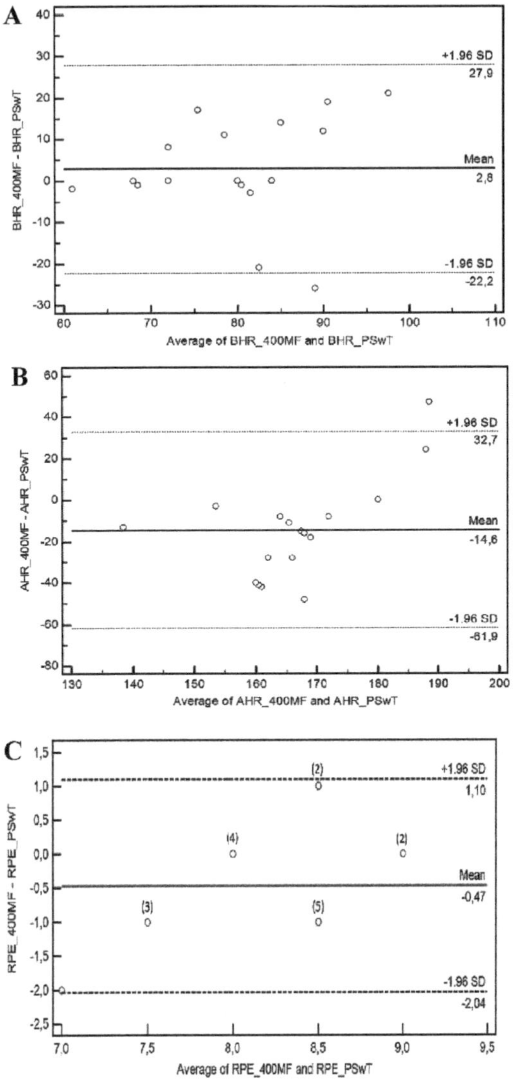

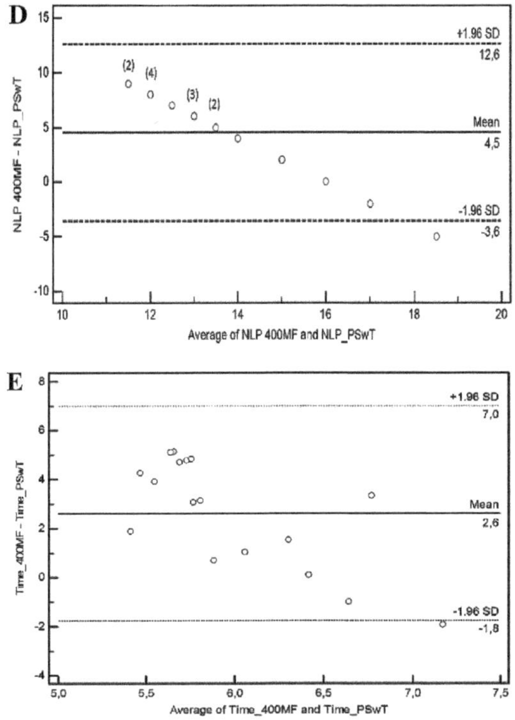

Figure 1–Plot of the bias (average of differences) and limits of agreement (± 1.96, IC 95%) between the variables analyzed from the simulation of the 400 meters freestyle test and the Progressive Swim Test, according to the Bland Altman analysis. Numbers between brackets represent the amount of overlapping results.

Plot of the bias (average of differences) and limits of agreement (± 1.96, IC95%) between the variables analyzed from the simulation of the 400 meters freestyle test and the Progressive Swim Test, according to the Bland Altman analysis. Numbers between brackets represent the amount of overlapping results.

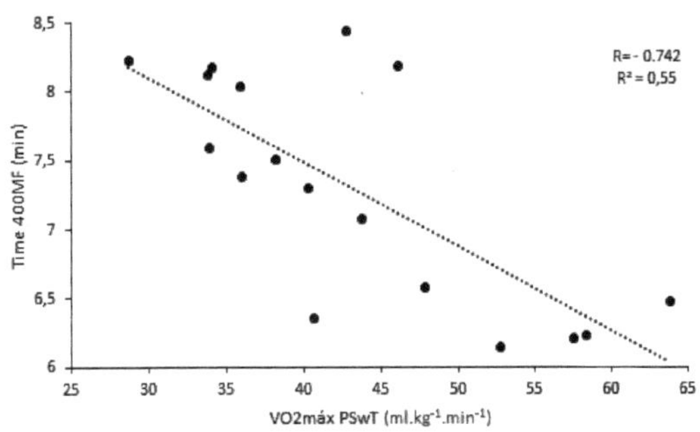

Figure 2–Relation between the VO2max estimated through the Progressive Swim Test and the performance in the 400 meters freestyle test. *$p < 0.01$.

Relation between the VO2max estimated through the Progressive Swim Test and the performance in the 400 meters freestyle test. * $p < 0.01$.

in a certain distance. A swimming test can be a good tool to evaluate competitive swimmers rather than recreational swimmers or for health purposes[11,25-27].

While verifying the reproducibility of the PSwT, Veronese da Costa, Costa, Carlos, Guerra, Silva, Barbosa[11] regarded the NLP as a predictor of the physical conditioning of the non-expert swimmers due to the fact the distance over a predetermined time was used as a criterion for exercise intensity in swimming[11]. By validating the equation which estimates the VO2max using the results obtained in the PSwT (i.e., through NLP, BM in kg and AHR), the test was found to be appropriate for non-expert adult swimmers as a way of assessing physical conditioning[12].

In the simulated 400 MF, it was observed that, even demanding the maximum performance possible, there were alterations in swimming intensity over the course of the test. This also occurred with Laffite, Vilas-Boas, Demarle, Silva, Fernandes, Louise Billat[29]. while analyzing the metabolic and technical parameters during the 400 MF test, noting that trained swimmers, even when controlled by a *visual light pacer* failed to remain stable, and to compensate for the decrease in *stroke length* (SL), increased their *stroke rate* (SR) in the last 100 meters[29]. In the PSwT this did not occur, for at any given moment, when the swimmer reached their threshold, they sought to keep performing at their best until they could not keep up with the increased intensity of the required protocol[11]. This can also be observed when comparing AHR in the 400 MF and the PSWT ($p < 0.01$), where non-expert swimmers reached

78% and 89% of HR_{max} respectively, whereas the swimmer had to be at least at 85% of their HR_{max} taking the VO2max as a parameter[7,28]. This was achieved in the PSWT by verifying the equation for estimating VO2max, with a mean value of 45.59 ± 9.32 ml/kg.min[-1][12].

In regards to the connection between the variables of the 400 MF test and the PSwT, it was not possible to correlate the distance of the simulated test with the NLP due to the fact that the 400 MF is predetermined (i.e., 16 swimming pools), whereas the NLP depends upon the physical conditioning of the swimmer in doing the maximum possible laps in progression[11,30,31]. In the AHR and the performance duration, values greater than $r = -0.60$, CV and SEM below 10% demonstrated that there was a correlation between the variables at the end of the tests and the values which occurred in the Bland Altman plot were within the level of magnitude demanded. However, the results between the 400 MF and the PSwT were inversely proportional, since to perform a simulated test in a shorter time, the non-expert swimmers exacted a level of effort which demanded their anaerobic capacity. At one point in the test, this led to the swimmers presenting a greater capacity for sustaining than the intensity through exercise, causing AHR to not be kept at its maximum[1,24]. During the PSwT, when the swimmer achieved their maximum performance, the test was completed, providing values in AHR and NLP consistent to what we intend to measure, the VO2max. The results obtained in continuous tests (in this case, the simulated 400 MF test) were a major concern in the development of the PSwT, where it was noted the tests which control the intensity of the swim would be advisable for non-expert swimmers[11,12].

As for the connection between the VO2max estimated through the PSwT and the performance in the simulated 400 MF test, the meaningful correlation presented between the variables ($r = -0.79$; $p < 0.01$) confirms the aforementioned test likely offers the same exercise physiological conditions for swimming, corresponding to the VO2max[1,22], with the particularity of accompanying the scaled intensity employed in the non-expert swimmers test[11,12]. Thus, the PSwT was proven reliable when evaluated on different days by different evaluators, presenting possibilities of application in the aquatic environment to be associated with a swimming test[11]. Additionally, it was compared to a direct oximetry method showing the same performance connection[12], and finally its equation was applied to a practical situation through the 400 MF test where using HR, distance, and time to determine the aptitude of non-expert swimmers, both obtained a high association[12,32,33].

The following were considered to be limitations of the study: (i) it was not possible to evaluate the biomechanical aspects during both tests, since when swimmers reached their maximum performance, they suffered alterations in the length and number of strokes; (ii) the results described here are valid only for non-expert swimmers, which means another researcher should refrain from applying this test to elite swimmers; (iii) it was not possible to evaluate the test's sensibility through an exercise program which could then utilize the test to verify aerobic power.

Conclusion

According to these data, the authors determined there is a negative association between a swimming test and a test which estimates the VO2max by verifying that the PSwT presented results of better approximation to the aerobic power of non-expert swimmers. Thus, the Progressive Swim Test is applicable for non-expert adult swimmers, becoming a new assessment tool which will contribute to the creation of more efficient training programs for seeking better physical conditioning of these participants.

References

1. Fernandes R, Vilas-Boas J. Time to Exhaustion at the VO2max Velocity in Swimming: A Review. J Hum Kinet. 2012; 32: 121–34.
2. Raffaelli C, Galvani C, Lanza M, Zamparo P. Different methods for monitoring intensity during water-based aerobic exercises. Eur J Appl Physiol. 2012; 112(1): 125–34.
3. Roschel H, Tricoli V, Ugrinowitsch C. Physical Training: Scientific and Practical Considerations. Rev Bras Educ Física e Esporte. 2011; 25: 53–65.
4. Corazza ST, Katzer JI. Creating and Validating a Test for Measuring Motor Performance of the Crawl Swimming Style. Eur J Cardiothorac Surg Off J Eur Assoc Cardiothorac Surg. 2000; 73(5): 73–8.
5. Michele R Di, Gatta G, Leo A Di, Cortesi M, Andina F, Tam E, et al. Estimation of the Anaerobic Threshold from Heart Rate Variability in an Incremental Swimming Test. J Strength Cond Res . 2012; 26(11): 3059–66.
6. Wakayoshi K, Yoshida T, Udo M, Kasai T, Moritani T, Mutoh Y, et al. A simple method for determining critical speed as swimming fatigue threshold in competitive swimming. Int J Sports Med. 1992; 13(5): 367–71.
7. Ribeiro JP, Cadavid E, Baena J, Monsalvete E, Barna A, De Rose EH. Metabolic predictors of middle-distance swimming performance. Br J Sports Med. 1990; 24(3): 196–200.
8. Fernandes RJ, Cardoso CS, Soares SM, Ascensão A, Colaço PJ, Vilas-Boas JP. Time limit and VO2 slow component at intensities corresponding to VO2max in swimmers. Vol. 24, International journal of sports medicine. 2003.
9. Hue O, Antoine-Jonville S, Galy O, Blonc S. Anthropometric and physiological characteristics in young afro-Caribbean swimmers. A preliminary study. Int J Sports Physiol Perform. 2013;(3):71–8.
10. Léger L, Boucher R. An indirect continuous running multistage field test: the Université de Montréal track test. Can J Appl Sport Sci J Can Des Sci Appl Au Sport. 1980; 5(2): 77–84.
11. Veronese da Costa A, Costa M, Carlos D, Guerra L, Silva A, Barbosa T. Reproducibility of an aerobic endurance test for non-expert swimmers. J Multidiscip Healthc. 2012; 5: 215.
12. Veronese da Costa A, Costa M, Oliveira S, Albuquerque F, Guimarães F, Barbosa T. Validation of an equation for estimating maximal oxygen consumption of nonexpert adult swimmers. Open access J Sport Med. 2013; 4: 19–25.

13. Faul F, Erdfelder E, Lang A-G, Buchner A. G*Power 3: a flexible statistical power analysis program for the social, behavioral, and biomedical sciences. Behav Res Methods. 2007; 39(2): 175–91.
14. Thomas S, Reading J, Shephard RJ. Revision of the Physical Activity Readiness Questionnaire (PAR-Q). Can J Sport Sci J Can des Sci du Sport. 1992; 17(4): 338–45.
15. Montpetit R, Smith H, Boie G. Swimming economy: How to standardize the data to compare swimming proficiency. J Swim Res. 1988; 4(1): 5–8.
16. Silva AJ, Machado Reis V, Marinho D, Carneiro AL, Novaes G, Aidar FJ. Swimming economy: determinant factors and assessment issues. Brazilian J Kinanthropometry Hum Perform. 2006; 8(3): 93–9.
17. Jackson AS, Pollock ML. Generalized equations for predicting body density of men. Br J Nutr. 1978; 40(3): 497.
18. Nevill AM, Metsios GS, Jackson AS, Wang J, Thornton J, Gallagher D. Can we use the Jackson and Pollock equations to predict body density/fat of obese individuals in the 21st century? Int J Body Compos Res. 2008;
19. Borg G, Ljunggren G, Ceci R. The increase of perceived exertion, aches and pain in the legs, heart rate and blood lactate during exercise on a bicycle ergometer. Eur J Appl Physiol Occup Physiol. 1985;4(4):43–9.
20. Wallace LK, Slattery KM, Coutts AJ. The ecological validity and application of the session-RPE method for quantifying training loads in swimming. J Strength Cond Res. 2009 J;23(1): 33–8.
21. Bland JM, Altman DG. Statistical methods for assessing agreement between two methods of clinical measurement. Vol. 1, Lancet. 1986.
22. Morais JE, Costa MJ, Mejias JE, Marinho DA, Silva AJ, Barbosa TM. Validation of predictive equations of the cross-sectional area of the human trunk. Rev Bras Cineantropometria Desempenho Hum. 2011; 13: 461–7.
23. Costill DL, Kovaleski J, Porter D, Kirwan J, Fielding R, King D. Energy expenditure during front crawl swimming: predicting success in middle-distance events. Int J Sports Med. 1985; 6(5): 266–70.
24. Fernandes RJ, Keskinen KL, Colaço P, Querido AJ, Machado LJ, Morais PA, et al. Time limit at V̇O2max velocity in elite crawl swimmers. Int J Sports Med. 2008; 29(2): 145–50.
25. Barbosa TM, Fernandes RJ, Keskinen KL, Vilas-Boas JP. The influence of stroke mechanics into energy cost of elite swimmers. Eur J Appl Physiol. 2008; 103(2): 139–49.
26. Deminice R, Papoti M, Zagatto AM, Prado MV do. Validity of 30 minutes test (T-30) in aerobic capacity, stroke parameters and aerobic performance determination of trained swimmers. Rev Bras Med do Esporte. 2007; 13: 195–9.
27. Figueiredo P, Zamparo P, Sousa A, Vilas-Boas JP, Fernandes RJ. An energy balance of the 200 m front crawl race. Eur J Appl Physiol. 2011; 111(5): 767–77.
28. Castro FA de S, Franken M, Silveira RP, Mota CB. Oxygen consumption in swimming: different methodologies and application possibilities. Brazilian J Sci Mov. 2010; 18(3): 88–93.
29. Laffite LP, Vilas-Boas JP, Demarle A, Silva J, Fernandes R, Louise Billat V. Changes in Physiological and Stroke Parameters During a Maximal 400-m Free Swimming Test in Elite Swimmers. Can J Appl Physiol. 2004; 29(S1): S17–31.
30. Dekerle J, Sidney M, Hespel JM, Pelayo P. Validity and reliability of critical speed, critical stroke rate, and anaerobic capacity in relation to front crawl swimming performances. Int J Sports Med. 2002; 23(2): 93–8.
31. Toubekis AG, Drosou E, Gourgoulis V, Thomaidis S, Douda H, Tokmakidis SP. Competitive performance, training load and physiological responses during tapering in young swimmers. J Hum Kinet. 2013; 8: 125–34.
32. Barbosa TM, Fernandes R, Keskinen KL, Colaço P, Cardoso C, Silva J, et al. Evaluation of the energy expenditure in competitive swimming strokes. Int J Sports Med. 2006; 27(11): 894–9.
33. Zacca R, Wenzel BM, Piccin JS, Marcilio NR, Lopes AL, de Souza Castro FA. Critical velocity, anaerobic distance capacity, maximal instantaneous velocity and aerobic inertia in sprint and endurance young swimmers. Eur J Appl Physiol. 2011; 110(1): 121–31.

Corresponding author

Adalberto Veronese da Costa
Physical Education College, BR 110,Km 48 (Campus, UERN), Costa e Silva Area, Mossoró, RN, Brazil
E-mail: adalberto.ef@gmail.com

20

Psychosocial correlates of organized physical activity in Portuguese urban youth

Adilson Marques
Universidade de Lisboa, Lisboa, Portugal
Universidade Nova de Lisboa, Lisboa, Portugal

Miguel Peralta
Universidade de Lisboa, Lisboa, Portugal

João Martins
Universidade de Lisboa, Lisboa, Portugal
Universidade Lusófona de Humanidades e Tecnologias, Lisboa, Portugal

Hugo Sarmento
Universidade de Coimbra, Coimbra, Portugal

Ash C. Routen
Loughborough University, Loughborough, United Kingdom

Francisco Carreiro da Costa
Universidade de Lisboa, Lisboa, Portugal
Universidade Lusófona de Humanidades e Tecnologias, Lisboa, Portugal

Abstract—This study aimed to explore the association between psychosocial factors and organized physical activity (PA) in urban children and adolescents. Data on organized PA, psychosocial variables, and demographic characteristics were collected via questionnaires. Logistic regression analyses were used to examine the relationship between psychosocial correlates and organized PA. Analyses were run separately for different age groups. Results showed that children and adolescents with a greater positive attitude toward PA were more likely to be involved in organized PA. Ego orientation was associated with organized PA at the age of 13–15 years. Task orientation was related to PA participation at the age of 13–15 and 16–18 years. Perception of competence was related to participation at the age of 10–12 and 13–15 years. These findings suggest that interventions to increase the level of participation in organized PA in youth should focus on increasing students' perceived physical competence, attitude toward PA, and establishing a strong motivational task/mastery climate.

Keywords: adolescents, children, correlates, physical activity

Introduction

Regular participation in physical activity (PA) in childhood is associated with numerous current and future health benefits, including improved bone mineral density, cardiovascular risk profiles, aerobic fitness, mental health, and body composition[1]. Therefore, national and international public health authorities unilaterally recommend that children and adolescents should accumulate at least 60 min or more of moderate-to-vigorous PA (MVPA) every day. However, despite these aforementioned health benefits and well established PA guidelines, recent data shows that the majority of young people are not sufficiently active to benefit their health[2,3]. Alongside, a pervasive finding in the literature is the decline in PA with age from late childhood/ early adolescence[4,5], which may be more marked among girls and those from lower socioeconomic groups[6,7].

It is clear that participation in PA is an important component of a healthy lifestyle[1], and therefore a more comprehensive understanding of the factors and contexts associated with participation in PA in young people is a research priority. The study of psychological and social correlates of PA (e.g., self-perceptions, attitude toward PA and physical education, goal orientation—ego and task orientation and parents' and peers' PA) is important because these are potentially modifiable factors, and could form a theoretical base on which to construct and implement effective programs to improve PA levels[8,9].

A range of psychological variables and their relationship to measures of PA have been extensively examined in the scientific literature[8,9]. For example, review studies in youth populations have shown that attitudes toward PA[10,11] and perception of competence[11,12] are positively correlated with PA in most, but not all cases[8]. Furthermore, positive motivation, best reflected by mastery and task goal orientation[13], has also emerged as a consistent correlate of PA in young people[10–12]. Additionally, findings on the relationship between parents' and children's PA are mixed, but there has been shown to be small and positive associations[14,15]. On the contrary, recent and specific reviews have demonstrated that friends' PA levels appear to have a significant influence on children's PA[16,17].

Acknowledging that PA decreases with age[4,5], it seems pertinent to examine what particular type or subcomponent of PA is most stable with age, and what psychosocial factors are related to this type of PA. Extant studies have shown that children and adolescents with the most stable PA behaviors are those who participate in greater levels of organized PA[18,19]. These investigations have corroborated the results of a longitudinal study by Telama[20] that monitored participants for 21 years and found that participation in organized PA enhanced the likelihood of being physically active as an adult. Nonetheless, despite the substantial evidence base on psychosocial correlates of PA in children, there is little evidence on correlates of organized PA among urban Portuguese children and adolescents. Considering that in recent decades Portugal has undergone a demographic transition from an eminently rural country to one where most of the population lives in urban areas, it is therefore critical to understand the habits of the young people that now are living in urban areas and the correlates of PA participation. Moreover, Portugal is now within a period of economic crisis and therefore understanding how psychosocial factors might be related to young people's organized PA participation in this national context is important.

Therefore the main aim of this cross-sectional study was to examine associations between hypothesized psychosocial correlates and organized PA in Portuguese urban children and adolescents. Based on extant literature, boys, older adolescents and those with a higher socioeconomic status are more likely to be involved in organized PA. Additionally, perceived competence, attitude toward physical activity, task orientation, and parents' and friends' perceived PA might be positively related to adolescent's organized PA.

Method

Participants

The study was conducted in six Portuguese public elementary schools in the urban area of Lisbon. These schools were selected as they are in locations that cover a range of socioeconomic groups, as well as having a range of facilities nearby for the practice of PA. The potential sample included 3315 children and adolescents. Of the 3215 children and adolescents enrolled in schools, 350 did not complete the questionnaire, and 148 were dropped from the analysis for missing gender data and being older than 18 years old. A final response rate of 84.5% was obtained and the sample therefore included 2617 students (1336 boys, 1281 girls) drawn from grade 5 to 12, aged 10–18 years old (13.3±2.5). Informed written consent was obtained from the students and their parents/guardians. The study received institutional ethical approval from the Ethics Committee of Faculty of Human Kinetics of the University of Lisbon.

Measures

Height was measured using a portable stadiometer (recorded to the nearest 0.5 cm). Weight was measured using electronic weighing scales (recorded to the nearest 0.5 kg), with participants wearing shorts and a t-shirt and without shoes. Body mass index (BMI) was calculated by dividing weight in kilograms by height in meters squared.

Socioeconomic status (SES) was assessed via parental occupation. Parents were classified as lower, middle, and upper class. The lower class category included skilled and unskilled manual workers, farmers, and fishermen; the middle class included service occupations such as non-professional health service workers, office clerks, and salespeople; the upper class consisted of business-owners, executives, university-educated specialists and professionals[21].

To determine students' participation in PA, a questionnaire listing 21 leisure time activities including participation in organized and non-organized PA was used. This instrument[22], has been used in a number of national and international studies[23,24]. Responses for participation in leisure time activities were dichotomous (yes or no). Test-retest reliability of the leisure time activity scale was assessed via repeat administrations within a 1-week interval in a sub-sample (n = 100), and was found to be high (ICC = 0.90–0.95). Parents' PA levels were measured using a single item for the mother and father, respectively[25], and responses were dichotomized as follows: "practice every week" or "do not practice." For the measurement of peer PA, students were asked how often their friends practice PA. Answers were given on a five-point scale (1 = never to 5 = daily).

Attitudes were measured using a single item for physical education and PA, respectively, as used in other studies[26,27]: "What do you think about your physical education lessons?," and "What do you think about practicing PA?" Answers were given on a five-point scale ranging from "I dislike it very much" to "I like it very much." These items have displayed high reliability, with intraclass correlation coefficients (1-week interval) of 0.9.

The importance attributed to being popular at school was assessed via two items: "How important is it for you to be popular among boys" and "How important is for you to be popular among girls" as used before in another study[25]. Responses were given using a five-point Likert scale. These items displayed high reliability, with intraclass correlation coefficients (1-week interval) of 0.9 for both questions. The internal consistency (Cronbach's alpha) of both items was acceptable ($\alpha = 0.7$) and a new variable was computed to create a popularity index.

Sports goal orientation was measured using the 12-item Task and Ego Orientation in Sport Questionnaire[28]. Answers were given using a four-point scale and good Cronbach's alpha coefficients were obtained for both ego ($\alpha = 0.9$) and task ($\alpha = 0.9$) subscales.

Physical competence was measured by Lintunen's Perceived Physical Competence Scale[29]. The six-items, using a five-point Likert scale, demonstrated good internal consistency ($\alpha = 0.9$). Perception of body image and perception of health were measured by a scale taken from a WHO study[26]. Perception of body image was assessed via three items, using a five-point Likert scale, and the internal consistency was acceptable ($\alpha = 0.7$). Student's perception of health status was assessed via a four-point scale ranging from "I am not feeling well" (= 1) to "I am very healthy" (= 4).

Statistical analysis

The sample was divided into three age groups, based on known developmental changes in adolescents[30]. Descriptive statistics were calculated for all variables in each age group, included percentages for nominal variables and mean and standard deviations for ordinal or scale variables. Chi-square and ANOVA tests were used to assess differences among age groups. The effect of the variables on organized PA participation was assessed using binary logistic regression. Adjusted odds ratio (OR) with 95% confidence intervals (CI) were calculated. Adjustments were performed for all studied variables. An OR greater than 1 reflects an increased likelihood of participation in organized PA. The analyses were stratified by age groups to evaluate potential differences. All statistical analyses were performed using IBM SPSS Statistics 20.0. The level of significance was set at 0.05.

Results

Table 1 summarizes the sample size and distribution as well as descriptive statistics for all measured variables according to age groups. More than half of the participants (56.5%) reported practicing organized PA. As age increased, the number of physically active participants decreased ($p < 0.001$). There were significant differences among age groups for attitude toward physical education, importance attributed to being popular among peers, and ego and task orientation.

Table 1. Descriptive characteristics by age group.

	Total		10–12 years		13–15 years		16–18 years		*p*[a]
	n	%	n	%	n	%	n	%	
Gender[b]									
Girls	1281	48.9	592	50.4	434	48,5	255	46.5	0.316
Boys	1336	51.1	583	49.6	460	51.5	293	53.5	
BMI[b]									
< 25	2069	79.1	936	79.7	675	75.5	458	83.6	0.069
25–29.9	145	5.5	56	4.8	44	4.9	45	8.2	
≥30	29	1.1	12	1.0	13	1.5	4	0.7	
SES[b]									
Low	722	27.6	412	35.1	206	23.0	104	19.0	<0.001
Medium	1187	45.4	531	45.2	422	47.2	234	42.7	
High	29	27.1	232	19.7	266	29.8	210	38.3	
Organized PA[b]									
Yes	1478	56.5	712	60.6	496	55.5	270	49.3	<0.001
No	1139	43.5	463	39.4	398	44.5	278	50.7	
Father PA[b]									
Yes	598	22.9	291	24.8	181	20.2	126	23.0	0.004
No	1678	64.1	688	58.6	609	68.1	381	69.5	
Mother PA[b]									
Yes	493	18.8	248	21.1	153	17.1	92	16.8	0.001
No	1839	70.3	750	63.8	664	74.3	425	77.6	
Peers PA[c]									
Never	49	1.9	23	2.0	17	1.9	9	1.6	<0.001
Sometimes	555	21.2	216	18.4	175	19.6	164	29.9	
Usually	1155	44.1	490	41.7	395	44.2	270	49.3	
Frequently	551	21.1	277	23.6	194	21.7	80	14.6	
Daily	291	11.1	162	13.8	106	11.9	23	4.2	
			M ± SD (min–max)						
Attitude toward PE	4.0±1.0 (1-5)		4.2±1.0 (1-5)		4.0±0.9 (1-5)		3.6±1.1 (1-5)		<0.001
Attitude toward PA	4.0±0.9 (1-5)		4.0±0.9 (1-5)		4.0±0.9 (1-5)		4.1±0.8 (1-5)		0.794
Popularity	2.4±0.9 (1-4)		2.4±0.9 (1-4)		2.5±0.8 (1-4)		2.3±0.8 (1-4)		0.004
Ego orientation	2.2±1.2 (1-4)		2.3±1.2 (1-4)		2.1±1.2 (1-4)		1.9±1.2 (1-4)		<0.001
Task orientation	2.7±1.4 (1-4)		2.8±1.3 (1-4)		2.7±1.4 (1-4)		2.6±1.5 (1-4)		0.040
Perception of competence	3.5±0.8 (1-5)		3.5±0.8 (1-5)		3.5±0.8 (1-5)		3.5±0.8 (1-5)		0.231
Perception of body image	3.5±0.8 (1-5)		3.5±0.8 (1-5)		3.5±0.8 (1-5)		3.4±0.8 (1-5)		0.165
Perception of health	3.1±1.0 (1-4)		3.1±1.0 (1-4)		3.1±1.0 (1-4)		3.0±0.8 (1-4)		0.196

BMI, body mass index; SES, socioeconomic status; PA, physical activity; PE, physical education

[a]Analysis of differences among age groups

[b]Tested by chi-square

[c]Tested by ANOVA

Table 2 presents the results for the crude logistic binary regression analysis. Girls were almost 50% less likely to participate in organized PA than boys in every age group. The medium SES was only related to adolescents' organized PA for those in the age 16–18 years group (OR = 2.11, 95% CI: 1.31–3.40, p = 0.002), while high SES was related to organized PA participation in the younger (OR = 1.43, 95% CI: 1.03–2.00, p = 0.035) and older (OR = 1.88, 95% CI: 1.16–3.05, p = 0.011) age groups. Perceived father PA (OR = 1.64, 95% CI: 1.23–2.20, p = 0.001) and mother PA (OR = 1.60, 95% CI: 1.20–2.20, p = 0.003) was positively related to organized PA for the younger age group. However, for the age 13–15 years group, only perceived mother PA was related to organized PA of adolescents (OR = 1.77, 95% CI: 1.23–2.56, p = 0.002), and in the age 16–18 years group only fathers PA was significantly related (OR = 1.83, 95% CI: 1.21–2.76, p = 0.004). As for the rest of the variables, all were positively related to organized PA in all age groups, with the strongest correlations found for attitude toward PA (OR = 2.48, 95% CI: 1.93–3.20, p < 0.001) and perceived physical competence (OR = 2.11, 95% CI: 1.64–2.72, p < 0.001) in the age 16–18 years group.

Table 2. Unadjusted logistic regression models examining correlates of PA by age groups.

	10–12 years	**13–15 years**	**16–18 years**
	Crude OR (95% CI)	**Crude OR (95% CI)**	**Crude OR (95% CI)**
Gender			
Boys	1.00 (ref)	1.00 (ref)	1.00 (ref)
Girls	0.51 (0.40-0.65)***	0.54 (0.41-0.71)***	0.53 (0.38-0.74)***
BMI			
< 25	1.00 (ref)	1.00 (ref)	1.00 (ref)
25-29.9	0.70 (0.41-1.21)	0.99 (0.54-1.83)	0.54 (0.29-1.03)
≥30	1.22 (0.36-4.10)	0.88 (0.29-2.64)	0.33 (0.03-3.17)
SES			
Low	1.00 (ref)	1.00 (ref)	1.00 (ref)
Medium	1.19 (0.92-1.54)	0.90 (0.64-1.25)	2.11 (1.31-3.40)**
High	1.43 (1.03-2.00)*	1.30 (0.90-1.90)	1.88 (1.16-3.05)*
Father PA			
No	1.00 (ref)	1.00 (ref)	1.00 (ref)
Yes	1.64 (1.23-2.20)***	1.28 (0.91-1.79)	1.83 (1.21-2.76)**
Mother PA			
No	1.00 (ref)	1.00 (ref)	1.00 (ref)
Yes	1.60 (1.20-2.20)**	1.77 (1.23-2.56)**	1.50 (0.95-2.37)
Peers PA	1.26 (1.12-1.41)***	1.37 (1.19-1.57)***	1.59 (1.28-1.97)***
Attitude toward PE	1.53 (1.34-1.73)***	1.41 (1.22-1.63)***	1.24 (1.07-1.45)**
Attitude toward PA	1.90 (1.64-2.19)***	2.27 (1.91-2.70)***	2.48 (1.93-3.20)***
Importance of being popular	1.20 (1.05-1.37)**	1.29 (1.10-1.52)**	1.38 (1.11-1.71)**
Ego orientation	1.62 (1.50-1.80)***	1.89 (1.67-2.15)***	1.85 (1.57-2.19)***
Task orientation	1.60 (1.45-1.76)***	1.77 (1.58-1.98)***	1.90 (1.63-2.21)***
Perception of competence	1.82 (1.55-2.13)***	2.03 (1.67-2.13)***	2.11 (1.64-2.72)***
Perception of body image	1.31 (1.14-1.51)***	1.33 (1.13-1.51)**	1.56 (1.24-1.95)***
Perception of health	1.19 (1.06-1.34)**	1.30 (1.14-1.50)***	1.60 (1.29-1.99)***

BMI, body mass index; SES, socioeconomic status; PA, physical activity; PE, physical education
*$p < 0.05$, **$p < 0.01$, ***$p < 0.001$

Table 3 shows results of the adjusted logistic binary regression analysis. Biological and demographic variables (gender, BMI and SES) were not related to organized PA participation in all age groups, or father and mother PA participation. Reported peer PA was related to adolescents' organized PA in the age 16–18 years group (OR = 1.35, 95% CI: 1.01–1.81, $p = 0.045$), while there was no relationship in the other two younger age groups. Children and adolescents with higher attitude scores were more likely to be involved in organized PA. This variable was correlated to organized activities in all age groups. Ego orientation was significantly associated with adolescents' organized PA in the age 13–15 years group (OR = 1.40, 95% CI: 1.00–1.94, $p = 0.047$). Moreover, task orientation was also related to PA participation in the age 13–15 years group (OR = 1.36, 95% CI: 1.03–1.79, $p = 0.030$), and the age 16–18 years group (OR = 2.14, 95% CI: 1.54–2.97, $p < 0.001$). Finally, perception of competence was related to participation in both the age 10–12 years (OR = 1.42, 95% CI: 1.07–1.88, $p = 0.016$) and the age 13–15 years group (OR = 1.72, 95% CI: 1.19–2.47, $p = 0.004$).

Table 3. Adjusted logistic regression models examining correlates of PA by age groups.

	10–12 years	13–15 years	16–18 years
	Adjusted OR (95% CI)	**Adjusted OR (95% CI)**	**Adjusted OR (95% CI)**
Gender			
Boys	1.00 (ref)	1.00 (ref)	1.00 (ref)
Girls	0.77 (0.55-1.88)	1.37 (0.91-2.07)	0.86 (0.51-1.45)
BMI			
< 25	1.00 (ref)	1.00 (ref)	1.00 (ref)
25-29.9	0.58 (0.29-1.17)	1.58 (0.71-3.51)	1.06 (0.45-2.46)
≥30	1.52 (0.31-7.46)	0.97 (0.21-4.47)	0.30 (0.02-5.36)
SES			
Low	1.00 (ref)	1.00 (ref)	1.00 (ref)
Medium	1.00 (0.69-1.43)	0.79 (0.49-1.29)	1.70 (0.91-3.17)
High	1.07 (0.69-1.67)	1.11 (0.66-1.87)	1.61 (0.84-3.10)
Father PA			
No	1.00 (ref)	1.00 (ref)	1.00 (ref)
Yes	1.20 (0.80-1.75)	0.82 (0.50-1.33)	1.32 (0.77-2.29)
Mother PA			
No	1.00 (ref)	1.00 (ref)	1.00 (ref)
Yes	1.15 (0.77-1.74)	1.51 (0.89-2.55)	1.14 (0.61-2.11)
Peers PA	1.09 (0.91-1.29)	1.09 (0.89-1.34)	1.35 (1.01-1.81)*
Attitude toward PE	1.14 (0.93-1.39)	0.99 (0.78-1.26)	0.85 (0.67-1.07)
Attitude toward PA	1.45 (1.16-1.82)**	1.95 (1.49-2.56)***	1.89 (1.34-2.67)***
Importance of being popular	0.86 (0.70-1.05)	1.08 (0.83-1.40)	1.18 (0.86-1.62)
Ego orientation	1.17 (0.87-1.58)	1.40 (1.00-1.94)*	0.72 (0.48-1.09)
Task orientation	1.27 (0.97-1.65)	1.36 (1.03-1.79)*	2.14 (1.54-2.97)***
Perception of competence	1.42 (1.07-1.88)*	1.72 (1.19-2.47)**	1.10 (0.70-1.72)
Perception of body image	0.79 (0.61-1.03)	0.91 (0.67-1.23)	1.18 (0.81-1.71)
Perception of health	1.04 (0.88-1.24)	1.00 (0.81-1.23)	1.18 (0.87-1.59)

BMI, body mass index; SES, socioeconomic status; PA, physical activity; PE, physical education
*$p < 0.05$, **$p < 0.01$, ***$p < 0.001$

Discussion

This study examined correlates associated with the children and adolescents' organized PA. Three major findings appeared. First, attitude toward PA was the only variable associated with organized PA across all age groups. Second, perception of physical competence was related to organized PA participation among children and younger adolescents. Third, gender and SES were not related to organized PA participation.

The prevalence of organized PA participation was close to 50% of the total sample. It was also found that PA participation decreased with age, confirming the decline observed in previous studies and so often referred to in the literature[4,5].

In the initial crude analysis, gender was correlated to organized PA. However, when the model was adjusted for all variables, gender was no longer a significant correlate. The difference in these findings between our study and other studies[9] might be related to the context of PA participation. Most previous studies measured total PA levels, and did not consider participation in a particular context. Specific to the particular context of organized PA, findings from existing literature do not show a pattern, as some studies show gender as a significant correlate[31], and others show that girls are less involved in organized PA[32].

Numerous studies report SES as a correlate of youth PA[31,33], while others conversely show no relationship[11]. The findings are inconsistent and do not present a clear picture regarding SES and PA in children and adolescents. The discrepancies in findings between studies might reflect the organization of sport/leisure activities in different countries. In some countries, participation in certain sporting activities is subject to payment of a fee, whereas in other countries participation is free of charge. Our results demonstrate in the crude analyses at least that medium and high SES was positively related to organized PA. Nonetheless, when the model was adjusted this association was no longer significant. It seems that SES in the presence of other psychosocial variables is not a strong correlate of organized PA.

Based on the social cognitive model[34] it is sensible to suggest that parental behavior presents a model for children's behavior. Crude analysis supported this idea, though it was not observed when the model was adjusted for all other variables. Although parents as role models have influence in their children's behavior, a review of correlates showed that parental PA practice is not related to their child's PA[8]. However, parents can influence their children to practice PA in other ways, such as logistic support, fees payment, and encouragement. These types of family support are likely to be related to the acquisition and maintenance of regular PA participation during childhood and adolescence.

Peers' PA remained a significant as predictor of organized PA participation for the older age group. As children and adolescents grow up, the influence of peers in their lives increases, while conversely, parental influence likely decreases[33].

In the unadjusted and adjusted model, attitude toward PA was one of the strongest correlates. In a previous study it was reported that attitude toward PA was positively related to school sport participation[36]. It appears therefore that young people who have a positive attitude toward PA are more willing to participate in PA regardless of the context. This is an important finding, and thus programs supporting positive attitudes toward PA are necessary to optimize PA adoption and adherence as a means to combat physical inactivity in childhood and adolescence. Attitude toward physical education was only related to older adolescents' organized PA. Previous research has indicated that adolescents who have positive attitudes toward PA and PE are reported to be more likely to participate in PA outside of school and demonstrate higher PA levels than those with less positive attitudes[37].

Ego and task orientation were predictors of organized PA. Both goals orientations were positively related to organized PA because they are orthogonal constructs, meaning that an individual can be both ego- and task-oriented. Studies have demonstrated that achievement goals have implications in youth sport involvement[38]. Ego orientation predisposes individuals to use an achievement situation as an opportunity to demonstrate their ability in front of others[39]. Considering that in the crude analysis, perception of competence and the importance attributed to being popular were also predictors of organized PA participation, it is understandable that ego orientation was found to be related to organized PA. However, task orientation is associated with intrinsic motivation and is considered a good predictor of PA involvement[28,40]. Our results showed that adolescents' organized PA participation could be predicted by task orientation. Therefore, educators, coach and parents should encourage adolescents to enhance task orientation, and value participation as much as the outcome.For the two younger age groups, perception of competence was significantly correlated with organized PA. It is considered an important facilitator of PA[41], and thus physical self-concept should be enhanced among children and adolescents. Physical education teachers and PA professionals should therefore focus their pedagogical interventions on increasing students' perceived competence and establishing a strong motivational task/mastery climate.

Importance of being popular, perception of body image, and perception of health had no relation with organized PA in the adjusted analyses. This suggests that children and adolescents' reasons for participating in organized PA are independent of their self-rated health and body image. However, in the crude analyses these variables were positively related to organized PA participation. It is plausible that when the model was adjusted, the perception of competence and attitude toward PA retained the variance explained by these variables, confirming the importance of these constructs for PA participation among children and adolescents[42].

Some limitations of the present study should be acknowledged. The cross-sectional design impedes the inference of causality in the relationships examined. Data from participation in organized PA were collected via self-report rather than via objective methods, e.g., accelerometry. Although the PA questions have previously been demonstrated to be both reliable and valid, they could be subject to bias due to recall error, for example. Participants were from schools in urban areas. This limits the variability in participation in organized PA settings and the ability to generalize to other locations, particularly rural areas. Despite its limitations, this study also contributes data to the literature regarding the prevalence of organized PA participation among children and adolescents from urban areas. Moreover, a strength of this study was the separate analysis of correlates among different age groups that may be related to children and adolescents' developmental changes.

Conclusion

The present study highlights different correlates of organized PA among different age groups of children and adolescents. Attitude toward PA was a factor correlated with organized PA throughout the different age groups examined. The PA participation of the adolescents aged 13–15 years was related to ego and task orientation, and perception of competence. For older adolescents aged 16–18 years, task orientation and a positive attitude toward physical education predicted organized PA participation. Gender and SES were not related to organized PA participation. These findings suggest that intervention to increase the level of participation in organized PA of children and adolescents should considered different strategies according to age group. The emphasis on which factors to target and the methods by which they are addressed should be modified according to the age groups.

References

1. Janssen I, Leblanc A. Systematic review of the health benefits of physical activity and fitness in school-aged children and youth. Int J Behav Nutr Phys Act. 2010; 7(40): 2-16.
2. Baptista F, Santos D, Silva A, Mota J, Santos R, Vale S, Ferreira J, Raimundo A, Moreira H, Sardinha LB. Prevalence of the Portuguese population attaining sufficient physical activity. Med Sci Sports Exerc. 2012; 44(3): 466-473.
3. Currie C, Zanotti C, Morgan A, Currie D, Looze M, RobertsC, Samdal O, Smith O, Barnekow V. Social determinants ofhealth and well-being among young people. Health Behaviourin School-aged Children (HBSC) study: international reportfrom the 2009/2010 survey Vol. Health Policy for Children andAdolescents, No. 6. Copenhagen: WHO Regional Office forEurope. 2012.
4. Cairney J, Veldhuizen S, Kwan M, Hay J, Faught BE. Biological Age and Sex-Related Declines in Physical Activity during Adolescence. Med Sci Sports Exerc. 2013; 46(4): 730-735.
5. Seabra A, Maia J, Mendonca D, Thomis M, Caspersen C, Fulton J. Age and sex differences in physical activity of Portuguese adolescents. Med Sci Sports Exerc. 2008; 40(1): 65-70.

6. Stalsberg R, Pedersen A. Effects of socioeconomic status on the physical activity in adolescents: a systematic review of the evidence. Scand J Med Sci Sports. 2010; 20(3): 368–383.
7. Telama R, Nupponen H, Rimpela A, Pere L. Secular trends in youth physical activity and parents' socioeconomic status from 1977 to 2005. Pediatr Exerc Sci. 2009; 21(4): 462-474.
8. Bauman A, Reis R, Sallis J, Wells J, Loos R, Martin B. Correlates of physical activity: why are some people physically active and others not? Lancet. 2012; 380(9838): 258-271.
9. Uijtdewilligen L, Nauta J, Singh A, Van Mechelen W, Twisk J, Van der Horst K, Chinapaw M. Determinants of physical activity and sedentary behavior in young people: a review and quality synthesis of prospective studies. Br J Sports Med. 2011; 45(11): 896-905.
10. Van der Horst K, Chin M, Twisk J, Van Mechelen W. A brief review on correlates of physical activity and sedentariness in youth Med Sci Sports Exerc. 2007; 39(8): 1241-1250.
11. Sallis J, Prochaska J, Taylor W. A review of correlates of physical activity of children and adolescents. Med Sci Sports Exerc. 2000; 32(5): 963-975.
12. Biddle S, Atkin A, Cavill N, Foster C. Correlates of physical activity in youth: a review of quantitative systematic reviews. Int Rev Sport Exerc Psychol. 2011; 4(1): 25-49.
13. Papaioannou, A., Zourbanos, N., Krommidas, C., & Ampatzoglou, G. The place of achievement goals in the social context of sport: a comparison of Nicholls' and Eliiot's models. In G. Roberts & D. Treasure (Eds.), Advances in Motivation in sport and exercise. 2012; (pp. 59-90). Champaign, IL: Human Kinetics.
14. Edwardson C, Gorely T. Parental influences on different types and intensities of physical activity in youth: A systematic review. Psychol Sport Exerc. 2010; 11(6): 522-535.
15. Gustafson S, Rhodes R. Parental correlates of physical activity in children and early adolescents. Sports Med. 2006; 36(1): 79-97.
16. Maturo C, Cunningham S. Influence of friends on children's physical activity: A review. Am J Public Health. 2013; 103(7): e23-e38.
17. Sawka K, McCormack G, Nettel-Aguirre A, Hawe P, Doyle-BakerP. Friendship networks and physical activity and sedentary behavior among youth: a systematized review. Int J Behav Nutr Phys Act. 2013; 10(1): 130-139.
18. Guagliano J, Rosenkranz R, Kolt G. Girls' physical activity levels during organised sports in Australia. Med Sci Sports Exerc. 2013; 45(1): 116-122.
19. Wichstrom L, von Soest T, Kvalem IL. Predictors of growth and decline in leisure time physical activity from adolescence to adulthood. Health Psychol. 2013; 32(7): 775-784.
20. Telama R, Yang X, Hirvensalo M, Raitakari O. Participation in organised youth sport as a predictor of adult physical activity: a 21-year longitudinal study. Pediatr Exerc Sci. 2006; 18(1): 76-88.
21. Raudsepp L, Viira R. Sociocultural correlates of physical activity in adolescents. Pediatr Exerc Sci. 2000; 12(1): 51-60.
22. Telama R, Naul R, Nupponen H, Rychtecky A, Vuolle P. (2002). Physical fitness, sporting lifestyles and olympic ideals: Crosscultural studies on youth sport in Europe. Schorndorf: Verlag Karl Hofmann.
23. Mota J, Almeida M, Santos R, José Ribeiro J, Santos M. Association of perceived environmental characteristics and participation in organised and non-organised physical activities of adolescents. Pediatr Exerc Sci. 2009; 21(2): 233-239.
24. Telama R, Nupponen H, Piéron M. Physical activity among young people in the context of lifestyle. Eur Phys Educ Rev. 2005; 11(2): 115-137.
25. Piéron M, Telama R, Naul R, Almond L. Etude du style de vie d'adolescents européens. Considérations théoriques, objetifs et méthodologie de recherche. Sports. 1997; 159/160: 43-50.
26. Aaro L, Wold B, Kannas L, Rimpela M. Health Behaviour in Schoolchildren. A WHO Cross-national Survey. Health Promot In. 1986; 1(1): 17-33.
27. Delfosse C, Ledent M, Carreiro da Costa F, Telama R, Almond L, Cloes M, Piéron M. Les attitudes de jeunnes européens à l'égard de l'école et du cours d'éducation physique. Sports. 1997; 159/160: 96-105.
28. Duda J. The relationship between task and ego orientation and the perceived purpose of sport among male and female high school athletes. J Sport Exerc Psychol. 1989; 11(3): 318–335.
29. Lintunen T. Perceived physical competence scale for children. Scand J Sports Sci. 1987; 9: 57-64.
30. Kail R. (2006). Children and their development. London: Pearson Education.
31. Garcia Bengoechea E, Sabiston CM, Ahmed R, Farnoush M.Exploring links to unorganised and organised physical activity during adolescence: the role of gender, socioeconomic status, weight status, and enjoyment of physical education. Res Q Exercise Sport. 2010; 81(1): 7-16.
32. Vilhjalmsson R, Kristjansdottir G. Gender differences in physical activity in older children and adolescents: the central role of organized sport. Soc Sci Med. 2003; 56(2): 363-374.
33. Seabra A, Mendonca D, Thomis M, Malina R, Maia J. Correlates of physical activity in Portuguese adolescents from 10 to 18 years. Scand J Med Sci Sports. 2011; 21(2): 318-323.
34. Bandura A. (1986). Social foundations of thought and action: A social cognitive theory. Englewood Cliffs, NJ: Prentice Hall.
35. Davison K, Jago R. Change in parent and peer support across ages 9 to 15 yr and adolescent girls' physical activity. Med Sci Sports Exerc. 2009; 41(9): 1816-1825.
36. Marques A, Martins J, Santos F, Sarmento H, Carreiro da Costa F. Correlates of school sport participation: a cross-sectional study in urban Portuguese students. Sci Sports. 2013; 29(4): 31-38.
37. Chung M, Phillips DA. The relationship between attitude toward physical education and leisure-time exercise in high school students. Physical Educator. 2002; 59(3): 126-138.
38. Xiang P, McBride RE, Bruene A, Liu Y. Achievement goal orientation patterns and fifth graders' motivation in physical education running programs. Pediatr Exerc Sci, (2007); 19(2): 179-191.
39. Hanrahan S, Cerin E. Gender, level of participation, and type of sport: differences in achievement goal orientation and attributional style. J Sci Med Sport. 2009; 12(4): 508-512.
40. Duda J. Motivation in sport settings: A goal perspective approach. In G. Roberts (Ed.), Motivation in sport and exercise. 1992; (pp. 57-92). Champaign, IL: Human Kinetics.
41. Welk GJ, Eklund B. Validation of the children and youth physical self-perceptions profile for young children. Psychol Sport Exerc. 2005; 6(1): 51-65.

42. Barr-Anderson D, Young D, Sallis J, Neumark-Sztainer D, Gittelsohn J, Webber L, Saunders R, Cohen S, Jobe J. Structured physical activity and psychosocial correlates in middle-school girls. Prev Med. 2007; 44(5):404-409.

Corresponding author

Adilson Marques
CIPER, Faculdade de Motricidade Humana,
Universidade de Lisboa, Estrada da Costa,
Cruz Quebrada, Portugal
Email: amarques@fmh.ulisboa.pt

Building an urban park increases the intention of adults to practice physical activity

Raphaelly Machado Felix
Vinicius Martins Farias
Mauren Lúcia de Araújo Bergmann
Gabriel Gustavo Bergmann
Universidade Federal do Pampa, Uruguaiana, RS, Brasil

Abstract — Physical activity levels in adults are low and strategies should be put in place to change this. The aim of this study was to investigate whether building an urban park can increase adult neighborhood residents' intentions to partake in physical activity. In total, 395 adults living near where the park was being built participated in the study. The following information was collected: sociodemographic characteristics, current physical activity levels, and intention to use the park for physical activity. Around 80% of the subjects intended to use the park for physical activity. This frequency was higher among those who were classified as physically active and gradually higher as the distance between the home of the subject and the park decreased ($p < 0.05$). The offer of a public leisure space can contribute positively to changing population behavior related to regular physical activity.

Keywords: physical Activity, leisure activity, urban parks

Introduction

It has been largely reported that regular practice of physical activity provides health benefits[1–5]. Despite evidence of the benefits of exercise, the prevalence of physical inactivity is high in Brazil and other developed countries, regardless of gender, age, socioeconomic status, and education[3]. Therefore, strategies should be developed to offer the population the opportunity to access and practice physical activity[2,3].

Urban parks are examples of public spaces that can be used for active recreation. Evidence indicates that the presence of these spaces contributes to increasing the physical activity level of the neighborhood residents[6,7]. However, it is important to highlight that the functional and physical characteristics of neighborhood parks can influence the choices and possibilities of leisure of individuals, but do not ensure their use for physical activity[8–10].

An important characteristic that has been identified is the inverse association between the distance from parks and their use for physical activity[11,12]. Although in Brazil some such efforts are being undertaken, information on this is scarce and mainly derived from large cities: there are no records of studies related to smaller cities[13]. Furthermore, the evidence available is from studies analyzing physical activity in existing urban and neighborhood parks. We have no knowledge of studies that have examined the effects of the construction of new public spaces for leisure on the intention of adults for using it for physical activity. This study investigated if the construction of an urban park with leisure purposes can contribute to increasing the intention of neighborhood residents to practice physical activity regularly.

Methods

Population and sample

An analytical observational population-based study was conducted with adult subjects (18–64 years old) from the city of Uruguaiana, Brazil, living in the Ipiranga neighborhood, where the completion of the Sports and Culture Park was expected by April 2015. The park was to be a large public space (1034.46 square meters of built area) with numerous recreational possibilities, including: sports court (indoor); skateboarding facilities; outdoor gym; walking path; running track; playground; table games area; reading areas; and venues for cultural events.

The following characteristics were considered for sampling: a) total neighborhood population of 5,328 individuals aged 18–64 years (Census, 2010); b) 95% confidence interval (CI 95%); c) acceptable sampling error of five percentage points; d) prevalence of 50%, and e) 10% increase to compensate for possible losses and refusals. After the adoption of these criteria, 395 individuals were selected.

The selection process was carried out in a multiphase probabilistic way. The six blocks distributed around the park were considered. All houses in the first block (which are located in parallel streets and facing the park) were selected. In the second block the selection process of the houses took place alternately, i.e., when a house was selected, the house immediately next door was left out of the study, and then the next one was again selected. The procedure was the same for the third, fourth, fifth, and sixth blocks: after selecting the first house, the next two, three, four, and five houses were disregarded, respectively. For the streets perpendicular to the park the selection criteria of the houses was the same as for the parallel streets, i.e., alternately and increasing the number of homes not selected as the distance from the park increases. When there was refusal to participate in the study, the house next door was automatically selected, starting the selection procedure of the nearby homes from this house. All individuals meeting the inclusion criteria from the selected households were invited to participate in the study, regardless of the number of people living in each house. The criteria for selecting the first house were: the researcher was positioned in front of the entrance gate of the park, the first house (corner) of the block to the right of the park was selected. This study was reviewed and approved by the Ethics Committee of the Federal University of Pampa (protocol number: 840.171).

Approach

The houses selected were visited on weekdays and weekends between 14:00 and 20:00. The researchers presented the objectives, procedures, and criteria for participation in the study. The subjects were interviewed after the explanation and the delivery of the free consent terms, receiving their agreement to sign the document and meeting all the inclusion criteria. The inclusion criteria were to reside next to the Sports and Culture Park in Uruguaiana/RS (up to six blocks away) and to be within the age group of interest (18–64 years old). Exclusion criteria were not being able to perform physical activity because of physical disabilities (self-declared) and having any cognitive limitations that made them unable to answer the instrument questions (cognitive limitations characterized as indicated by a relative, guardian or caregiver).

Variables and data collection instruments

The instrument for data collection consisted of demographic and socioeconomic information, and current practice and intention of practicing physical activity. The demographic information collected was gender (male or female), age (years complete). and distance from the Sports and Culture Park (less than a block away, one, two, three, four, five, or six blocks). Socioeconomic information included family income (number of minimum wages) and education (incomplete primary education, complete primary education, incomplete secondary education, complete secondary education, incomplete higher education and college degree). In order to measure physical activity levels the long version of the International Physical Activity Questionnaire (IPAQ) was used[14]. For the analysis the only information used was from the leisure time physical activity and the results were categorized into two groups: subjects with less than 150 minutes of moderate to vigorous physical activity per week (<150 MVPA) and those with 150 or more minutes of moderate to vigorous physical activity per week (≥150 MVPA).

In order to identify the intention of practicing physical activity a tool for behavior change stages was used[15]. Briefly, the individuals who claimed to practice regular physical activity or not (yes or no) were identified. In case of a positive response, whether the practice has being carried out for more or less than six months was ascertained. In case of negative answer, whether there was an intention to begin or not was ascertained. If so, whether there was an intention to begin within the next 30 days or not. In addition, a question of intention to practice physical activity in the Sports and Culture Park (after the completion of its construction) was inserted.

Data analysis

Variables were initially described using mean and standard deviation (age), and absolute and relative frequencies (other variables) followed by interval confidence of 95% (IC95%). To test the possible association between physical activity levels, distance from the park and the intention of using it (after its completion) for the practice of physical activity, the chi-square test was used for heterogeneity and trend, respectively. To test these associations adjusted for sex, age, socioeconomic status. and educational level, binary logistic regression was used. The significance level adopted was 0.05 and all analyses were performed using SPSS software version 20.0.

Results

The description of the variables analyzed is presented in Table 1. An average age of 42.05 years old was observed, the majority of the sample were female (64.3%). and 77.7% of the subjects were not sufficiently active in leisure activities. Just over one-quarter of the sample stated they were active. However, 78.5% planned to practice physical activities in the Sports and Culture Park. Many of the samples claimed to live with one minimum wage and more than one-third did not complete elementary school.

Table 1. Description of the variables analyzed from adults aged between 18–65 years, living in the city of Uruguaiana (Brazil) near the Sports and Culture Park.

Variable	N	% (CI95%)
Gender		
Female	254	64,3 (58,4-70,2)
Male	141	35,7 (27,8-43,6)
Age	395	X=42,05 (SD=13,880)
Household income		
Less than one minimum wage	15	3,8 (0-13,50)
One minimum wage	169	42,8 (35,3-50,3)
Two minimum wages	134	33,9 (25,9-41,9)
Three minimum wages	53	13,4 (4,2-22,6)
Four minimum wages	21	5,3 (0,43-14,9)
Five minimum wages or more	3	0,8 (0-10,9)

Variable	N	% (CI95%)
Education level		
Incomplete primary education	155	39,2 (31,5-46,9)
Complete primary education	71	18,0 (9,1-26,9)
Incomplete secondary education	35	8,9 (0-18,3)
Complete secondary education	103	26,7 (17,6-34,6)
Incomplete higher education	17	4,3 (0-13,9)
College Degree	14	3,5 (0-13,1)
Distance between from the park		
Less than one block	47	11,9 (2,6-21,2)
One block	58	14,7 (5,6-23,8)
Two blocks	79	20,0 (11,2-28,8)
Three blocks	57	14,4 (5,3- 23,5)
Four blocks	54	13,7 (4,5-22,9)
Five blocks	65	16,5 (7,5-25,5)
Six blocks	35	8,9 (0-18,3)
LPA in leisure (IPAQ)	395	
<150 MVPA	307	77,7 (73,0-82,4)
≥150 MVPA	88	22,3 (13,6-31,0)
LPA self-declared	395	
Inactive	283	71,6 (66,3-76,9)
Active	112	28,4 (20,0-36,8)
Change of behavior stage		
Started for over 6 months		
Yes	94	83,9 (76,5-91,3)
No	18	16,1 (0-33,1)
Intend to start in the next months		
Yes	159	53,2 (48,5-63,9)
No	124	43,8 (35,1-52.5)
Intend to start in the next 30 days		
Yes	112	70,4 (61,9-78,9)
No	47	29,6 (16,5-42,7)
Intend to use the park for physical activity		
Yes	306	78,5 (74,4-82,6)
No	84	21,5 (17,4-25,6)

n: absolute number of individuals in each variable and category; %: relative frequency; CI95%: confidence interval of 95%.

Table 2 shows the frequency of individuals who intend to use the park for physical activity according to the levels of physical activity in leisure, self-reported physical activity levels, and distance from the park. The frequency of individuals who intend to use the park were significantly higher between those who attending the recommendation for physical activity in leisure (150 minutes or more of MVPA) and who self-reported as active than those who have not reached the recommendation for physical activity and who self-reported as inactive ($p < 0.05$). Regarding the distance from the park, as the distance increases, the frequency of individuals who intend to use it for physical activity decreases ($p < 0.05$).

Table 2. Frequency of individuals who intend to use the park to practice physical activity, according to the level of physical activity in leisure estimated by IPAQ and self-declared, and by the distance from the park.

	Intend to use the square for physical activity		
Variável	**N**	**% (CI95%)**	**p**
LPA (IPAQ)	390		0,010
≥150	87	88,5 (81,8-95,2)	
<150	303	75,6 (70,8-80,4)	
LPA self-declared	390		0,000
Inactive	279	73,8 (79,0-68,6)	
Active	111	90,1 (95,7-84,5)	
Distance from the park	390		0,030
Less than one block	47	87,2 (96,8-77,6)	
one block	56	83,9 (93,5-74,3)	
two blocks	79	82,3 (90,7-73,9)	
three blocks	57	75,4 (86,6-64,2)	
four blocks	53	67,9 (80,5-55,3)	
five blocks	64	73,4 (84,2-62,6)	
six blocks	34	79,4 (93,0-65,8)	

n: absolute number of individuals in each level and category; %: relative frequency of individuals who intend to use the park in each category; CI95%: confidence interval of 95%; p: value for p.

The results from bivariate analysis were confirmed after adjustment for gender, age, education, and household income. Individuals who were most active (estimated by the IPAQ and self-declared) and residing closest to the park had increased odds (p <0.05) relative to the intention of using it for physical activity (Table 3).

Table 3. Adjusted association between the level of physical activity in leisure estimated by IPAQ, the level of self-declared physical activity, distance from the Sport and Culture Park and the intention to use it for physical activity in adults (Uruguaiana/RS, 2014).

		OR adjusted (CI95%)
*LPA (IPAQ)**		
	≥150	2.14 (1.03–4.45)
	<150	1
*LPA self-declared**		
	Inactive	1
	Active	2,95 (1,47-5,93)
*Distance from the park*** (raise by the number of blocks)		0,87 (0,76-0,99)

OR: odds ratio; CI95%; confidence interval of 95%; LPA: Level of physical activity; ≥150–150 or more minutes of physical activity of moderate to vigorous intensity per week; <150: less than 150 minutes of physical activity of moderate to vigorous intensity per week; *adjusted for distance from the park, gender, age, education, and family income; **adjusted for level of physical activity in leisure (IPAQ), self-declared level of physical activity, gender, age, education, and family income.

Discussion

In this study we identified that the construction of an urban park can encourage an increased level of physical activity of the neighborhood residents. The results indicated that most of the subjects, regardless of their current level of physical activity, intended to use the park to practice physical activity after its construction. Furthermore, the distance from the park influenced its use. As the distance increased, the frequency of participants who intended to use it decreased.

These results are considered important as they indicate that the construction of a neighborhood park with spaces and facilities for physical activity increases the chance of inactive individuals to become active and also assists individuals who are active to remain this way. The results corroborate other studies identifying that the construction of urban and neighborhood parks play a key role in facilitating the practice of physical activity[11,16].

The environmental characteristics appear to influence individual behavior change, including the practice of physical activity[7,17–19]. The existence of parks close to home or within walking distance appears to help make it more attractive for exercising[8,20].

Although the existence of parks increases the chances for the local population to engage in physical activity, the distance between these and the residences should be considered. Those living further away from parks use them less often and tend to have lower physical activity levels. In this sense, the present study results are in line with those reported by other authors[11,12]. In one of these studies the authors suggest that parks with designated areas for physical activity should be located less than a kilometer away from every residence[11]. This reinforces the hypothesis that the existence of a park nearby is a facilitator for the promotion of physical activity in leisure and reflects directly on discussions about public policies.

Whereas there is currently still little information from studies in Brazil, this study provides an important contribution to a better understanding of the associations between the existence of urban and neighborhood parks and the level of physical activity of adults. However, some possible repercussions about the limitations of this study should be discussed. Physical activity levels were measured with a questionnaire that—while it is an internationally validated instrument used in several studies for this purpose—has limitations due to the subjectivity of the answers, in addition to the interviewee recall bias. The outcome variable of this study, intention to practice physical activity in the park, also brings limitations to the interpretation of the results. It measured the perspective regarding the intention of using the park. However, it did not guarantee that the participants will actually do so. To overcome this limitation, a new study should be conducted after the construction of the park.

In conclusion, urban and neighborhood parks can be facilitators for the practice of physical activity during leisure time. In addition, the proximity of parks is associated with people's intention of using them for physical activity. Joint actions with the government should be planned in order to provide alternatives so that the level of physical activity of the population increases.

References

1. Harrison RA, Mcelduff P, Edwards R. Planning to win: health and lifestyles associated with physical activity amongst 15, 423 adults. Public Health. 2006; 120:206-212.
2. Sallis J, Cervero RB, Ascher W, Henderson KA, Kraft MK, Kerr J. An ecological approach to creating active living communities. Annu Rev Public Health. 2006; 27:297-322.
3. Lee I-M, Shiroma EJ, Lobelo F, Puska P, Blair SN, Katzmarzyk PT. Effect of Physical Inactivity on Major Non Communicable Diseases Worldwide: an analyses of burden of disease and life expectancy. Lancet. 2012; 380:219-229.
4. Nahas MV, Duca GFD. Atividade física e doenças crônicas: evidências e recomendações para um estilo de vida ativo – 1ed – Florianópolis, UFSC/Núcleo de Pesquisa em Atividade Física e Saúde, 2011.
5. Pucci GC, Rech CR, Fermino RC, Reis RS. Associação entre atividade física e qualidade de vida em adultos: revisão sistemática. Rev. Saúde Pública. 2012; 46:166-79.
6. Kaczynski AT, Henderson KA. Parks and recreation settings and active living: a review of associations with physical activity function and intensity. J Phys Act Health. 2008; 5(4):619-632.
7. Cohen DA, Mackenzie TL, Sehgal A, Williamson S, Golinelli D, Lurie N. Increasing Physical Activity in Parks: Results of a Randomized Controlled Intervention Trial Using Community-Based Participatory Research. Am J Prev Med. 2013; 45(5):590-597.
8. Santos ES. Reflexões sobre a utilização de espaços públicos para o lazer esportivo. *RA´E GA*, 2006; *11*:25-33.
9. Silva DAS, Petroski EL, Reis RS. Barreiras e facilitadores de atividades físicas em frequentadores de parques públicos. Motriz, 2009; 15(2):219-227.

10. Silva MC, Barbosa ASA, Costa TE. Condições de espaços públicos destinados a prática de atividades Físicas na cidade de Pelotas/RS/Brasil. Rev. bras. ativ. fís. saúde. 2012; 17(1):28-32.
11. Cohen DA, Han B, Derose KP, Williamson S, Marsh T, Mackenzie TL. Contribution of Public Parks to Physical Activity. Am J Public Health. 2007; 97 (3):509-514.
12. Mccormack GR, Rock M, Toohey AM, Hignell D. Characteristics of urban parks associated with park use and physical activity: A review of qualitative research. Health Place 2010;16:712-26.
13. Fermino RC, Reis RS, Cassou AC. Fatores individuais e ambientais associados ao uso de parques e praças por adultos de Curitiba-PR, Brasil. Rev Bras Cineantropometria Desemp Humano. 2012; 14(4):377-389.
14. Matsudo S, Araújo T, Marsudo V, Andrade D, Andrade E, Oliveira LC et al Questinário internacional de atividade física (IPAQ): estudo de validade e reprodutibilidade no Brasil. Rev Bras Ativ Fís Saúde. 2001; 6(2):05-18.
15. Marcus BH, Banspach SW, Lefebvre RC, Rossi JS, Carleton RA, Abrams DB Using the stages of change model to increase the adoption of physical activity among community participants. Am J Health Promot. 1992; 6:424-429.
16. Hino AAF, Reis RS, Sarmiento OL, Parra DC, Brownson RC. The built environment and recreational physical activity among adults in Curitiba, Brazil. Prev. Med. 2011; 52(6):419-422.
17. Andersen RE, Franckowiak SC, Snyder J, Bartlett SJ, Fontaine KR. Can Inexpensive Signs Encourage the Use of Stairs? Results from a Community Intervention. Ann Intern Med. 1998; 129(5):363-369.
18. Kanh EB, Ramsey LT, Brownson RC, Heath GW, Howze EH, Powell KE, et al. The effectiveness of interventions to increase physical activity. A systematic review. Am J Prev Med.2002; 22:73-107.
19. Petroski EL, Silva DAS, Reis RS, Pelegrini A. (Estágios de mudança de comportamento e percepção positiva do ambiente para atividade física em usuários de parque urbano. Motricidade. 2009; 5(2):17-31.
20. Bedimo-Rung AL, Mowen AJ, Cohen DA. Activity and public health: A conceptual model. Am J Prev Med. 2005; 28:159-168.

Corresponding author

Gabriel Gustavo Bergmann
Address: UNIPAMPA - Campus Uruguaiana
Email: gabrielbergmann@unipampa.edu.br

An After-School, high-intensity, interval physical activity programme improves health-related fitness in children

Sergio Reloba Martínez
Luis Javier Chirosa Ríos
Ignacio Martín Tamayo
Universidad de Granada, Granada, España

Laura Guerrero Almeida
Universidad de Sevilla, Sevilla, España

Miguel Angel López-Gomez
Universidad de Granada, Granada, España

Christian Campos Jara
Universidad Andrés Bello, Santiago, Chile

Abstract— Health problems related to a low level of physical activity (PA) in children and adolescents have prompted research into extracurricular PA programs. This study was designed to determine the effects of two different levels of PA on the health-related fitness of school children. Ninety-four girls and boys (7–9 years) were randomly assigned to a control group (CG) or intervention group (IG). Over a 12 week study period, children in the CG participated in a similar PA program to that of a standard school physical education program while those in the IG completed a high intensity interval training (HIIT) program. Both programs involved two 40 minute extracurricular sessions per week. Our findings indicate that the HIIT intervention improved motor capacity (speed/agility), Vpeak, $VO_{2\,m}ax$ and excess post-exercise oxygen consumption (EPOC) ($p < 0.05$) along with the musculoskeletal capacity of the lower trunk (mean propulsive velocity and standing long jump, $p < 0.05$). The PA program had no effect on anthropometric variables or hand-grip strength. The data indicate that a 12 week strength training program using workloads adapted to children may significantly improve several markers of health and physical fitness compared to a standard school PA program.

Keywords: children, physical condition, aerobic training, high intensity, health, Alpha-fitness

Introduction

Concern about growing sedentary behaviour, overweight and obesity[1,2] along with reduced physical activity (PA) among children[3,4] has recently prompted a series of investigations designed to assess the benefits of extracurricular PA programs[5-7]. Such studies have indicated beneficial effects of PA interventions on various health and fitness markers[8-12] as well as diminishing sedentary habits[13,14].

However, authors such as Leek[15] and Myer and Faigenbaum[16] have argued that these PA interventions currently do not guarantee that young people attain the levels of health and PA recommended by the different organizations and authors. This has sparked an exponential increase in research on the impact of extracurricular PA[9,16,17-26].

As may be inferred from the vast amount of literature available on the topic, most PA interventions involve moderate-intensity aerobic PA, or so-called moderate-intensity training (MIT), and are based on working techniques similar to those of a traditional school physical education (PE) program[9,17-20]. However, over the past 10 years, several complementary studies have started to emerge that suggest that high-intensity intermittent aerobic exercise, otherwise known as high-intensity interval training (HIIT), adapted for children and preadolescents[21-25] shows a beneficial effect on cardiovascular health and fitness[16,26]. This type of PA program has been proposed as an alternative to the conventional school PE syllabus.

For HIIT, Baquet, Van Praagh and Berthoin[27] suggested a relative exercise intensity of ≥80% of the maximum heart rate to produce significant changes in the maximal oxygen consumption ($VO_{2\,m}ax$) of prepubertal children. Myer and Faigenbaum[16] targeted neuromuscular development and motor skills to improve the health of young children while Naclerio and Faigembaum[28] highlighted the efficacy of high-intensity exercise in improving the health and fitness of school children. Other authors have also described positive effects of HIIT programs on growth and development[29-31], along with improved postural control and stability[32], a spontaneous increase in PA during the day[33], and a reduced risk of injury while playing sport[16].

Despite the well-established beneficial effects of MIT and in smaller measure, HIIT, to the best of our knowledge no study has compared the effects of both training strategies on the health-related fitness of children. In addition, the different variables and training protocols such as duration, frequency, volume and intensity assessed along with intervening factors such as nutrition education[17, 34, 35] and healthy habits[13, 36] hinder indirect comparisons between the two PA intervention strategies.

This study was designed to determine the effects of a moderate-intensity PA and a high-intensity interval PA program on the health-related fitness of school children. As markers of health and fitness, we used the Alpha-fitness battery of tests designed for children and adolescents[37-39] along with several other frequently used markers. A further objective of this study was to assess the use of the Alpha-fitness test battery and of the indicators, $VO_{2m}ax$, excess post-exercise oxygen consumption (EPOC) and mean propulsive velocity of the lower trunk (MVprop) in school children.

Methods

Subjects

The study participants were 52 boys and 42 girls, aged 7–9 years (mean 8.2 ± 0.7 years) randomly assigned to a control group (CG, n = 56; 34 boys) that took part in an extracurricular moderate-intensity aerobic PA program or an intervention group (IG, n = 38; 18 boys) that participated in a similar duration high-intensity interval training (HIIT) PA program The age range selected was based on criteria that identify the onset of neuromuscular coordination in children[28]. The sample selection criteria were: 1) belonging to the second cycle of primary school education (ages from 7 to 9); and 2) Having a higher attendance than 90% in the programs over 90% of program assistance The exclusion criteria were: 1) any illness suggesting possible difficulty in completing the study in the 3 months prior to its onset; and/or 2) any medical or orthopaedic problem that could impair completion of the exercise program. All the participants (and their parents or legal guardians) were informed of the procedures involved and possible risks and/or benefits. The study protocol was approved by the Bioethics Committee of the Universidad de Granada (Granada, Spain) and adhered to the tenets of the Declaration of Helsinki. All parents/legal guardians signed a written consent form.

Experimental design

The study consisted of a pre-posttest with natural groups that had similar characteristics. The extracurricular intervention was performed during the two hours per week of physical education (PE) on the primary school timetable. The groups did not engage in regular PE classes. Instead, they followed the two programs offered. Five groups were randomly assigned to either program.

The following indicators of fitness and health were used as dependent variables: maximum oxygen consumption ($VO_{2m}ax$); peak velocity (Vpeak); hand-grip; – grip; jumping ability; lower trunk mean propulsive velocity (MVprop); excess post-exercise oxygen consumption (EPOC); percentage of fat mass (% body fat); body mass index (BMI); and waist circumference. PA practised by the participants was employed as an independent variable.

Data acquisition and measurements

To compare the two interventions, the following tests were performed before and after each program. All the participants took part in several practice sessions before each set of tests.

Alpha-fitness. An explanation of the tests that were performed follows. a) *Maximum oxygen consumption ($VO_{2m}ax$).* As a measure of aerobic capacity, $VO_{2m}ax$ was determined in the 20 m shuttle run test. For the test, subjects ran 20 m (there and back) in time with an acoustic signal. The signal sets a starting velocity of 8 km/h, which thereafter increases by 1 $km \cdot h^{-1}$ each minute. The test ends when the subject cannot keep up with the rhythm set. The authors of the Alpha-fitness test battery express the test results as the "stage' completed by the subject. However, we indirectly calculated $VO_{2m}ax$ by entering the maximum velocity recorded for each subject in the equation described by Leger, Mercier, Gadoury and Lambert[40] for children under 18 years of age. b) *Peak velocity (Vpeak).* As a further measure of aerobic capacity, we determined Vpeak as the maximum velocity recorded before the child abandoned the 20 m shuttle run test. c) *Speed/agility.* As a measure of motor capacity, speed/agility was determined in the 4x10 m shuttle run test. In this test, the subject runs 10 m, picks up a cone, returns to the starting line, switches the cone for another cone and continues the process until he/she covers 4 x 10 m. The result is expressed in seconds. d) *Hand-grip.* Hand strength (right and left) was measured by dynamometry in kilograms. e) *Jumping ability.* The distance jumped in a standing long jump was recorded in centimetres. Starting with the legs at shoulders' width, the subjects were instructed to jump as far as possible, landing with their feet together. f) *Waist circumference.* As a measure of central body fat, waist circumference was measured in centimetres.

Body composition analyser. Body composition was assessed through bioimpedance and measured using Tanita® *Body Composition* Monitor model BF-350. This instrument provides body fat and body mass index (BMI) when height is introduced.

T-force System platform. Lower trunk mean propulsive velocity (MVprop) was measured using this force platform (T-Force System, Ergotech, Murcia, Spain) when subjects performed 5 half-squat repetitions using a lightweight wooden barbel with no added weights. The children were given instructions carefully and encouraged verbally to undertake the concentric phase of the athletic movement as quickly as possible. Feedback was provided by an observer, who informed the subject of the velocity reached in each repetition. Six practice sessions were performed before the test.

HR monitor equipped with the corresponding software (Bodyguard, Firstbeat SPORTS software, Jyväskylä, Finland). Excess post-exercise oxygen consumption (EPOC) was estimated after the 20 m shuttle run test from the variation produced in heart rate (HR).

All participants were assigned to stage I of Tanner's development stage[41, 42]

Training interventions

Intervention group (IG)

Subjects in the IG participated in an interval training program for 12 weeks, which consisted of 2 sessions of 40 minute duration per week. Each session involved 20 minutes of high-intensity intermittent exercises (around 10–20 s) and 20 minutes of sports activities as described in prior studies by Faigenbaum and Myer[33], Behringer, Vom Heede, Yue, Mester[29], Baquet, Van Praagh, Berthoin[27] and Baquet, Guinhouya, Dupont, Nourry, Berthoin[26]. Following a standard warm-up, sessions commenced with several sets of half-squats followed by sprints and a training circuit consisting of jumps, speed/agility tasks, carrying weights, pulling exercises, etc. Activities were performed as games or in a competitive manner and participants were constantly encouraged verbally to perform the high-intensity exercises with maximum effort. The details of the HIIT performed in each session are provided in Table 1. Workloads and stimuli in each session were carefully designed for maximum efficiency[16].

Control group (CG)

The CG subjects underwent the same 12 week extracurricular training program, but instead of completing 20 minutes of interval exercises they took part in 20 minutes of moderate-intensity aerobic exercises and games; this was also followed by 20 minutes of sport.

Table 1. Details of the first 20 minutes of each high-intensity interval training (HIIT) session carrying weights, pulling exercises

Session	HIIT PROGRAM	Session	HIIT PROGRAM
1	Half-squats 3×5: (barbel 1; IRR 2 min)	7	Half-squats 3×7: (barbel 3; IRR 2 min)
2	Sprint 3×15 m.: IRR 2.5 min Reaction rate activities	8	Sprint 4×20 m.: IRR 2 min Reaction rate activities
3	Circuit with times -S1: Jump with feet together to stand (50cm high) ×2 -S2: In Zic-zac activities 4 signal cones velocity -S3: Long jump with stride ×2 -S4: Sprint 3m	9	Circuit with times -S1: Jump with feet together to stand (50cm high) ×3 -S2: In Zic-zac activities 6 signal cones velocity -S3: Long jump with stride ×3 -S4: Sprint 4m
4	Half-squats 3×6: (barbel 2; IRR 2 min)	10	Half-squats 3×9: (barbel 3; IRR 2 min)
5	Sprint 3×15 m.: IRR 2.5 min Reaction rate activities	11	Sprint 4×25 m.: IRR 2min.
6	Circuit with times -S1: Sprint 1 m combined with pulling exercices -S2: Jump with feet together 4 hoops 30cm distance -S3: Shot put 2 kg at the greatest horizontal distance -S4: Sprint 3m	12	Reaction rate activities Circuit with times -S1: Sprint 2m combined with pulling exercices -S2: Jump with feet together 4 hoops 50cm distance -S3: Shot put 3kg at the greatest horizontal distance -S4: Sprint 4m

IRR: inter-repetition rest period; m: metres; barbel 1: cushioned 2 kg bar; barbel 2: cushioned 2.5 kg bar; barbel 3: cushioned 3 kg bar.; *S: Station;* All sessions include a formal initial meeting, which included familiarization with the exercises provided in the session.

Statistical Analysis

Data are provided as means and their corresponding standard deviations (M ± SD). The homogeneity of the two study groups in terms of the anthropometric and health-related fitness variables recorded at baseline was confirmed by one-way ANOVA. Intervention effects were assessed through ANOVA of pre/post intervention data by examining PA intervention and measurement time point as the independent variables along with their interactions. Significant interactions were subjected to Bonferroni correction. All statistical tests were performed using the software package SPSS version 20.0 for Windows (Chicago, IL, USA). Significance was set at $p<0.05$.

Results

The means and standard deviations of the health-related fitness and anthropometric variables recorded before and after the intervention are provided in Tables 2 and 3. The effects of each intervention on the health-related fitness variables are illustrated in Figures 1 and 2, and Tables 4 and 5.

The HIIT intervention led to improved motor capacity (speed/agility), Vpeak, $VO_{2\,m}ax$ and EPOC, along with improved musculoskeletal capacity of the lower trunk (MVprop and standing long jump). As may be observed in Tables 2 and 3, differences in means following the intervention were higher in the GI than in the CG. Both PA programs had no effect on anthropometric or hand strength measurements.

Table 2. Health-related fitness variables (M ± SD) recorded before and after a 12 week extracurricular, moderate-intensity training (MIT) or high-intensity interval training (HIIT) program.

		IG	CG	Total
Vpeak (Km/h)	Before	9.4 ± 0.55	9.5 ± 0.45	9.4 ± 0.43
	After	10.6 ± 1.11	10.1 ± 0.56	10.3 ± 0.94
VO2 max (indirect) (ml/kg/min)	Before	46.4 ± 2.51	47.0 ± 2.50	46.8 ± 2.50
	After	51.5 ± 4.91	49.6 ± 3.59	50.4 ± 4.26
EPOC (ml/kg)	Before	23.7 ± 12.83	23.2 ± 14.82	23.4 ± 13.97
	After	37.2 ± 27.41	25.8 ± 23.84	30.3 ± 25.80
Speed/agility (s)	Before	15.84 ± 1.29	15.45 ± 1.72	15.61 ± 1.60
	After	14.79 ± 1.43	15.56 ± 1.65	15.24 ± 1.60
Standing long jump (cm)	Before	139.7 ± 16.53	138.7 ± 14.85	139.10 ± 15.46
	After	149.3 ± 20.34	139.3 ± 21.87	143.31 ± 21.73
MVprop (m/s)	Before	1.18 ± 0.19	1.11 ± 0.24	1.14 ± 0.22
	After	1.21 ± 0.23	0.99 ± 0.27	1.08 ± 0.28
Dynamometry left hand (kg)	Before	12.8 ± 2.20	13.7 ± 3.23	13.3 ± 2.89
	After	13.5 ± 3.38	13.7 ± 4.38	13.6 ± 3.99
Dynamometry right hand (kg)	Before	14.0 ± 2.71	14.7 ± 3.41	14.4 ± 3.15
	After	14.4 ± 3.58	14.4 ± 4.52	14.4 ± 4.14

Vpeak: peak velocity; $VO_{2\,m}$ax: maximum oxygen consumption; EPOC: excess post-exercise peak oxygen consumption; MVprop: mean propulsive velocity

Table 3. Anthropometric variables (M ± SD) recorded before and after a 12-week, extracurricular, moderate-intensity training (MIT) or high-intensity interval training (HIIT) program.

		IG	CG	Total
Body mass index (kg/m^2)	Before	17.8 ± 3.4	18.1 ± 3.7	18.0 ± 3.6
	After	18.8 ± 3.6	18.8 ± 3.6	18.8 ± 3.6
Body fat (%)	Before	18.7 ± 7.9	19.8 ± 8.9	19.3 ± 8.5
	After	22.5 ± 8	22.5 ± 9.1	22.5 ± 8.6
Waist circumference (cm)	Before	61.2 ± 8.7	62.9 ± 7.9	62.2 ± 8.2
	After	62.9 ± 8.5	62.4 ± 6.7	62.6 ± 7.5

No significant differences were detected when Vpeak values between the two interventions were compared ($F_{1,79}$=1.927; η^2=0.024;1-β=0.279; p=0.169) though differences were observed between pre – and post-intervention values ($F_{1,79}$=155.88; η^2=0.664; 1-β=1.000; p=0.001) and for the interaction between time point and intervention ($F_{1,79}$ =12.306; η^2=0.135; 1-β=0.934; p=0.001). When Vpeak values between the CG and IG were compared, no significant differences were recorded before the intervention (p=0.627), but differences did emerge after the intervention (p=0.002). In addition, both groups showed significant effects of the intervention when pre – and post-intervention data were compared (IG p=0.001; CG p=0.001).

$VO_{2\,m}$ax values differed significantly, both according to the measurement time point ($F_{1,79}$ =129.697; η^2=0.621;1-β =0.9999; p=0.001) and its interaction with the intervention ($F_{1,79}$ =15.370; η^2=0.163; 1-β=0.972; p=0.001). No differences in $VO_{2\,max}$ were recorded according to the type of intervention ($F_{1,79}$ =0.757; η^2=0.009; 1-β=0.138; p=0.387). Paired comparisons revealed an effect of the time point (pre – vs post-intervention) in both groups (IG p=0.001; CG p=0.001) along with differences between groups in post-intervention $VO_{2\,m}$ax values (p=0.044), but not pre-intervention values (p=0.207).

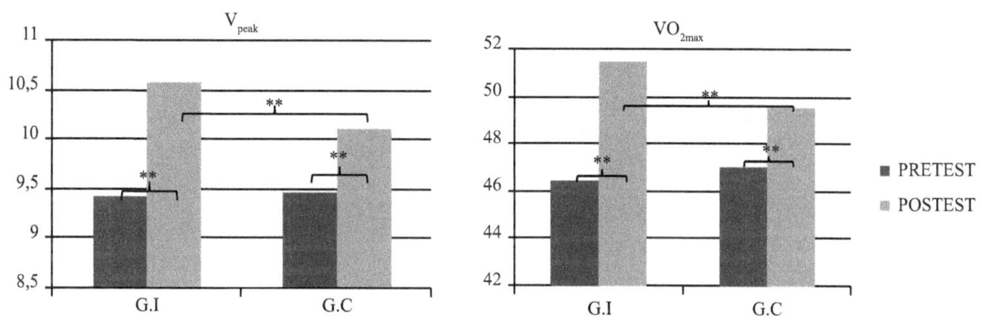

Figure 1. Vpeak and $VO_{2\,m}$ax values recorded in the 20 m shuttle sprint test before and after the control and high-intensity interval training programs (** p<.01; *p<.05).

EPOC values varied according to the measurement time point and the interaction time point x intervention. No effects were observed of the intervention type (see Table 4). Pre-intervention EPOC values failed to vary between the groups (p=0.560), but post-intervention values varied (p=0.050). No differences in pre – and post-intervention EPOC values were recorded in the CG (p=0.534), but differences were detected in the IG (p=0.001).

Table 4. Statistics obtained for excess post-exercise oxygen consumption

	$F_{1,79}$	η^2	1-β	p		Pairwise comparisons		
EPOC						CG/IG	CG	IG
Before/After	16.254	0.171	0.978	0.001**	Before	0.560		
PA intervention	1.323	0.016	0.206	0.254	After	0.050*		
Interaction	10.534	0.118	0.894	0.002	Before/ After		0.534	0.001**

(** p<.01; *p<.05)

Similarly, when we compared the results of the 4x10 m speed/agility test, significant effects were observed of the measurement time point ($F_{1,85}$ =11.398; η^2=0.018;1-β =0.916; p=0.001) and of the interaction time point x intervention ($F_{1,85}$ =17.483; η^2=0.171; 1-β=0.985; p=0.001). No effects of the intervention were noted ($F_{1,85}$=0.291; η^2=0,003;1-β =0.083; p=0.591). In the Bonferroni test comparisons, speed/agility showed no inter-group differences before the intervention (p=0.219), but did differ after the intervention (p=0.027). Differences between the two time points were not observed in the CG (p=0.533), yet were detected in the IG (p=0.001).

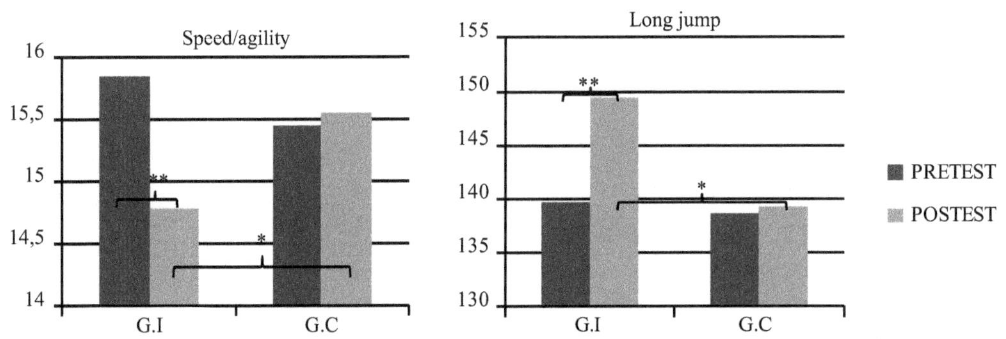

Figure 2. Speed/agility and standing long jump values recorded in the Alpha fitness test battery before and after the control and high-intensity interval training programs (** p<.01; *p<.05)

Standing long jump results differed significantly according to both the measurement time point ($F_{1,90}$ =8.019; η^2=0.082; 1-β =0.800; p=0.006) and the interaction time point x intervention ($F_{1,90}$ =6.095; η^2=0.063; 1-β =0.685; p=0.015). No effects of the intervention were detected ($F_{1,90}$ =2.237; η^2=0.024;1-β =0.316; p=0.138). Bonferroni test comparisons revealed no differences between the CG and IG in pre-intervention long jump results (p=0.768), yet differences in post-intervention results were observed (p=0.036). No differences in before/after long jump distances were detected in the CG (p=0.772), but these emerged in the IG (p=0.001) (see Figure 2). MVprop varied according to the intervention and the interaction time point x intervention. After the intervention, this variable decreased in the CG to provide before/after differences (p=0.001) whereas MVprop showed a slight increase in the IG (see Tables 2 and 5).

Table 5. Statistics obtained for lower trunk musculoskeletal capacity

	$F_{1,81}$	η^2	1-β	P		Pairwise comparisons		
MVprop						CG/IG	CG	IG
Before/After	3.763	0.044	0.483	0.056	Before	0.227		
PA intervention	8.658	0.097	0.828	0.004**	After	0.001**		
Interaction	8.390	0.094	0.816	0.005**	Before/ after		0.001**	0.531

** p<.01; *p<.05

No significant effects were produced on the dynamometer results of the measurement time point (left hand $F_{1,90}$=0.927, η^2=0.010;1-β=0.159, p=0.338; right hand $F_{1,89}$=0.012, η^2=0.0001, 1-β=0.051, p=0.912), intervention (left hand $F_{1,90}$=0.728, η^2=0.008;1-β=0.135, p=0.396; right hand $F_{1,89}$=0.257, η^2=0.003, 1-β=0.079, p=0.613) or interaction time point x intervention (left hand $F_{1,90}$=0.953, η^2=0.010, 1-β=0.162, p=0.332; right hand ($F_{1,89}$=0.486, η^2=0.005, 1-β=0.106, p=0.488).

The anthropometric variables examined increased both in the IG and CG (see Table 3). Significant differences in BMI values were observed for the different measurement time points ($F_{1,83}$=22.550; η^2=0.214; 1-β=0.997; *p*=0.001), yet no changes were observed according to intervention type ($F_{1,83}$=0.021; η^2=0.0001;1-β=0.052; *p*=0.885) or the interaction between time point and intervention ($F_{1,83}$=0.101; η^2=0.001;1-β=0.061; *p*=0.752). The percentage of body fat varied similarly according to the time point ($F_{1,83}$=55.488; η^2=0.401;1-β=0.9999; *p*=0.001), but not according to the intervention ($F_{1,83}$=0.002; η^2=0.0001;1-β=0.050; *p*=0.965) or the interaction time point x intervention ($F_{1,83}$=0.060; η^2=0.001;1-β=0.057; *p*=0.807). Waist circumference failed to vary significantly according to the time point ($F_{1,83}$=3.720; η^2=0.043;1-β=0.479; *p*=0.057), intervention ($F_{1,83}$=0.001; η^2=0.0001;1-β=0.050; *p*=0.970), or interaction time point x interaction ($F_{1,83}$=2.447; η^2=0.029;1-β=0.340; *p*=0.122).

Discussion

The main findings of this study were that a 12 week extracurricular strength training program consisting of controlled workloads adapted for children was more able to improve several health-related fitness variables than the effects of a more conventional lower intensity PA program. The high-intensity interval activities undertaken in the training intervention led to significant improvements in Vpeak, $VO_{2\,m}$ax, EPOC and lower trunk MVprop as well as in the performance of speed/agility tests and long jump.

All the variables recorded after a 20 m shuttle run test was significantly improved in the intervention group. The effects produced on both Vpeak and $VO_{2\,m}$ax resemble those described in a large number of studies[22, 26, 43, 44]. Despite improvements in post-intervention $VO_{2\,m}$ax values recorded in both our intervention and control groups, the greatest effects were produced in the IG to the extent that significant post-intervention differences were observed with respect to the CG despite even lower pre-intervention values (see Figure 1). These findings are consistent with the conclusions arrived at by Baquet, Van Praagh, Berthoin[27], who reported that the $VO_{2\,m}$ax improvement produced in response to the aerobic PA generally undertaken by children in this age group is reduced in comparison to the effects of high-intensity short-duration activities on the cardiovascular health of children. In effect, intermittent exercises performed at maximum intensity may be observed in a child's spontaneous activity[45]. In a study by Bailey, Olson, Pepper, Porszasz, Barstow, Cooper[46], it was found that the mean duration of the physical activities of children between the ages of 6 and 10 years was no more than 3 seconds (under 15 seconds in 95% of cases) and that intensities were high. Many authors have attributed the lower anaerobic performance of children to a non fully-developed glucose metabolism pathway[47,48,] thus, contraindicating high-intensity PA. However, the results of several studies seem to challenge this idea[49-51]. Accordingly, Van Praagh and Doré[51] argued that lower blood and muscle lactate concentrations in children may be explained by the lower muscle mass involved in physical exercise. According to Ratel et al.[45], there is no sound physiological evidence to indicate that high-intensity exercise could be harmful for children and these authors endorsed this type of program based on their observation of appreciable effects on both the aerobic and anaerobic capacity of prepubertal children. These findings are in line with the present results. The Vpeak and $VO_{2\,m}$ax improvements observed are related to the EPOC values attained by our subjects. During the stage of recovery following exercise, calorie intake increases and this increase is maintained until all metabolic processes return to their baseline state. In our study, EPOC were recorded during the rapid stage of oxygen consumption within the initial hour of recovery[52, 53]. The highest post-intervention EPOC levels recorded in the IG may be related to a greater metabolic disruption[54] as a consequence of the increased oxygen consumption or $VO_{2\,m}$ax, during the 20m sprint. Descriptive studies in adults such as those of Bahr, Grønnerød, Sejersted[55] and Laforgia, Withers, Shipp, Gore[56] have shown that the intensity at which an exercise is executed (3 x 2 min on a cycle ergometer at 108% VO_{2m}ax; 20 x 1 minute sprints at 105% $VO_{2\,m}$ax, respectively) will affect excess post-exercise oxygen consumption significantly. In a review of the effects of the exercise intensity, duration and modality on excess post-exercise oxygen consumption, Borsheim and Bahr[52] reported that high-intensity activities significantly increase EPOC values, thus, supporting the results of our intervention. Despite the frequent use of this variable in adults, as far as we know no such data are available for children precluding any comparisons.

Besides the beneficial cardiovascular effects observed, our HIIT program also led to better agility/velocity levels (see Figure 2). Other authors have also described a link between cardiovascular status and other fitness-related factors including agility/velocity[26, 57-59]. In contrast, Ardoy et al.[60] observed no such improvement in pairwise comparisons in two experimental groups despite high-intensity exercise in one of the groups reflected by a high mean heart rate.

Among the factors related to muscular-skeletal capacity, we detected significant improvements in the explosive force generated in the legs, both in the standing long jump test and in the variable MVprop. Thus, following the intervention, subjects in the IG covered a significantly longer distance in the long jump compared to those in the CG (see Figure 2). These data are consistent with those reported by Baquet, Guinhouya, Dupont, Nourry, Berthoin[26], Secchi, García, España-Romero, Castro-Piñero[59] and Cuenca-García et al.[37], which the beneficial effects of a HIIT program on lower trunk strength. The mean propulsive velocity, MVprop, was unaffected by the intervention, most likely because of the instability experienced doing squat exercises at this age.

Our study has several limitations. For the post-intervention tests, our CG subjects had less practice at the half-squats than their peers in the IG. In addition, the HIIT intervention should have included exercises designed to improve upper limb strength. Finally, owing to the time available for the PA sessions, HR data could not be obtained during the strength training exercises such that the work intensity during the proposed strength training program could not be determined accurately.

In conclusion, the findings of our study indicate that short-duration high-intensity neuromuscular exercises are an effective option to improve the health-related physical fitness of school children. To date, this kind of program has only been implemented in sports' clubs and teams in which population bias exists due to the level of motor competence. Hence, this type of training program in an education setting, whether curricular or extracurricular, would be a powerful tool to improve the physical fitness of children, regardless of their unwillingness to participate in sport. More work in the field is needed with special emphasis on aspects such as motivation levels during longer-duration programs and levels of adherence to such programs.

References

1. Janssen I. Physical activity guidelines for children and youth. APNM. 2007; 32: 109–121.
2. Ortega F, Ruiz J, Castillo M, Moreno L, Gonzalez-Gross M, Wärnberg J. et al. Bajo nivel de forma física en los adolescentes españoles. Importancia para la salud cardiovascular futura (Estudio AVENA). Rev Esp Cardiol. 2005; 58(8): 898-909.
3. Reverter J, Plaza D, Jové C, Hernández V. Actividad físico-deportiva extraescolar en alumnos de primaria: el caso de Torrevieja (Alicante). Retos. 2014; 25: 48-52.
4. Troiano RP, Berrigan D, Dodd KW, Masse LC, Tilert T, McDowell M. Physical activity in the United States measured by accelerometer. Med Sci Sports Exerc. 2008; 40(1): 181-188.
5. Escalante Y, Saavedra J, García-Hermoso A, Domínguez A. Improvement of the lipid profile with exercise in obese children: A systematic review. PrevMed. 2012; 54: 293-301.
6. García-Cantó E, Pérez JJ. Programa para la promoción de actividad física saludable en escolares murcianos. Retos. 2014; 25: 131-135
7. González J, Portolés A. Actividad física extraescolar: relaciones con la motivación educativa, rendimiento académico y conductas asociadas a la salud. RIPED. 2014; 1 (9): 51-65.
8. Annesi J, Faigenbaum A, Westcott W, Smith A, Unruh J, Hamilton F. Effects of the Youth Fit For Life protocol on physiological, mood, self-appraisal, and voluntary physical activity changes in African American preadolescents: Contrasting after-school care and physical education formats. Int J Clin Hlth Psyc. 2007; 3: 641-659.
9. Cordova A, Villa G, Sureda A, Rodriguez-Marroyo JA, Sanchez-Collado P. Actividad física y factores de riesgo cardiovascular de niños españoles de 11-13 años. Rev Esp Cardiol. 2012; 65 (7): 620-626.
10. Hasselstrøm H, Karlsson M, Hansen S, Grønfeldt V, Froberg K, Andersen L. A 3-Year Physical Activity Intervention Program Increases the Gain in Bone Mineral and Bone Width in Prepubertal Girls but not Boys: The Prospective Copenhagen School Child Interventions Study (CoSCIS). Calc Tiss Res. 2008; 83: 243-250.
11. Hogg J, Diaz A, Cid M, Mueller C, Grace E, Cheruvu S. et al. An after-school dance and lifestyle education program reduces risk factors for heart disease and diabetes in elementary school children. J Pediatr Endocr Met. 2012; 25(5-6): 509–516.
12. Resaland GK, Anderssen LB, Mamen A, Anderssen SA. Effects of a 2-year school-based daily physical activity intervention on cardiorespiratory fitness. The Sogndal school-intervention study. Scand J Med Sci Spor. 2011; 21: 302-309.
13. Colín-Ramírez E, Castillo-Martínez L, Orea-Tejeda A, Vergara-Castañeda A, Keirns-Davis C, Villa-Romero A. Outcomes of a school-based intervention (RESCATE) to improve physical activity patterns in Mexican children aged 8-10 years. Health Educ Res. 2010; 25 (6): 1042-1049.
14. Wright K, Giger JN, Norris K, Suro Z. Impact of a nurse-directed, coordinated school health program to enhance physical activity behaviours and reduce body mass index among minority children: A parallel-group, randomized control trial. Int J Nurs Stud. 2012; 50 (6): 727–737
15. Leek D, Carlson J, Cain K, Henrichon S, Rosenberg D, Patrick K. et al. Physical Activity During Youth Sports Practices. Arch Pediatr Adolesc Med. 2010; 4 (165): 294-299.
16. Myer GD, Faigenbaum AD. Exercise is sports medicine in youth: Integrative neuromuscular training to optimize motor development and reduce risk of sports related injury. Kronos. 2010; 10 (1): 39-48.
17. Ben Ounis O, Elloumi M, Zouhal H, Makni E, Denguezli M, Amri M, Lac G, Tabka Z. Effect of individualized exercise training combined with diet restriction on inflammatory and igf-1/igfbp-3 in obese children. Ann Nutr Metab. 2010; 56: 260-266.
18. Kriemler S, Zahner L, Schindler C, Meyer U, Hartmann T, Hebestreit H, Brunner-La Rocca H, Van Mechelen W, Puder J. Effect of school based physical activity programme (KISS) on fitness and adiposity in primary schoolchildren: cluster randomised controlled trial. BMJ. 2010; 340: 1-8.
19. Sandercock G, Cohen D, Griffin M. Evaluation of a multicomponent intervention to improve weight status and fitness in children: Upstarts. Pediatr Int. 2012; 6 (54): 911-917.
20. Sigmund E, El Ansari W, Sigmundová D. Does school-based physical activity decrease overweight and obesity in children aged 6¿ 9 years? A two-year non-randomized longitudinal intervention study in the Czech Republic. BMC Public Health. 2012; 1 (12): 570-583.
21. Faigenbaum A, Westcott W, LaRosa R, Long C. The Effects of Different Resistance Training Protocols on Muscular Strength and endurance development in children. Pediatrics. 2005; 1 (104): 1-7.
22. Gamelin FX, Baquet G, Berthoin S, Thevenet D, Nourry C, Nottin S, Bosquet L. Effect of high intensity intermittent training on heart rate variability in prepubescent children. Eur J Appl Physiol. 2009; 105: 731-738.
23. Nourry C, Deruelle F, Guinhouya C, Baquet G, Fabre C, Bart F, Berthoin S, Mucci P. High-intensity intermittent running training improves pulmonary function and alters exercise breathing pattern in children. Eur J Appl Physiol. 2005; 94(4): 415-23.
24. Rosenkranz R, Welk G, Dzewaltowski D. Environmental correlates of objectively measured physical activity and sedentary behaviour in after-school recreation sessions. JPAH. 2011; 8: 214-221.
25. Yu C, Sung YT, So R, Lui KC, Lau W, Lam P, Lau E. Effects of Strength Training on Body Composition and Bone Mineral Content in Children Who Are Obese. J Strength Cond Res. 2005; 19(3): 667-672

26. Baquet G, Guinhouya C, Dupont G, Nourry C, Berthoin S. Effects of a short-term interval training program on physical fitness in prepubertal children. J Strength Cond Res. 2004; 18(4): 708-713
27. Baquet G, Van Praagh E, Berthoin S. Endurance Training and Aerobic Fitness in Young People. Sports Med. 2003; 33(15): 1127-1143.
28. Naclerio F, Faigenbaum A. Integrative neuromuscular training for youth. Kronos. 2011; 10 (1): 49-56.
29. Behringer M, Vom Heede A, Yue Z, Mester J. Effects of resistence training in children an adolescents: a metaanálisis. Pediatrics. 2010; 126 (5): 199-210.
30. Faigenbaum A, Myer GD. Resistence training among young athletes: safety, efficacy an injury prevention effects. Br J Sports Med. 2009; 44: 56-63
31. Slining M, Adair LS, Goldman BD, Borja JB, Bentley M. Infant overweight is associated with delayed motor development. J Pediatric. 2010; 157: 20-25.
32. Mickle KJ, Munro BJ, Steele JR. Gender and age affect balance performance in primary school-aged children. J Sci Med Sport. 2011; 14: 243-248.
33. Faigenbaum A, Myer GD. Resistance training and paediatric health. Kronos. 2011; 10 (1): 31-38.
34. Donnelly J, Jacobsen D, Whatley J, Hill J, Swift L, Cherrington A, Polk B, Tran Z, Reed G. Nutrition and physical activity program to attenuate obesity and promote physical and metabolic fitness in elementary school children. Obes Res. 2012; 3 (4): 229-243.
35. Gortmaker S, Lee R, Mozaffarian R, Sobol A, Nelson T, Roth B, Wiecha J. Effect of an After-School Intervention on Increases in Children's Physical Activity. Med Sci Sport Exer. 2012; 44(3): 450-457.
36. McMinn D, Rowe DA, Murtagh S, Nelson NM. The effect of a school-based active commuting intervention on children's commuting physical activity and daily physical activity. Prev Med. 2012; 15 (54): 316-318.
37. Cuenca-García M, Jiménez-Pavón D, España-Romero V, Artero E, Castro-Peñero JC, Ortega F, Ruiz JR, Castillo M. Condición física relacionada con la salud y hábitos de alimentación en niños y adolescentes: propuesta de addendum al informe de salud escolar. Rev Invest Ed. 2011; 9 (2): 35-50.
38. Serra-Paya N, Ensenyat A, Real J, Castro-Viñuales I, Zapata A, Galindo G, Solé-Mir E, Bosch-Muñoz J, Mur JM, Teixido C. Evaluation of a family intervention programme for the treatment of overweight and obese children (Nereu Programme): a randomized clinical trial study protocol. BMC Public Health. 2013; 13: 1-14.
39. Torrijos-niño C, Martínez-Vizcaino V, Pardo-Guijarro MJ, García-Prieto JC, Arias-Palencia NM, Sánchez-López M. Physical Fitness, Obesity, and Academic Achievement in Schoolchildren. J Pediatr. 2014; 1 (165): 104-109.
40. Leger LA, Mercier D, Gadoury C, Lambert J. The multistage 20 metres shuttle run test for aerobic fitness. J Sport Sci. 1988; 6: 93-101.
41. Muñoz MT, Pozo J. Pubertad normal y sus variantes. Pediatr Integral. 2011; 15 (6): 507-518.
42. Tanner JM. The measurement of maturity. Trans Eur Orthod Soc. 1975; 45-60.
43. Baquet G, Berthoin S, Dupont G, Blondel N, Fabre C, Van Praagh E. Effects of high intensity intermittent training on peak VO (2) in prepubertal children. Int J Sports Med. 2012; 23(6): 439-44
44. Berthoin S, Baquet G, Dupont G, Van Praagh E. Critical velocity during continuous and intermittent exercises in children. Eur J Appl Physiol. 2006; 98: 132-138.
45. Ratel S, Lazaar N, Dore E, Baquet G, Williams C, Berthoin S. et al. High-intensity intermittent activities at school: controversies and facts. J Sport Med Phys Fit. 2004; 44: 272-280.
46. Bailey R, Olson J, Pepper S, Porszasz J, Barstow T, Cooper D. The level and tempo of children´s physical activities: an observational study. Med Sci Sport Exer. 1995; 7 (27):1033-1041.
47. Falgairette G, Bedu M, Fellman N, Van Praagh E, Coudert J. Bioenergetic profile in 144 boys aged from 6 to 15 years with special reference to sexual maturation. Eur J Appl Physiol. 1991; 62: 151-156.
48. Van Praag E, Doré E. Short-term muscle power during growth and maturation. Sports Med. 2002; 32: 701-708.
49. Armstrong N, Welsman JR, Kirby BJ. Performance on the Wingate anaerobic test and maturation. Pediatr Exerc Sci. 1997; 9: 253-261.
50. Petersen SR, Gaul CA, Stanton MM., Hanstock CC. Skeletal muscle metabolism during short-term, high-intensity exercise in prepuberal and pubertal girls. J Appl Physiol. 1999; 21 (87): 51-56.
51. Van Praagh E, Bedu M, Falgairette G, Fellmann N, Coudert J. Oxygen uptake during a 30-s supramaximal exercise in 7 to 15-year-old boys. In: R Frenkl, 1 editor. Children and exercise XV. Budapest: Natl Inst for health promotion. 1991; 281-287.
52. Børsheim E, Bahr R. Effect of Exercise Intensity, Duration and Mode on Post-Exercise Oxygen Consumption. Sports. 2003; 14 (33): 1037-1060.
53. Lamont LS, Romito R, Rossi K. Fat-free mass and gender influences the rapid-phase excess postexercise oxygen consumption. Appl Physiol Nutr Me. 2010; 35 (1): 23-26.
54. Earnest CP, Scott CB. Resistance Exercise Energy Expenditure is Greater with Fatigue as Compared to Non-Fatigue. JEPonline. 2011; 14 (1): 1-10.
55. Bahr R, Grønnerød O, Sejersted OM. Effect of supramaximal exercise on excess postexercise O2 consumption. Med Sci Sport Exercise. 1992; 1 (24): 66-71.
56. Laforgia J, Withers T, Shipp J, Gore J. Comparison of energy expenditure elevations after submaximal and supramaximal running. J. Appl. Physiol. 1997; 2 (82): 661–666.
57. Ara I, Rodriguez V, Perez-Gomez J, Jimenez-Ramirez J, Serrano-Sanchez JA, Dorado C, Calbet J. Influence of extracurricular sport activities on body composition and physical fitness in boys: a 3-year longitudinal study. Int J Obesity. 2006; 30: 1062-1071.
58. Ortega F, Ruiz JR, Castillo MJ, Moreno LA, González-Gross M, Wärnberg J, Gutiérrez À. Bajo nivel de forma física en los adolescentes españoles.Importancia para la salud cardiovascular futura (Estudio AVENA). Rev Esp Cardiol. 2005; 58(8): 898-909.
59. Secchi JD, García C, España-Romero V, Castro-Piñero J. Condición física y riesgo cardiovascular futuro en niños y adolescentes argentinos: una introducción de la batería ALPHA. Arch Argent Pediatr. 2014; 112 (2): 132-140

60. Ardoy D, Fernández-Rodríguez JM, Ruiz JR, Chillón P, España-Romero V, Castillo M, Ortega F. Mejora de la condición física en adolescentes a través de un programa de intervención educativa: Estudio EDUFIT. Rev Esp Cardiol. 2011; 64 (6): 484-491.

Corresponding author

Sergio Reloba Martínez
Doctor en Educación física Departamento Educación Física y deportiva, Facultad de Ciencias de la Actividad física y la Salud. Universidad de Granada (España).
Email: Reloba.s@gmail.com

23

Fear of Failure in Sport: A Portuguese Cross-cultural Adaptation

Marco Correia
António Rosado
Sidónio Serpa
Universidade de Lisboa, Lisboa, Portugal

Abstract— The Performance Failure Appraisal Inventory (PFAI) is a multidimensional measure of threat appraisals associated with one's fear of failure. Whilst emerging research has supported the validity and reliability of the PFAI with North American and British sport participants, its psychometric proprieties remain untested within Portuguese samples. This study examined the psychometric proprieties of the PFAI with a sample of 556 Portuguese athletes. A confirmatory factor analysis was employed to test whether the proposed multi-factorial structure of the PFAI fits well the Portuguese data. All factors displayed good internal consistency, convergent validity, and discriminant validity. Multi-group analysis revealed cross-validity and the models' invariance. The correlations between fear of failure and sport anxiety measures revealed evidence of its concurrent validity. The PFAI appears to be a psychometrically sound measure and a valid and reliable tool for assessing fear of failure in Portuguese sport contexts.

Keywords*:* fear of failure, cross-cultural validation, confirmatory factor analysis

Introduction

Sport represents an important achievement domain and the existence of pressure to achieve top sporting performances can produce an increase in fear of failure among athletes[1].

In sport, limited research has shown fear of failure to be associated with cases of burnout[2], youth sport drop out, barriers to sport participation[3], athletes' drug abuse[4], and athletic stress[5].

Conroy, Willow, and Metzler[6] proposed a multidimensional model of fear of failure (The Performance Failure Appraisal Inventory–PFAI), grounded in Lazarus's cognitive-motivational-relational theory of emotions and consistent with other multidimensional models of fear of failure[7]. For the PFAI authors, one of the greatest advantages of this instrument over alternatives fear of failure measures[8–11] may be its superior substantive foundation.

The Performance Failure Appraisal Inventory was developed by Conroy[6,12] to measure individuals' beliefs in specific aversive consequences of failing. This inventory comprises 25 items that measure five dimensions of threat appraisals associated with fear of failure: (1) fear of shame and embarrassment; (2) fear of devaluing one's self-estimate; (3) fear of having an uncertain future; (4) fear of important others losing interest; and (5) fear of upsetting important others.

The PFAI is the first fear of failure measure developed from the meta-theory of emotions and it examines fear of failure as a function of person-environment interaction (rather than a state or trait) and acknowledges the individual nature of perceptions of failure, rather than assuming it to be the same for all performers[13].

Conroy[6] views fear of failure as the dispositional predisposition to appraise threat, to the achievement of personally meaningful goals, when one fails. Individuals with a higher fear of failure have learnt to associate failure with aversive consequences and typically perceive failure in evaluative situations as threatening. They also believe that aversive consequences will occur following a failure.

Confirmatory factor analysis conducted by Conroy[6] revealed satisfactory goodness of fit indexes for the five dimensions when tested as a five correlated-factor model as well as a higher-order factor model.

Research using PFAI, showed good psychometric proprieties including internal consistency, factorial validity, and temporal stability[6,14-16]. However, according to our knowledge, no author has verified the convergent and discriminant validity of each factor till date.

To our knowledge, the PFAI has been applied in sport and exercise contexts mainly with North American athletes[14–17]. There were, however, three other studies conducted outside the USA. Specifically, Sideridis and Kafetsios[18] examined fear of failure in high school and college students in an educational setting in Greece. While Sagar and Jowett[13] examined the psychometric proprieties of the PFAI with British sport participants, and two years later, the same authors[19] explored the effects of personal and contextual factors such as age, gender, sport type, and level of sport participation on athletes' fear of failure.

The aim of this study was to conduct a cross-cultural adaptation of the PFAI. More specifically, we intended to analyze the factor structure as it was proposed by the PFAI's authors. Furthermore, into a more refined analysis, we tested the model to determine the following: its internal consistency, convergent, and discriminant validity; the invariance of the structure with a cross-validation strategy; and to explore its concurrent validity with Portuguese athletes.

Having a reliable measure that can provide individual beliefs of perceptions of failure in a sport context is essential since sport is a highly evaluative situation in one of the most popular achievement domains.

Method

Participants and data collection

A total of 556 athletes distributed in two convenience samples participated in the study. They competed in a variety of individual (e.g., athletics, climbing, surfing, tennis, orienteering, and swimming) and team sports (e.g., soccer, volleyball, and basketball) at club and school level, from different competition levels. The mean age of the first sample ($n = 350$) was 15.65 years old ($SD = 2.45$) and approximately two-thirds were males (72%). Regarding the second sample ($n = 206$), the mean age of the participants was 15.29 years old ($SD = 2.47$) and the great majority were males (79.6%).

Prior to data collection, the study was reviewed by the University Ethics Board. Upon approval, participants were recruited. Clubs, sport associations and schools were contacted by e-mail or by telephone and were invited to participate.

Once club and school authorizations were provided, letters and parental consent forms were sent home to parents for participants under the age of 18 informing them of the nature of the study and requesting their permission for their child's participation. All participants, including minors, signed consent forms.

Measures

The Performance Failure Appraisal Inventory[6] is a multidimensional measure of threat appraisals associated with one's fear of failure. Participants were asked to rate how strongly they believed each of the 25 aversive consequences of failure were likely to occur to them following a failure. The measure assessed the strength of their beliefs about possible consequences of failure across five domains: experiencing shame and embarrassment, devaluing one's self-estimate, having an uncertain future, important others losing interest, and upsetting important others. Items were answered on a five-point Likert scale ranging from 1 (*do not believe at all*) to 5 (*truly believe*).

The Portuguese version of the Sport Anxiety Scale–SAS-2[20] translated and adapted by Cruz and Gomes[21] has three subscales (somatic anxiety, worry, and concentration disruption) consisting of five items each. This scale was used for concurrent validity proposes. The 15 items of the SAS-2 were designed to reflect possible responses that young athletes may have before, or while, they compete in sports. For each item, athletes indicated how they typically felt, based upon a five-point Likert scale, ranging from 1 (*not at all*) to 5 (*very much*).

PFAI Translation Procedures

Once approval was obtained from the original scale author, the translation of the PFAI was performed using a five-stage process (e.g., *translation, synthesis, back-translation, review of content validity,* and *pre-testing*)[22].

Data Analysis

Data were analyzed using AMOS 22.0 and a confirmatory factor analysis (CFA) was performed to assess the psychometric proprieties of the PFAI instrument. The maximum likelihood (ML) method was used since it is considerably more insensitive to variations in sample size and kurtosis and tends to be more stable, demonstrating higher accuracy in terms of empirical and theoretical fit compared to other estimators[23]. Standardized factor loadings, standard residuals, and modification indices were analyzed to screen for possible model misspecification.

In order to confirm the factorial structure of the PFAI model, an analysis was conducted using the Conroy, Willow, and Metzler[6] model. Given that this is a second-order model, we selected a two-step confirmatory strategy (as suggested by Byrne[24], Kline[25], Schumaker and Lomax[26]). Initially, a test was conducted on the first-order model and after, in a second step, we tested the second-order model.

The appropriateness of the model was tested using a variety of goodness-of-fit indexes. Specifically, the measurement model was assessed with the chi-square (χ^2) statistical test, the ratio of χ^2 to its degrees of freedom (χ^2/df), comparative-of-fit-index (CFI), goodness-of-fit index (GFI), parsimony comparative-of-fit-index (PCFI), parsimony goodness-of-fit index (PGFI), and root mean square error of approximation (RMSEA). The χ^2 value has been identified as potentially problematic due to sample size sensitivity, but its value is reported since it represents the only true inferential statistic of model testing[27]. Given its sensitivity to sample size, the χ^2/df was also used as a measure of model fit[28]. Research practices using these indices state that values for the χ^2/df should be less than 3, PCFI and PGFI above .60, while values above .90 for the CFI and GFI, and below .05 for the RMSEA represents a good fit[29–33].

Internal consistency (reliability) of the constructs was assessed through composite reliability and we followed the recommendations of Fornell and Larcker[34] to calculate composite reliability (CR), in which it is recommended that values $\geq .7$ indicates a proper value of CR.

Convergent validity was evaluated through the average variance extracted (AVE), whereby the values of AVE $\geq .5$ are appropriate indicators of convergent validity[35].

Discriminant validity was established when AVE for each construct went beyond the squared correlations between that construct and any other[35]. In order to verify PFAI's factorial invariance, cross-validation procedures were used with a multi-group analysis strategy[36–38].

A multi-group analysis was conducted to compare the first sample with the second sample in order to access cross-validity. The model's invariance was tested by comparing the unconstrained model with constrained models (factor loadings fixed and variances/co-variances fixed). Factorial invariance was accepted when the models did not differ significantly ($p > 0.05$), according to the qui-square statistic[39,40]. As the qui-square difference tests represent an excessively stringent test of invariance, we also considered Cheung and Rensvold's[41] suggestion that a difference of CFI of less than or equal to .01 is an indication that the constrained parameters are invariant.

Concurrent validity was analyzed by Pearson's correlation coefficients between the PFAI's and the SAS's dimensions as well as their total score values[42].

Results

Preliminary Analysis

Preliminary analyses were performed on the data in order to scan for evidence of non-normality, univariate and multivariate outliers, and patterns of missing data. No missing values were found within the data.

The assumption of normality for confirmatory factor analysis was examined using measures of skewness and kurtosis. Absolute values of skewness ranged from – 0.132 to 2.211 (SD = 0.56) and absolute values of kurtosis ranged from – 1.324 to 4.842 (SD = 1.42). According with these values, we decided that the data was approximately univariately normal, since items with absolute values of skewness lower than 3 and kurtosis lower than 7 did not deviate enough from the normal distribution[43].

Results revealed that data violated the assumption of a multivariate Gaussian distribution since Mardia's (1970) values have been noted as a sign of multivariate kurtosis[44,45]. Based upon the Mahalanobis distance statistic, 14 multivariate outliers were identified from the sample and were consequently removed. Thus, it was decided to adjust the p value of the chi-square statistic with the bootstrapping procedure of Bolen and Stine[46].

Evaluation of Model Fit

At first, not all estimated factor loadings exceeded the cut-off point of .50,[39] ranging from .10 to .81. The goodness-of-fit indices produced for this first order measurement model also indicated poor fit [χ^2 = 748.088, B-S p < 0.01; χ^2/df = 2.82, PCFI = .74, PGFI = .69, CFI = .84, GFI = .85, RMSEA = .07] showing that the hypothesized measurement model is inconsistent with observed data, which is interpreted as evidence against the adequacy of measuring the model. This poor fit is specifically perceived in the values of the CFI and GFI that were below the cut-off point of .90.[39].

Post hoc model adjustments were conducted in an effort to develop a better fitting model due to the lack of support from CFA. The results in the original model (first-order model) indicated that not all items loaded significantly on its construct. Since nonsignificant parameters can be considered unimportant to the model, in the interest of scientific parsimony, all scale items that showed unacceptable factor loadings were removed[24]. Furthermore, examination of the modification indices (MI) suggested that an improved model resulted in the elimination of specific items, following the intent of Chartrand, Robbins, Morril, and Boggs[47] to create "*pure measures of each factor*" (p. 495) by allowing items to load on only one factor. According to Byrne[24], large MI argues the presence of factor cross-loadings (i.e., a loading on more than one factor) and error covariances, respectively.

The indices of fit indicated a noteworthy improvement of the hypothesized first-order model, as reported in Table 1.

Table 1. PFAI's Re-specified 1st Order Model – Factor Loadings, Z-values, Composite Reliability (CR), and Average Variance Extracted (AVE)

PFAI factors/items	Loadings	Z-value	CR	AVE
FSE			.789	.558
Item 18	.638	11.939		
Item 25	.736	14.441		
Item 24	.852	17.239		
FDSE			.754	.511
Item 15	.576	10.037		
Item 04	.708	13.480		
Item 07	.837	16.062		
FUF			.768	.624
Item 02	.772	14.351		
Item 08	.807	15.017		
FIOLI			.766	.521
Item 11	.715	13.563		
Item 21	.727	13.864		
Item 23	.724	13.778		
FUIO			.774	.540
Item 03	.560	10.136		
Item 14	.762	14.910		
Item 19	.852	16.950		

Note. FSE = fear of experiencing shame and embarrassment; FDSE = fear of devaluing one's self-estimate; FUF = fear of having an uncertain future; FIOLI = fear of important others losing interest; FUIO = fear of upsetting important others.

Evidence of discriminant validity was accepted since none of the squared correlations exceeded the AVE values for each associated construct[34].

After these procedures, the model adjusted to the data. The results demonstrated an acceptable fit [χ^2 = 146.63, B-S p < 0.001; χ^2/df = 2.19, PCFI = 0.70, PGFI = 0.60, CFI = 0.96, GFI = 0.94, RMSEA = 0.06]. Composite reliability values ranged from .75 (fear of devaluing one's self-estimate) to .79 (fear of shame and embarrassment), indicating that the constructs were internally consistent[35]. Evidence for convergent validity was obtained since AVE values ranged from .51 (fear of devaluing one's self-estimate) to .62 (fear of having an uncertain future), being greater than the recommended standard of .50.[34]

Conroy[6] hypothesized a higher-order factor model, whereby the five dimensions of fear of failure were incorporated under a general factor. The second-order measurement model showed an overall acceptable fit to the data [χ^2 = 176.32, B-S p < 0.001; χ^2/df = 2.42, PCFI = 0.75, PGFI = 0.64, CFI = 0.94, GFI = 0.93, RMSEA = 0.07].

Cross-validity

Cross-validation procedures were used[38] in order to study the adequacy of model replication. More specifically, a cross validation technique using a multi-group analysis with two equivalent samples in their characteristics ($n_{testing}$ sample = 350; $n_{validation}$

sample = 206) and then a technique of parameter-invariance to verify the equivalence between the two groups[36].

As exposed in Table 2, the fit of the unconstrained model [Model A: $\chi^2(134) = 210.77$ (B-S $p < .001$), PCFI = 0.71, PGFI = 0.60, CFI = 0.96, GFI = 0.92, RMSEA = 0.041] was acceptable. The fit of this model provides the baseline value against which all subsequently specified invariance models are compared[24]. The models with constrained factor loadings [Model B: $\chi^2(143) = 216.05$ (B-S $p < .001$), PCFI = 0.75, PGFI = 0.62, CFI = 0.96, GFI = 0.92, RMSEA = 0.039], and with constrained variances/covariances [Model C: $\chi^2(158) = 234.87$ (B-S $p < .001$), PCFI = 0.83, PGFI = 0.69, CFI = 0.96, GFI = 0.91, RMSEA = 0.04], showed a satisfactory fit. The qui-square statistic showed no significant differences between Model A and Model B [χ^2dif (9) = 5.28; $p = .81$], and also no significant differences between Model A and Model C [χ^2dif (24) = 24.10; $p = .46$]. There were no differences in the CFI values for all model comparisons. Thus, the results demonstrated the model's invariance in both samples, indicating that the factorial structure of the scale was stable in the two independent samples.

Table 2. Results of the Multi-Group Analysis across the Unconstrained Model and the Constrained Models of the PFAI (Testing Sample: n = 350; Validation Sample: n = 206)

Multi-group models	χ^2	df	$\Delta\chi^2$	Δ *df*	B-S p	CFI	GFI	PCFI	PGFI	RMSEA
Model A	210.77	134	-	-	-	.96	.92	.71	.60	.041
Model B	216.05	143	5.28*	9	<.01	.96	.92	.75	.62	.039
Model C	234.87	158	24.1*	24	<.01	.96	.91	.83	.69	.038

Note. χ^2= chi-square; *df* = degrees of freedom; $\Delta\chi^2$= chi-square difference; Δ*df*=degrees of freedom difference; B-S p = Bolen-Stine *p*-value; CFI = comparative fit index; PCFI = parsimony comparative fit index; GFI = goodness of fit index; PGFI = parsimony goodness of fit index; RMSEA = root mean square error of approximation.
**p*-value > .5.

Concurrent Validity

The results presented in Table 3, related to the correlations used to examine the relationships among the PFAI and SAS-2, reveal that the PFAI and SAS-2 sub-scales were positively correlated. The fear of failure scores were also positively related to concentration disruption, somatic anxiety, worry, and total sport anxiety scores.

Table 3. Correlation Matrix between Performance Failure Appraisal Inventory (PFAI) and Sport Anxiety Scale–2 (SAS-2)

	FSE	FDSE	FUF	FIOLI	FUIO	FF
SAS–Concentration disruption	.34*	.42*	.41*	.26*	.27*	.45*
SAS–Worry	.49*	.49*	.33*	.29*	.42*	.54*
SAS–Somatic anxiety	.32*	.40*	.31*	.18*	.20*	.38*
SAS–Total score	.50*	.56*	.44*	.32*	.39*	.56*

Note. FSE = fear of experiencing shame and embarrassment; FDSE = fear of devaluing one's self-estimate; FUF = fear of having an uncertain future; FIOLI = fear of important others losing interest; FUIO = fear of upsetting important others; FF = fear of failure total score.
*Bolen-Stine $p < .01$

Discussion

This study aimed to investigate a cross-cultural adaptation of the PFAI originally developed by Conroy[6] and to test its factorial validity in a Portuguese sport setting.

The construct of fear of failure has been mainly tested and used in North American and British populations, but it was yet to be explored within the Portuguese population.

The confirmatory factorial analysis performed on the PFAI with a sample of 556 athletes provided some support to the five-factor structure proposed by Conroy[6]. Conversely, some items revealed unacceptable factor loadings in their different sub-scales and were eliminated, generating a more effective model. The items elimination procedure was done since it minimized content redundancy and shortened the questionnaire significantly, which is very convenient in competitive sport settings, without affecting its content broadness and relevance. As such, the scale modifications resulted in a shorter questionnaire containing 14 items, representing the original five factors originally developed by Conroy[6].

The confirmatory factorial analysis using the re-specified model showed an acceptable fit of the data. The first-order construct showed composite reliability, convergent validity, and discriminant validity for each factor. A second-order model was tested and the analysis revealed an adequate fit for this final model.

The model's invariance in two independent samples was supported, indicating cross validity. With this outcome, it is assumed that the instrument is operating exactly the same way and that the underlying construct being measured (i.e., fear of failure) has the same theoretical structure for both groups.

PFAI's concurrent validity has been ascertained with the Sport Anxiety Scale-2 (SAS-2), pointing to its high concurrent validity. PFAI scores have exhibited appropriate concurrent validity with measures of worry, sport anxiety, cognitive disruption, and somatic anxiety[6,48]. In this regard, it is important to acknowledge that fear of failure is a subclass of performance anxiety constructs in sport[6], so it was not surprising that fear of failure was strongly related to sport anxiety. This result is similar to previous findings where fear of failure has been associated with dispositional performance anxiety (worry, concentration disruption, somatic anxiety)[6,15,16]. These results provide an additional outcome for the validity of the PFAI as an adequate tool for research.

All dimensions of the PFAI showed a statistically significant relationship with this second-order construct, with the strongest predictor being fear of important others losing interest (.82), followed immediately by fear of experiencing shame and embarrassment (.78) and fear of having an uncertain future (.78).

Finally, there are limitations that need to be acknowledged. First, there was a large age range in the present study, representing a wide variety of sport experiences. Therefore, future studies should collect stratified samples of sport populations and sport experiences to better understand the fear of failure among athletes. Second, the PFAI does not assess all possible fear of failure appraisals, such as the beliefs of failure associated with (a) wasting one's efforts, (b) losing a special opportunity, or (c) experiencing tangible losses[12]. Furthermore, there may be other beliefs concerning aversive consequences of failure not identified by Conroy[12] or even existing cross-cultural differences that may provide different beliefs of aversive consequences of failure. On this behalf, it should be pertinent to include a qualitative inquiry in order to provide a holistic understanding of the athlete's fears of failure. Third, the present study is a cross-sectional survey and, as such, its findings do not inform us whether athletes' fear of failure appraisals levels oscillate over time in accordance with different events that take place in a sporting season or throughout a sport career. Future research will benefit from longitudinal designs over a sporting season and career, also essential for attaining predictive validity of the PFAI's Portuguese version. Fourth, the differences between our sample and the original sample used by Conroy[6] could provide dissimilar interpretations. The sample from the original study was composed uniquely with college students, having a considerably higher mean age, comparatively with our sport leagues and federations sample. Therefore, it will be essential to examine in future studies the different characteristics such as athletes' age and as well as gender, sport type, and performance level associated with fear of failure.

Conclusions

The PFAI is a valuable instrument for researchers and practitioners (e.g., sport coaches, coaching scientists, and psychologists) who want to assess fear of failure in such diverse settings as sport, exercise, and education[13]. The role of the PFAI in sport settings is vital, and this study provided a distinctive utility to scholars and coaches since from a practical point of view, it can be employed as a diagnostic tool in the assessment with implications for treatment and prevention of fear of failure, providing a precious help identifying individuals' maladaptive appraisals (or threat appraisals) associated with failure.

References

1. Hosek V, Man F. Training to reduce anxiety and fear in top athletes. In: D. Hackfort D, & C. D. Spielberger CD, editors (Eds.)., Anxiety in sport: An international.
2. Rainey DW. Stress, burnout, and intention to terminate among umpires. J Sport Behav. 1995; 18(4): 312-323.
3. Orlick TD. The athletic dropout: A high price of inefficiency. Canadian Association for Health, Physical Educational Recreat J. 1974. Nov./Dec.: 21-27.
4. Anshel MH. Causes of drug abuse in sport: A survey of intercollegiate athletes. J Sport Behav. 1991; 14: 283-307.
5. Gould D, Horn T, Spreeman J. Sources of stress in junior elite wrestlers. J Sport Psychol. 1983; 5: 159-171.
6. Conroy DE, Willow JP, Metzler JN. Multidimensional fear of failure measurement: The Performance Failure Appraisal Inventory. J Appl Sport Psychol. 2002; 14: 76-90.
7. Birney RC, Burdick H, Teevan RC. Fear of failure. New York: Van Nostrand. 1969.
8. Alpert R, Haber RN. Anxiety in academic achievement situations. J Abnorm Soc Psychol. 1960; 10: 207-215.
9. Passer MW. Fear of failure, fear of evaluation, perceived competence, and self-esteem in competitive-trait-anxious children. J Sport Psychol. 1983; 5: 172-188.
10. Sadd S, Lenauer M, Shaver PR, Dunivant N. Objective measurement of fear of success and fear of failure: A factor analytic approach. J Consulting Clinical Psychol. 1978; 46: 405-416.
11. Willis JD. Three scales to measure competition-related motives in sport. J Sport Psychol. 1982; 4: 338-353.
12. Conroy DE. Progress in the development of a multidimensional measure of fear of failure: The Performance Failure Appraisal Inventory (PFAI). Anxiety Stress Coping. 2001; 14: 431-452.
13. Sagar SS, Jowet S. Validation of a multidimensional measure of fear of failure in a British sample: The Performance Failure Appraisal Inventory (PFAI). Int J Coaching Sci. 2010; 4(1): 49-63.
14. Conroy DE, Metzler JN. Patterns of self-talk associated with different forms of competitive anxiety. J. Sport Exerc Psychol. 2004; 26: 69-89.
15. Conroy DE, Coatsworth JD, Kaye MP. Consistency of fear of failure score meanings among 8–18-year-old female athletes. Educational Psychol. Measurement. 2007; 67(2): 300-310.
16. Kaye MP, Conroy DE, Fifer AM. Individual differences in incompetence avoidance. J. Sport Exercise Psychol. 2008; 30: 110-132.
17. Athanas EH. Fear of failure, division and experience as predictors of state anxiety in USFA epee fencers [master's thesis]. [Statesboro (GA)]: Georgia Southern University; 2007. 75 p.
18. Sideridis G, Kafetsios K. Parental bonding, fear of failure and stress during class presentations. Int J Behav Development. 2008; 32(2), 119-130.
19. Sagar S, Jowet S. The effects of age, gender, sport type and sport level on athletes' fear of failure: Implications and recommendations for sport coaches. Int J Coaching Science. 2012; 6(2): 61-82
20. Smith RE, Smoll FL, Cumming SP, Grossbard JR. Measurement of multidimensional sport performance anxiety in children and adults: The Sport Anxiety Scale-2. J Sport Exerc Psychol. 2006; 28: 479-501.
21. Cruz JF, Gomes AR. Escala de Ansiedade no Desporto (EAD-2)–Versão para investigação [The Sport Anxiety Scale-2]. Braga (Portugal): Universidade do Minho; 2007.

22. Beaton DE, Bombardier C, Guillemin F, Ferraz MB. Guidelines for the process of cross-cultural adaptation of self-report measures. Spine. 2000; 25(24): 3186-3191
23. Olsson UH, Foss T, Troye SV, Howell RD. The performance of ML, GLS and WLS estimation in structural equation modeling under conditions of misspecification and nonnormality. Structural Equ Modeling. 2000; 7: 557-595.
24. Byrne BM. Structural equation modeling with Amos: Basic concepts, applications, and programming. New York: Taylor and Francis Group; 2010.
25. Kline RB. Principles and practices of structural equation modeling. 3rd ed. New York: The Guilford Press; 2011.
26. Schumacher RE, Lomax RG. A beginner's guide to structural equation modeling. Mahwah: Lawrence Erlbaum Associates; 1996.
27. Markland D. The golden rule is that there are no golden rules: A commentary on Paul Barrett's recommendations for reporting model fit in structural equation modeling. Pers Individ Differences. 2007; 42: 851-858.
28. Thompson B. Exploratory and confirmatory factor analysis: Understanding concepts and applications. Washington: American Psychological Association; 2004.
29. Arbuckle J. AMOS18 reference guide (version 18). Chicago: Statistical Package for the Social Sciences; 2009.
30. Bentler PM, Bonett DG. Significance tests and goodness of fit in analysis of covariance structures. Psychol Bull. 1980; 88: 588-606.
31. Blunch NJ. Introduction to structural equation modeling using SPSS and AMOS. Thousand Oaks: SAGE; 2008.
32. Kline RB. Principles and practice of structural equation modeling. New York: Guilford. 1998.
33. Marsh HW. Application of confirmatory factor analysis and structural equation modeling in sport/exercise psychology. In: Tenenbaum G, Eklund RC, editors. Handbook of sport psychology. New York: Wiley; 2007. p. 774-798.
34. Fornell C, Larcker D. Evaluation structural equations models with unobservable variable and measurement error. J Marketing Res. 1981; 18(3): 39-50.
35. Hair J, Anderson R, Tatham R, Black W. Multivariate data analysis. Upper Saddle River: Prentice Hall. 2009.
36. Brown T. Confirmatory factor analysis for applied research. New York: The Guildford Press. 2006.
37. Davey A, Savla J. Statistical power analysis with missing data: A structural equation modeling approach. New York: Taylor and Francis Group. 2010.
38. Schumaker RE, Lomax RG. A beginner's guide to structural equation modeling 2nd ed. Mahwah: Psychology Press. 2004.
39. Loehlin JC. Latent variable models: An introduction to factor, path, and structural equation analysis. Mahwah: Lawrence Erlbaum Associates. 2003.
40. Marôco J. [Structural equation modeling: Theoretical foundations, software and aplications]. Lisboa, Portugal: Report Number; 2010. 374 p. Portuguese.
41. Cheung G, Rensvold R. Evaluating goodness-of-fit indexes for testing measurement invariance. Structural Equ Modeling: A Multidisciplinary Journal. 2002; 9(2): 233-255.
42. Campbell D, Fiske D. Convergent and discriminant validation by the multitrait multimethod matrix. Psychol Bull. 1959; 56(2): 81-105.
43. Kline RB. Beyond significance testing: Reforming data analysis methods in behavioral research. Washington: American Psychological Association. 2004.
44. Bentler PM, Wu EJC. EQS/Windows user's guide. Los Angeles: BMDP Statistical Software. 1993.
45. Walker DA. A confirmatory factor analysis of the Attitudes Toward Research scale. Multiple Linear Regression Viewpoints. 2010; 36: 17-26.
46. Bollen KA, Stine RA. Bootstrapping goodness-of-fit measures in structural equation models. In: Bollen K, Long J, editors. Testing structural equation models. Newbury Park: Sage Focus Edition; 1993. p. 111-135.
47. Chartrand JM, Robbins SB, Morrill WH, Boggs K. Development and validation of the Career Factors Inventory. J Counseling Psychol. 1990; 37: 491-501.
48. Conroy DE, Metzler JN, Hofer SM. Factorial invariance and latent mean stability of performance failure appraisals. Factorial Equ Modeling. 2003; 10(3): 401-422.

Appendix

(Questionário Multidimensional do Medo de Falhar no Desporto)

Medo de Sentir Vergonha e Embaraço (MSVE)
9. Quando estou a falhar, é embaraçoso quando estão outras pessoas a assistir.
13. Quando estou a falhar, preocupo-me com o que os outros pensam de mim.
14. Quando estou a falhar, preocupo-me que os outros pensem que não me estou a esforçar.

Medo de Desvalorizar a Autoestima (MDAE)
8. Quando não estou a ter sucesso, fico em baixo muito facilmente.
3. Quando estou a falhar, culpo a minha falta de talento/jeito.
4. Quando estou a falhar, tenho medo de não ter talento/jeito suficiente.

Medo de Ter um Futuro Incerto (MFI)
1. Quando estou a falhar, o meu futuro parece-me incerto.
5. Quando estou a falhar, perturba o meu "plano" para o futuro.

Medo que Outros Importantes Percam Interesse (MOPI)
6. Quando não estou a ter sucesso, as pessoas ficam menos interessadas por mim.
11. Quando não estou a ter sucesso, algumas pessoas perdem definitivamente o interesse por mim.
12. Quando não estou a ter sucesso, o meu valor diminui para algumas pessoas.

Medo de Preocupar Outros Importantes (MPOI)
2. Quando estou a falhar, preocupo as pessoas que são importantes para mim.
7. Quando estou a falhar, aqueles que são importantes para mim não ficam contentes.

10. Quando estou a falhar, aqueles que são importantes para mim ficam desapontados.

Note. Item numbers are provided to identify the sequence of administration.

Corresponding author

Marco Estêvão Correia
Faculdade de Motricidade Humana, Universidade de Lisboa
Estrada da Costa, 1495-688, Cruz Quebrada, Portugal
Email: marc.correia@gmail.com / mcorreia@fmh.ulisboa.pt

24

Patellofemoral pain and sports practice: reduced symptoms and higher quality of life in adolescent athletes as compared to non-athletes

Danilo de Oliveira Silva
Maira Bergamaschi Coura
Marina Waiteman
Juliana Pradela
Marcella Ferraz Pazzinatto
Universidade Estadual Paulista "Júlio de Mesquita Filho", Presidente Prudente, SP, Brasil

Fernando Henrique Magalhães
Universidade de São Paulo, São Paulo, SP, Brasil

Fábio Mícolis de Azevedo
Universidade Estadual Paulista "Júlio de Mesquita Filho", Presidente Prudente, SP, Brasil

Abstract—Patellofemoral pain (PFP) is common in athletes and physically active individuals and it is one of the most frequent knee disorders among adolescents. However, the impact of the severity of PFP symptoms on quality of life (QOL) has been barely investigated. Thus, we aimed to compare the level of PFP and the self-reported QOL between adolescent athletes and non-athletes, and to explore the relationship between the severity of PFP symptoms and QOL. Fifty-six adolescents with PFP (22 athletes and 34 non-athletes) were asked to fulfill the Anterior Knee Pain Scale (AKPS) and the QOL dimension of the Knee Outcome in Osteoarthritis Survey (KOOS). Between groups comparisons indicated that adolescent non-athletes presented higher severity of PFP symptoms and lower QOF as compared with adolescent athletes. Significant correlations between the severity of PFP and QOL were found for both groups, regardless of the athletic status.

Keyword: adolescent; quality of life; knee; physical activity; athletic performance.

Introduction

Patellofemoral pain (PFP) is often observed in athletes and subjects physically active and it is one of the most common knee disorders among adolescents (Molgaard, Rathleff, & Simonsen, 2011; Rathleff, Roos, Olesen, Rasmussen, & Arendt-Nielsen, 2013). Population-based studies have indicated that the prevalence of PFP among adolescents aged 15–19 years old is 7%, while long-standing knee pain is frequently reported by this population with average pain duration of more than three years (Molgaard *et al.*, 2011; Rathleff, *et al.*, 2013). Thus, it seems that PFP may be present among even younger (<15 years old) adolescents. Besides long-standing pain, adolescents with PFP usually report important reductions in function and health-related quality of life (QOL) as compared to asymptomatic adolescents (Rathleff, *et al.*, 2013).

PFP has also been associated with increased levels of physical activity practice (Fairbank, Pynsent, Vanpoortvliet, & Phillips, 1984). For instance, higher levels of knee pain were reported by those who participated in pain-exacerbating activities during the preceding days (Thomeé, Augustsson, Karlsson, & Thomee, 1999). In this direction, athletes with PFP may be more exposed to symptoms aggravation and consequently have greater reduction in the QOL as compared to non-athletes. Injuries in athletes result in high health care costs and impose a significant physiological and psychosocial health impact (McLeod, Bay, Parsons, Sauers, & Snyder, 2009). Psychosocial examination is an important component of a sports injury appraisal because reduced QOL due to knee pain may demotivate the participation in professional sports activities (Cheung, Zhang, & Ngai, 2013). Despite these facts, the impact of QOL in association with sport-related injury remains an issue that has been barely investigated in the field of sports medicine.

The progression of PFP to more severe orthopedic disorders such as knee osteoarthritis and anterior cruciate ligament injury has been a matter of debate (Crossley, 2014; Myer *et al.*, 2014). Therefore, early identification of risk factors related to PFP may be critical for the prevention of PFP in young and highly active athletes. To the best of our knowledge, this is the first study that explores the association between the severity of PFP and QOL in adolescent athletes and non-athletes with PFP. Such information has the potential to provide insights in order to formulate adequate rehabilitation strategies for adolescent with PFP considering psychosocial approaches.

Therefore, the aims of this study were (1) to compare the level of PFP symptoms and the self-reported QOL between adolescent athletes and non-athletes with PFP, and (2) to explore the relationship between the level of PFP symptoms and QOL in adolescent athletes and non-athletes with PFP. In view of the literature briefly reviewed above, we hypothesized that adolescent athletes would report a greater level of PFP and reduced QOL as compared to non-athletes. In addition, we expected the severity of PFP symptoms to be associated with decreased QOL in both groups.

Methods

This was a cross-sectional study that compared adolescent athletes aged between 12 to 18 years old diagnosed with PFP with a control group of non-athletes with PFP. The study was approved by the Sao Paulo State University Human Ethics Committee (number: 037518/2015). Before completing the survey, the participants' parent or guardian signed an informed consent form with the participant's agreement.

Participants

Fifty-six adolescents were recruited and allocated in two groups. The group of adolescent athletes (N = 22; 14 Males and 8 Females) were recruited via athletic trainer and coach contacts at a sport center complex. The athletes were regularly involved in training and competition activities of the following modalities: basketball, volleyball, handball and soccer (Table 1). Adolescent non-athletes (N = 34; 23 Males and 11 Females) were recruited from 4 local high schools. In order to obtain this sample, we screened 80 adolescent athletes (total population of adolescent athletes available at the sport center complex of the city) and 180 adolescent non-athletes (the maximum number of adolescents that was possible to assess). Therefore, the rate of adolescent athletes and non-athletes with PFP corresponded to 27.5% and 18.8%, respectively. Thus, the presented study included a higher number of adolescent non-athletes as compared with athletes (due to the higher number of non-athletes that could be screened initially). Anthropometric data of the two groups can be found in Table 2. Participants were recruited between June and November 2015. In order to achieve homogeneity of the sample, only participants involved in recreational physical activity were included in the group of non-athletes. To be classified as physically active, the participants had to be fulfill the International Physical Activity Questionnaire (IPAQ) Scoring Protocol short form. The two criteria used for classification as physically active were: a) vigorous activity at least 3 days per week, or b) moderate activity at least 5 days per week (IPAQ Research Committee, 2005).

Table 1. Sports modality practiced by the adolescents with patellofemoral pain of athletes group.

Sport	Male	Female	Total
Basketball	8 (57.14%)	3 (37.50%)	11 (50.00%)
Handball	3 (21.42%)	1 (12.50%)	4 (18.18%)
Soccer	3 (21.42%)	-	3 (13.63%)
Volleyball	-	4 (50.00%)	4 (18.8%)
Total	14 (100%)	8 (100%)	22 (100%)

The number of participants in each modality of sport and the respective percentage (%).

Table 2. Summary of subject demographics.

	Adolescent Athletes	**Adolescents Non-athletes**	
Data	Mean ± SD	Mean ± SD	p-value
Age (years)	14.45 ± 1.29	13.85 ± 1.18	0.168
Body Mass (kg)	68.11 ± 12.52	66.88 ± 13.45	0.356
Height (m)	1.77 ± 0.10	1.73 ± 0.08	0.095
Previous month pain (VAS)	4.31 ± 1.35	5.23 ± 1.77	0.044*
Symptoms duration (Months)	19.45 ± 12.51	22.03 ± 17.06	0.545
AKPS score	84.73 ± 10.85	77.47 ± 10.17	0.017*
KOOS-QOL score	77.84 ± 18.77	67.87 ± 17.36	0.047*
Gender	15 males/ 7 females	23 males/ 11 females	-

Abbreviation: Mean ± SD = Mean and Standard Deviation; VAS = Visual Analogue Scale; AKPS = Anterior Knee Pain Scale; KOOS-QOL = Knee Outcome in Osteoarthritis Survey, Quality of Life dimension. The percentage of females in the Adolescent Athletes group is 46.66% and in the Adolescent Non-Athletes group is 47.82%

*Statistically significant difference between groups.

Adolescents of both groups were diagnosed with PFP if they met the following criteria (Rathleff, *et al.*, 2013): insidious onset of anterior knee or retropatellar pain for at least the past 6 weeks; pain provoked by at least 2 of the following activities: prolonged sitting or kneeling, squatting, running, or stair walking; tenderness on palpation of the posterior surface of the patella; and worst pain intensity in the previous month of at least 3 cm on a 10 cm visual analog scale. Exclusion criteria were concomitant injury or pain from the hip, lumbar spine, or other knee structures; previous knee surgery; patellofemoral instability; knee joint effusion; use of physiotherapy for treating knee pain within the previous year; currently undergoing medical treatment; or daily or weekly use of anti-inflammatory drugs. Participants of the group of non-athletes were excluded if involved in sports competition.

Procedure

All included participants completed two self-administered questionnaires: Anterior Knee Pain Scale (AKPS) and Knee Outcome in Osteoarthritis Survey (KOOS). The surveys were administered in a classroom (non-athletes group) or at the sport center complex (athletes group) and took approximately 30 minutes to be completed. The participants were assisted by a trained physical therapist.

Instruments

The AKPS is a 13-item questionnaire that evaluates subjective symptoms and functional limitations associated with PFP and can be used to assess the severity of PFP (Cheung *et al.*, 2013). The questionnaire score ranges from 0 to 100, with the maximum total score of 100 indicating no disability and 0 indicating the worst symptoms and restrictions of daily life functions. This tool has been validated for subjects with PFP and has been reported to demonstrate high test–retest reliability (Crossley, Bennell, Cowan, & Green, 2004).

The KOOS was constructed on the basis of the literature review and expert panel (Roos, Roos, Lohmander, Ekdahl, & Beynnon, 1998). The KOOS is a 42-item questionnaire that covers five dimensions reported separately: pain, symptoms, activities of daily living, sport and recreation function, and knee-related quality of life. This tool has been validated and also demonstrates high test–retest reliability (Singh, Luo, Landon, & Suarez-Almazor, 2014). Each dimension has its own score ranging from 0 to 100. The dimension of interest in this study was the knee-related QOL, with higher scores indicating better QOL and lower scores indicating worse QOL.

Statistical Analysis

Statistical analyses were performed using the Statistical Package for Social Sciences (SPSS) version 18.0 (SPSS Inc., Chicago IL). Descriptive statistics for sample characteristics were expressed using mean (standard deviation). To determine the normality and homogeneity of the data, Shapiro-Wilk's and Levene's tests were used, respectively (Field, 2013). The severity of PFP and QOL were compared between groups using independent-samples t test. A Pearson product–moment correlation matrix was used to examine the relationships between severity of PFP and QOL in each group.

Results

The data were found to be normally distributed for all variables. In addition, equal variances were assumed in the Levene's test for all variables (F-value < 1.22; p-value > 0.274). Therefore, parametric tests could be used for comparisons, despite the higher number of participants in the group of adolescent non-athletes (Field, 2013). There were no significant differences between the groups for body mass, age or height (Table 2). The adolescent athletes with PFP scored higher in the AKPS as compared with the adolescent non-athletes (p = 0.017) with PFP. Additionally, the athletes with PFP scored higher in the QOL dimension of the KOOS as compared with the non-athletes (p = 0.044).

Our findings indicated a significant positive relationship between the severity of PFP and the QOL in both groups, that is, the worse the symptoms of PFP the worse the QOL of adolescents with PFP, regardless of their athletic status (Table 3).

Table 3. Correlations between level of patellofemoral pain and quality of life (one of the five dimensions of KOOS) in adolescent athletes and non-athletes.

Anterior Knee Pain Scale	KOOS-QOL	p-value
Athlete	r = 0.671*	< 0.001
Non-athlete	r = 0.781*	< 0.001

Abbreviation: KOOS-QOL = Knee Outcome in Osteoarthritis Survey - Quality of Life dimension; r = Pearson product–moment correlation matrix value.

*Statistically significant correlation.

Discussion

As previously mentioned, PFP is one of the most common diagnoses in sports medicine, accounting for nearly 25% of all identified knee injuries (De Oliveira Silva, Briani, Pazzinatto, Ferrari, Aragão, Albuquerque, *et al.*, 2015a; Pazzinatto *et al.*, 2015; Silva *et al.*, 2015). It is a common problem, encompassing a variety of symptoms without a single identifiable cause (De Oliveira Silva, Briani, Pazzinatto, Ferrari, Aragão, & de Azevedo, 2015b; Witvrouw *et al.*, 2014). Multiple intrinsic anatomic factors are combined with extrinsic environmental factors thereby leading to a knee pain disorder that can be difficult for clinicians and researchers to comprehend (Briani *et al.*, 2015; Herbst *et al.*, 2015). Despite the importance and high-incidence of PFP, there are some lacks in the currently established literature, which our study aimed to examine. For instance, previous studies in this field have focused on females with PFP aged 18-35 years old (Boling *et al.*, 2010; De Oliveira Silva *et al.*, 2015a; Silva *et al.*, 2015), while few studies have investigated the male population. Therefore, a notably strengthening of our study was the inclusion of males and females adolescent athletes and non-athletes with PFP. The impact of PFP on QOL is another point that has been barely investigated and hence our findings extend the current knowledge.

We hypothesized that: 1) adolescent athletes would report a greater level of PFP symptoms and reduced QOL as compared to non-athletes and 2) the level of PFP would be positively associated with QOL in both groups. Contrastingly, our findings indicated that adolescent athletes reported lower severity of PFP symptoms and greater QOL as compared to non-athletes. On the other hand, our second hypothesis was confirmed as the level of PFP was positively associated with QOL in both groups. Our results indicate that the severity of PFP is strongly correlated with an important component of health status as QOL. These findings reinforce the necessity of including patient's self-reported measures to assess the effects of PFP across a broad spectrum of health status, so as to provide a more global and complete assessment of these individuals.

A large amount of biomechanical and physiological alterations have been observed in individuals with PFP.

For instance, many retrospective studies have shown that adults with PFP present hip muscle weakness as compared to controls (Cant, Pineux, & Pitance, 2014; Fredericson & Yoon, 2006; Razeghi, Etemadi, Taghizadeh, & Ghaem, 2010). However, these studies did not determine whether alterations such as muscle weakness are causes or effects of PFP. In a recent prospective study, Herbst *et al.* (2015) showed that, before developing PFP, adolescents actually demonstrated greater hip strength than those who remained healthy. The authors speculated that the adolescents with PFP probably developed greater hip abductor strength to compensate for an increased hip adduction patterns, which is an alteration that have been widely reported in individuals with PFP during functional activities (Barton, Levinger, Menz, & Webster, 2009; Lankhorst, Bierma-Zeinstra, & van Middelkoop, 2013; Nakagawa, Moriya, Maciel, & Serrão, 2012). As long as the greater hip abduction strength was able to correct the increased hip adduction kinematics, the participants remained asymptomatic. When this compensatory behavior failed, the participants developed PFP. Therefore, it is reasonable to speculate that similar mechanisms may have played a role in the present study, which may explain, at least in part, the rejection of our first hypothesis. That is, the adolescent athletes with PFP may have developed compensatory behaviors for longer periods due to the high-intensity training and well-prepared musculoskeletal system, thereby attenuating the severity of PFP symptoms and its impact on QOL. However, future prospective studies are needed in order to better explore this conjecture.

A matter of frequent investigation in PFP is the impact of biomechanical alterations on physical function and the severity of PFP (De Oliveira Silva, Briani, Pazzinatto, Ferrari, Aragão, & de Azevedo, 2015c). However, the relationship between the severity of PFP symptoms and its corresponding impact on the QOL has been neglected. We have found a significant relationship between the level of PFP and QOL for both groups (athletes and non-athletes), with increased PFP symptoms associated with decreased QOL. The present results provide evidence that PFP severity leads to negative health-related consequences that may affect areas of the adolescent's life other than their athletic and physical activities. Similar to our results (Cheung *et al.*, 2013) showed a significant association between the level of PFP and QOL in 19 adult professional athletes representative of the national track and field team of China. Thus, it seems that the relationship between QOL and PFP may be persistent over time, thereby leading to long-lasting impairments in the health status of physically-active subjects with PFP.

Poorly managed musculoskeletal injuries during adolescence may lead to some significant and disabling long-term health problems such as knee osteoarthritis (Crossley, 2014; McLeod *et al.*, 2009). Utting, Davies, & Newman, 2005 demonstrated that a substantial number of patients with patellofemoral arthritis had suffered with PFP during their adolescence. Moreover, many of these patients reported symptoms of PFP 20 years prior to their arthroplasty surgery, thereby suggesting that the problem had been continuous throughout their life and that PFP developed during adolescence might have contributed to the later establishment of patellofemoral osteoarthritis (Utting *et al.*, 2005). Therefore, considering the relationships found in our study, it seems imperative to develop treatment strategies to recover physical function and health status in adolescents with PFP as soon as possible, regardless if they are athletes or not.

Conclusion

In summary, adolescent non-athletes presented greater level of PFP and lower QOL as compared with adolescent athletes, suggesting that the involvement in sports training and competition by adolescent athletes with PFP did not contribute to the aggravation of PFP and decrease in QOL. Furthermore, the severity of PFP symptoms was significantly associated with reduced QOL in both groups of adolescents with PFP, regardless of their athletic status, providing evidence that PFP might lead to negative consequences to adolescent's psychosocial health.

References

Barton, C. J., Levinger, P., Menz, H. B., & Webster, K. E. (2009). Kinematic gait characteristics associated with patellofemoral pain syndrome: a systematic review. *Gait & Posture*, *30*(4), 405–16. doi:10.1016/j.gaitpost.2009.07.109

Boling, M., Padua, D., Marshall, S., Guskiewicz, K., Pyne, S., & Beutler, A. (2010). Gender differences in the incidence and prevalence of patellofemoral pain syndrome. *Scandinavian Journal of Medicine & Science in Sports*, *20*(5), 725–730. doi:10.1111/j.1600-0838.2009.00996.x.Gender

Briani, R. V., De Oliveira Silva, D., Pazzinatto, M. F., De Albuquerque, C. E., Ferrari, D., Aragão, F. A., & De Azevedo, F. M. (2015). Comparison of frequency and time domain electromyography parameters in women with patellofemoral pain. *Clinical Biomechanics*, *30*(3), 302–307. doi:10.1016/j.clinbiomech.2014.12.014

Cant, J. Van, Pineux, C., & Pitance, L. (2014). Hip muscle strength and endurance in femeles with patellofemoral pain: a systematic review with meta-analysis. *The International Journal of Sports Physical Therapy*, *9*(5), 564–582.

Cheung, R. T. H., Zhang, Z., & Ngai, S. P. C. (2013). Different relationships between the level of patellofemoral pain and quality of life in professional and amateur athletes. *PM & R*, *5*(7), 568–572. doi:10.1016/j.pmrj.2012.12.007

Crossley, K. (2014). Is patellofemoral osteoarthritis a common sequela of patellofemoral pain? *British Journal of Sports Medicine*, *48*, 409–410. doi:10.1136/bjsports-2014-093445

Crossley, K. M., Bennell, K. L., Cowan, S. M., & Green, S. (2004). Analysis of outcome measures for persons with patellofemoral pain: which are reliable and valid? *Archives of Physical Medicine and Rehabilitation*, *85*(5), 815–822. doi:10.1016/S0003-9993(03)00613-0

De Oliveira Silva, D., Briani, R., Pazzinatto, M., Ferrari, D., Aragão, F., & Azevedo, F. (2015)c. Vertical ground reaction forces are associated with pain and self-reported functional status in recreational athletes with patellofemoral pain. *Journal of Applied Biomechanics*, *31*(6), 409 – 414. doi:10.1123/jab.2015-0048

De Oliveira Silva, D., Briani, R. V., Pazzinatto, M. F., Ferrari, D., Aragão, F. A., Albuquerque, C. E., … Azevedo, F. M. (2015)a. Reliability and differentiation capability of dynamic and static kinematic measurements of rearfoot eversion in patellofemoral pain. *Clinical Biomechanics*, *30*(2), 144–148. doi:10.1016/j.clinbiomech.2014.12.009

De Oliveira Silva, D., Briani, R. V., Pazzinatto, M. F., Ferrari, D., Aragão, F. A., & de Azevedo, F. M. (2015)b. Reduced knee flexion is a possible cause of increased loading rates in individuals with patellofemoral pain. *Clinical Biomechanics*, *30*(9), 971–975. doi:10.1016/j.clinbiomech.2015.06.021

Fairbank, J. C. T., Pynsent, P. B., Vanpoortvliet, J. a, & Phillips, H. (1984). Mechanical Factors in the Incidence of Knee Pain in Adolescents and Young-Adults. *Journal of Bone and Joint Surgery-British Volume*, *66*(5), 685–693.

Field, A. (2013). *Discovering statistics using IBM SPSS statistics.* (4th ed.). London.

Fredericson, M., & Yoon, K. (2006). Physical examination and patellofemoral pain syndrome. *American Journal of Physical Medicine & Rehabilitation / Association of Academic Physiatrists*, *85*(3), 234–43. doi:10.1097/01.phm.0000200390.67408.f0

Herbst, K. a., Barber Foss, K. D., Fader, L., Hewett, T. E., Witvrouw, E., Stanfield, D., & Myer, G. D. (2015). Hip Strength Is Greater in Athletes Who Subsequently Develop Patellofemoral Pain. *The American Journal of Sports Medicine*, *43*(11), 2747–2752. doi:10.1177/0363546515599628

IPAQ Research Committee. Guidelines for data processing and analysis of the International Physical Activity Questionnaire(IPAQ), Short Form. (2005).

Lankhorst, N. E., Bierma-Zeinstra, S. M. a, & van Middelkoop, M. (2013). Factors associated with patellofemoral pain syndrome: a systematic review. *British Journal of Sports Medicine*, *47*(4), 193–206. doi:10.1136/bjsports-2011-090369

McLeod, T. C. V., Bay, R. C., Parsons, J. T., Sauers, E. L., & Snyder, A. R. (2009). Recent injury and health-related quality of life in adolescent athletes. *Journal of Athletic Training*, *44*(6), 603–610. doi:10.4085/1062-6050-44.6.603

Molgaard, C., Rathleff, M. S., & Simonsen, O. (2011). Patellofemoral pain syndrome and its association with hip, ankle, and foot function in 16- to 18-year-old high school students: a single-blind case-control study. *Journal of the American Podiatric Medical Association*, *101*(3), 215–222. doi:101/3/215 [pii]

Myer, G. D., Ford, K. R., Di Stasi, S. L., Barber Foss, K. D., Micheli, L. J., & Hewett, T. E. (2014). High knee abduction moments are common risk factors for patellofemoral pain (PFP) and anterior cruciate ligament (ACL) injury in girls: Is PFP itself a predictor for subsequent ACL injury? *British Journal of Sports Medicine*, *0*, 1–7. doi:10.1136/bjsports-2013-092536

Nakagawa, T. H., Moriya, É. T. U., Maciel, C. D., & Serrão, A. F. V. (2012). Frontal plane biomechanics in males and females with and without patellofemoral pain. *Medicine and Science in Sports and Exercise*, *44*(9), 1747–55. doi:10.1249/MSS.0b013e318256903a

Pazzinatto, M. F., Silva, D. O., Briani, R. V., Ferrari, D., Aragão, F. A., Albuquerque, C. E., & Azevedo, F. M. (2015). Reliability of electromyography parameters during stair deambulation in patellofemoral pain syndrome. *Motriz: Revista de Educação Física*, *21*(2), 207–213.

Rathleff, M. S., Roos, E. M., Olesen, J. L., Rasmussen, S., & Arendt-Nielsen, L. (2013). Lower mechanical pressure pain thresholds in female adolescents with patellofemoral pain syndrome. *The Journal of Orthopaedic and Sports Physical Therapy*, *43*(6), 414–21. doi:10.2519/jospt.2013.4383

Razeghi, M., Etemadi, Y., Taghizadeh, S., & Ghaem, H. (2010). Could hip and knee muscle strengthening alter the pain intensity in patellofemoral pain syndrome ? *Iranian Red Crescent Medical Journal*, *12*(2), 104–110.

Roos, E. M., Roos, H. P., Lohmander, L. S., Ekdahl, C., & Beynnon, B. D. (1998). Knee Injury and Osteoarthritis Outcome Score (KOOS)--development of a self-administered outcome measure. *The Journal of Orthopaedic and Sports Physical Therapy*, *28*(2), 88–96. doi:10.2519/jospt.1998.28.2.88

Silva, D. O., Briani, R. V., Ferrari, D., Pazzinatto, M. F., Aragão, F. A., & Azevedo, F. M. (2015). Ângulo Q e pronação subtalar não são bons preditores de dor e função em indivíduos com síndrome da dor femoropatelar. *Fisioterapia E Pesquisa*, *22*(2), 169–175. doi:10.590/1809-2950/14031522022015

Singh, J. A., Luo, R., Landon, G. C., & Suarez-Almazor, M. (2014). Reliability and clinically important improvement thresholds for osteoarthritis pain and function scales: A multicenter study. *Journal of Rheumatology*, *41*(3), 509–515. doi:10.3899/jrheum.130609

Thomeé, R., Augustsson, J., Karlsson, J., & Thomee, R. (1999). Patellofemoral pain syndrome: a review of current issues. *Sports Medicine*, *28*(4), 245–262.

Utting, M. R., Davies, G., & Newman, J. H. (2005). Is anterior knee pain a predisposing factor to patellofemoral osteoarthritis? *The Knee*, *12*(5), 362–5. doi:10.1016/j.knee.2004.12.006

Witvrouw, E., Callaghan, M. J., Stefanik, J. J., Noehren, B., Bazett-Jones, D. M., Willson, J. D., … Crossley, K. M. (2014). Patellofemoral pain: consensus statement from the 3rd International Patellofemoral Pain Research Retreat held in Vancouver, September 2013. *British Journal of Sports Medicine*, *48*(6), 411–4. doi:10.1136/bjsports-2014-093450

Authors' note

Danilo de Oliveira Silva, Maira Bergamaschi Coura, Marina Waiteman, Juliana Pradela, Marcella Ferraz Pazzinatto, Fábio Mícolis de Azevedo are affiliated with the University of São Paulo State, School of Science and Technology, Physical Therapy Department, Presidente Prudente, Brazil.

Fernando Henrique Magalhães is affiliated with the School of Arts, Sciences, and Humanities, University of Sao Paulo, Sao Paulo, Brazil

Acknowledgment

To São Paulo Research Foundation (FAPESP) for a scholarship (2015/15575-4). The financial sponsors played no role in the design, execution, analysis and interpretation of data, or writing of the study.

Corresponding author

Fernando Henrique Magalhães
Avenida Arlindo Bettio, 1000, School of Arts, Sciences and Humanities (EACH-USP), São Paulo, SP, 03828-000, Brazil.
Email: fhmagalhaes@usp.br

25

The effect of the maintaining the ball possession on the intensity of games

Felipe Lovaglio Belozo
Eliel Calazans Ferreira
Cristian J. R. Lizana
Guilherme Grandim
Universidade de Campinas, UNICAMP, Campinas, SP, Brasil

João Claudio Machado
Universidade Federal do Amazonas, UFAM, Manaus, AM, Brasil

René Brenzikofer
Denise Vaz Macedo
Milton Shoiti Misuta
Alcides José Scaglia
Universidade de Campinas, UNICAMP, Campinas, SP, Brasil

Abstract—The use of small-sided games (SSG) for soccer training has increased considerably in recent years. Tactical principles can influence the intensity and the movement of soccer players during training. The aim of this study was to evaluate the influence of maintaining possession of the ball on the intensity and the time of motion characteristics of players during training in games. Eleven athletes of the U-20 category of a professional club in São Paulo, Brazil, participated in this study. To check the influence of the tactical principle, we used a game control and an experimental game in three different field dimensions and number of players. The results show that possession of the maintenance rule influences the intensity of the games ($p<0.05$). However, it is concluded that the rule is fundamental for training through games.

Keywords: soccer, training, small-sided games.

Introduction

Soccer is one of the most popular sports in the world, despite its creation spanning over hundreds of years, there are still many doubts about its physiological, technical, biomechanical and psychological requirements. These questions may be explained by the fact that its initial training was influenced and developed through individual sports (Aguiar, Botelho, Lago, Macas, & Sampaio, 2012). However, with the technological and scientific developments applied to soccer, it has been recognized the need to develop training and evaluations that respect the principle of specificity (Bangsbo, Norregaard, & Thorso, 1991; Hoff, Wisloff, Engen, Kemi, & Helgerud, 2002; Kelly, Gregson, Reilly, & Drust, 2013; Kemi, Hoff, Engen, Helgerud, & Wisloff, 2003; Stolen, Chamari, Castagna, & Wisloff, 2005). In recent years, studies with small-sided games (SSG) have increased considerably; several studies point out the importance of the training of soccer players through SSG, since they are able to develop the technical, physical and tactical aspects in addition to respecting the specificity of the training (Bloomfield, Polman, O'Donoghue, & McNaughton, 2007; Dellal *et al.*, 2008; Eniseler, 2005; Hill-Haas, Dawson, Impellizzeri, & Coutts, 2011; Impellizzeri *et al.*, 2006; Rampinini *et al.*, 2007; Reilly, 2005; Scaglia, Reverdito.R., Leonardo, & Lizana, 2013).

In sports training, the monitoring of the training intensities is essential. Nowadays, it is possible to know the internal responses (heart rate and lactate concentration [La]) and the external responses, such as the distances covered in official games and in training (Gabbett & Mulvey, 2008; Hill-Haas, Rowsell, Dawson, & Coutts, 2009; Spencer *et al.*, 2004). Several studies have been examining the lactate concentration [La] to control the individual loads of athletes during research studies (Aguiar, Botelho, Goncalves, & Sampaio, 2013; Coutts, Rampinini, Marcora, Castagna, & Impellizzeri, 2009; Eniseler, 2005; Harrison, Gill, Kinugasa, & Kilding, 2013; Koklu, Sert, Alemdaroglu, & Arslan, 2013). However, it is known that lactate concentration, according to the studies of Bangsbo (1994), has a strong correlation with the latest efforts prior to blood collection. Thus, to assess the movement of the players on the field, the General Positioning System (GPS) is the most largely used tool in practices and well recognized in the research field because of its speed in data visualization (Hill-Haas, Coutts, Dawson, & Rowsell, 2010; Hill-Haas *et al.*, 2011; Hill-Haas *et al.*, 2009). On the other hand, methodological limitations exist since it is necessary to be careful with the data on collective activities with changes of direction and velocities above 20 km/h, where the accuracy is not high for a critical analysis (Coutts & Duffield, 2010; Johnston *et al.*, 2012). Those speeds in small- and medium-sized games are often not reached, however, on official fields, these velocities are frequently reached.

Another tool used to assess the movement of the players is the video analysis through shooting with digital cameras (Gabbett & Mulvey, 2008). According to Barros (2007), the kinematic analysis for soccer players can offer useful information on their movement in games. Thus, the videogrammetry, because of its accuracy of data, has been reported to be an excellent tool for the study of the movement of players (Figueroa, Leite, & Barros, 2003). One of the most studied variables is the total distance covered. However, it is not enough to know only the total distance, but rather at what intensity they are covered, since athletes can cover the same distance at different intensities (Bangsbo, 1994; Gabbett & Mulvey, 2008). Consequently, it is believed that the Ventilatory Threshold (VT) of each athlete is a great variable to characterize individually the intensity of different games. Through the videogrammetry and the functions developed in the Matlab system, we can know the velocity ranges that athletes travel during games and, when correlating them with the ventilatory threshold (VT) test proposed by Lourenço *et al.*,(2011), individually establish four different intensity ranges (low intensity, moderate intensity, moderate/high and high intensity). Without knowing the velocity of the VT (VVT) of each athlete, it becomes difficult to carry out a controlled individualized training, since for some players the effort can be of high intensity, while for others, only of moderate intensity.

Several studies point out that the rules, the size of the field, the absence of goalkeepers and the number of players directly influence the intensity and time motion characteristics of the athletes during the SSG (Brandes, Heitmann, & Muller, 2012; Castellano, Casamichana, & Dellal, 2013; Coutts *et al.*, 2009; Hill-Haas, Coutts, Rowsell, & Dawson, 2009; Hodgson, Akenhead, & Thomas, 2014; Kelly *et al.*, 2013; Koklu *et al.*, 2013). However, there are many variables in a single game, it is difficult to identify which directly interferes in the intensity and movement of the players. Therefore, the aim of this study was to examine the influence of the rules, with the tactical principle of maintaining ball possession, in the control of the intensity of efforts and time motion characteristics of players during training in small-, medium- and large-sided games. The application of this work is to determine the effect of the rules change on the intensity and time motion characteristics of soccer players, since the manipulation of these rules should be well planned by the coaching staff to avoid negative adjustments on the team.

Methods

Experimental design

The design protocol lasted 12 days for each set of experimental analysis. In the first and second days, anthropometric assessment and the incremental treadmill test to determine the VT proposed by Lourenço *et al.*, (2011) were assessed. In the third, fourth, fifth and sixth days, the athletes went through a period of familiarization to the games used in the research, they practiced the games for ten minutes before the training sessions. In the seventh and ninth days, in the afternoon, the athletes were submitted to 3x3+G and 6x6+G SSG only with the official FIFA rules. In the eighth and tenth days, following the same schedules as the previous collections, the 3x3+G and 6x6+G SSG happened, respectively, with the effort rule to promote the tactical principle of maintaining possession (MP). In the eleventh and twelfth days, the 10x10+G control and 10x10+G experimental games were carried out. The control and experimental games were placed on alternate days avoiding an adaptation of the athletes to the MP rules. The game collections occurred in the first two days of the week allowing a resting period to the athletes to the championship game that happened on Saturday mornings.

Subjects

Eleven junior soccer players of the U-20 category (age 18±1.2) belonging to a federated Club in São Paulo, Brazil, all with a minimum of five years of experience in the sport, accepted to participate in the study. The measures of body mass (BM) and height (HT) were performed in a digital scale equipped with stadiometer, brand Welmi®. For fat percentage (F%), we chose to register the subscapular, tricipital, biceptal, pectoral, suprailiac, midaxillary, abdominal, thigh and calf skinfolds using an adipometer (brand Lange®). The calculations were done through the Jackson and Pollock Protocol (1978). The characterization of the sample can be seen in Table 1. This study was approved by the Research Ethics Committee of the School of Medical Sciences of UNICAMP, on 11/Feb/2012 (Opinion No. 208.298 and CAAE: 10855212.2.0000.5404).

Table 1. Characterization of the sample.

Subjects (n=11)	Body mass (Kg)	Height (cm)	Fat mass (%)	Vel. Vo2max (Km/h)	Vel. Threshold (Km/h)
Values	66.58± 7.75	174.04 ± 6.93	10.90 ± 2.90	16.50± 1.19	10.82± 3.22

Procedures

Description of the small-sided games: For the analysis of the games, we adopted two fields: control and experimental, with different sizes and number of players. The formats of the games used are described in Table 2. The games on the control field were carried out without external rules, only with the FIFA ones, including the offside rule; in the experimental field, some external rules were inserted to facilitate the tactical principle of maintaining the ball possession. They are:

- Only two touches on the ball, and every extra touch means a point to the opponent;
- Taking the ball from one sideline to the other one means one point;

- Exchanging five passes in the offensive field (after the midfield) means two points;
- Goal (only allowed after the exchange of five passes) means eight points.

The rule that limits the number of touches on the ball, despite being a rule that contrasts with that one which determines the number of passes required for shot on the opponent's goal (Almeida, Ferreira, & Volossovitch, 2012), when used together in a game, do not mischaracterize the prevalence of positional attacks, where teams tend to maintain the ball possession, as can be seen in the study of Lizana *et al.*,(2015). The dynamic of soccer matches has increased over the last years; therefore, the teams and players must seek not only maintain ball possession, but also search to quickly circulate the ball for the purpose of unbalancing the defense organization of the opponent´s team.

Table 2. Format of the fields where the games took place.

	Format		
	3x3+G	**6x6+G**	**10x10+G**
Size	27x18m	32x52m	105x64
Total Area	486m	1664m	6720m²
Area per player	61m²	119m²	305m²
Goal	Official	Official	Official
Game Time	30min	30min	30min

G - indicates the presence of goalkeepers.

Among the different matrices games proposed by Scaglia *et al.* (2013), the conceptual games allow manipulation of the structural references (ball, size of the field and targets) and functional (operational principles and rules of action). These changes emphasize the training of tactical principles, technical aspects and the various physical and physiological responses proposed by the coaching staff within the pedagogical and organizational planning previously, and so it could not faithfully respect the logic of the competitive game.

Therefore, coaches and/or members of the coaching staff must understand how the handling of certain constraints in low games, the rules may influence the modeling of specific tactical behavior, taking into account the playing style defined by the coach (Clemente, Couceiro, Martins, Ivanova, & Mendes, 2013). In this study the conceptual games were used to emphasize the tactical principle of maintenance of ball possession (Bayer, 1994).

The teams were separated by the coaching staff so that the teams were balanced in relation to player positions (defense, midfield and attack) and also in relation to the technical and physical quality of the players. To reduce the variability between subjects, the same teams faced each other in the control and experimental field on the three field dimensions. Altogether, twenty field athletes participated in the research study; however, we have considered only the players who participated in all games for the statistical analysis. To ensure that there was no interference in the intensity of the games, a statistical analysis was made in relation to the total distance covered between the voluntary players and the sample. No significant difference was found between the groups ($p<0.05$).

Incremental treadmill test: Ventilatory Threshold was determined by the incremental treadmill test proposed by Lourenço *et al.* (2011), in which, at the beginning of the test, the athletes performed a three-minute warm-up running at 8–8.5 km/h on the treadmill (Inbrasport ATL, 2000). The initial speed was 9 km/h and slope of 1%. The increase was 0.3 km/h every 25 seconds. The test was performed until voluntary exhaustion, during which it was continuously monitored the variables: heart rate (Polar RS100), oxygen consumption (VO_2), carbon dioxide production (VCO_2) and respiratory exchange ratio (RER). The cardiorespiratory parameters (VO_2, VCO_2 and RER) were measured breath by breath through a gas analyzer (CPX/D Med Graphics, St. Paul, MN). Immediately after exhaustion, the participants underwent a recovery test, in which the speed of the treadmill was decreased every minute to 60%, 55%, 50%, 45% and 40% of the maximum velocity reached.

For the visual determination of the VT, we used the V-slope method, which consists in the characterization of VT by loss of linearity of VCO_2/VO_2. The respiratory compensation point (RCP) was also determined by visual inspection, which consists in the loss of linearity of the VE/VCO2 ratio. Therefore, we collected the variables Ventilatory threshold (VT), Velocity of the ventilatory threshold ($_V$VT), Heart rate of the ventilatory threshold (HRvt), VO2max, Velocity of VO_2max ($_V VO_2$max), VO_2max heart rate (VO_2maxHR), which allows us to establish four training ranges, stratified by the low intensity below the Threshold, the moderate intensity between VT1 and peak respiratory compensation (PRC), the moderate/high between PRC and Ventilatory Threshold2 and the high intensity above the Ventilatory Threshold2 (VT2).

Data collection and kinematics analyses: The footage of the games was recorded with digital video cameras, with the NTSC standard and 30 Hz of acquisition rate. The cameras were positioned on the highest point of the bleachers, in a fixed position during the entire game, in order to fit the entire playing field. After filming, the sequences of images from each camera were transferred to the computer's hard drive (computer Intel® Core ™ i7-2600k, 3.40GHz, RAM memory, 16 GB, video card NVIDIA GeForce 9500 GT). The file format used is the AVCHD (Advanced Video Codec High Definition) with the resolution of 1080 lines per 1980 columns.

The study of the movement of the soccer players was carried out independent of the size of the body or rotational movements hence it is important that the description of the position of the player is made from the location of a single point (Misuta, Menezes, Figueroa, Cunha, & Barros, 2005). Obtaining the position of the player on the field consists primarily in knowing the relationship between the screen coordinates (x, y) and the reference system associated with the field. Thus, the calibration of each camera was made from at least four known points in the coordinate system associated with the field and their corresponding coordinates in the image. The calibration and two-dimensional (2D) reconstruction method used was proposed by Abdel-Aziz, Karara (1971), named DLT (Direct Linear Transformation).

Through this screening, it was obtained the physical variables: total distance covered, maximum velocities and partial distance, divided into velocity ranges according to the assessment of VT. The functions to determine the physical variables were developed in the Matlab 7.0 system.

Statistical analysis

The Matlab 7.0 system was used for the elaboration of the functions related to the physical variables, such as total distance covered, maximum velocities, intervals between high intensity efforts, amount of high intensity efforts and distances covered at different velocity ranges according to the assessment of the VT of the athletes. The values are expressed as mean and standard deviation. The distribution of the data normality was verified by the Shapiro-Wilk test. After confirming that the data was parametric, we used the *t*-Student test and the value of $p<0.05$ was considered statistically significant. The data were analyzed paired, comparing the variables within the same field size.

Results

Ventilatory Threshold

Figure 1 illustrates a significant difference between the control and experimental fields; on the 3x3+G control games, the athletes covered an average of 141.5±55.3m at high intensity, and just 101.6±55.6m on the experimental games. In the 6x6+G games, the total distance covered at high intensity was 389±179.6m (on the control field) and 175.8±65.3 m (on the experimental field). For the 10x10+G fields, it was found that the average of the total distance covered at high intensity was 560.5±165.9 m for the control field and 361±135.1 m for the experimental field. The distances covered below the VT, regarded as of low intensity, were significantly increase between the 10x10+G control and experimental games, in which the athletes covered 2182.8± 169.3m in the control field and 2302.8±203.1 m in the experimental field.

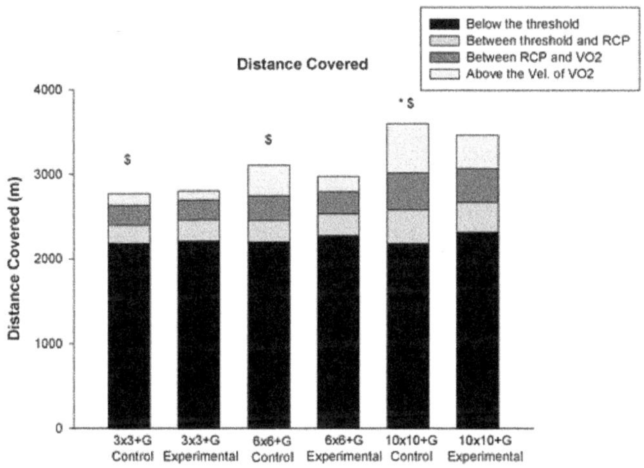

Figure 1. Comparison between the distances covered at different velocity ranges between the control and experimental fields.

$ points to a significant difference in the distances covered at hight intensity between the control and experimental fields ($p<0,05$).
*demonstrate significant differences in the distances covered at low intensity between the control and experimental fields ($p<0,05$).Insert here Figure 1

Figure 2 presents the significant increase in the distance of the high intensity efforts between the 6x6+G control and experimental games, in which the distance of the efforts was 10.7±1.15m in the control field and 9.4±1.0m in the experimental field ($p<0.05$). Similarly, we found in the 10x10+G games, in which the distance was 14±1.71m in the control field and 11.8±1.56m in the experimental field. In the 3x3+G games, no significant difference was seen in the distance of the high intensity efforts. At maximum velocity, there is a significant increase between the 3x3+G control and experimental games, in which the maximum velocity was of 7.15±0.4m/s in the control field and 6.4±0.3m/s in the experimental field. Higher maximum velocity was also found in the 6x6+G games for control field, which was 8.2±0.7m/s and 6.9±0.6m/s in the control field and in the experimental field, respectively. In the 10x10+G games, no significant difference was found for the maximum velocity.

In relation to the amount of high intensity efforts, we can verify a significant increase between the control and experimental fields for the 3x3+G and 6x6+G games. The athletes performed on average 29.2±9.4 high intensity efforts in the 3x3+G control game, and 23.4±10.4 in the 3x3+G experimental game ($p<0.05$). This difference was also verified in the 6x6+G games, in which the athletes performed on average 45.8±18.5 high intensity efforts in the control field and 31.8±9.3 in the experimental field ($p<0.05$). In the 10x10+G fields, no significant difference was found regarding the amount of high intensity efforts. There was no significant difference between the intervals of high intensity efforts and the total distance covered in any of the games analyzed.

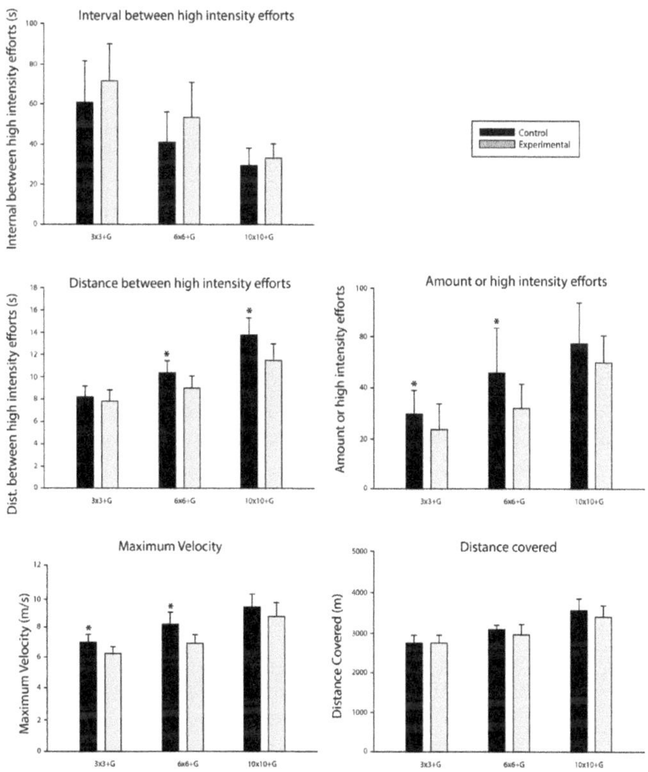

Figure 2. Comparison of the physical variables between the control and the experimental fields in the same field size.

*significant differences between the control and experimental fields ($p<0,05$).

Discussion

The aim of this study was to evaluate the influence of a single variable, i.e. the rule with the tactical principle of maintaining ball possession, in the control of the intensity of efforts and time motion characteristics of players during training in small-, medium- and large-sided games. The results indicate that there is a significant increase in the total distance covered at high intensity in the control field in relation to the experimental field in all fields evaluated, and they also point to significant increase in the distances of high intensity efforts, maximum velocity, and also in the number of such efforts. It is important to note that every time we refer to high intensity actions, we are analyzing the sprints; however, as the literature conceptualizes them above 18 km/h (Hill-Haas, Dawson, Coutts, & Rowsell, 2009; Koklu *et al.*, 2013), we prefer to classify the efforts according to the threshold test. Thus, every effort above the velocity of VO_2max was classified as a high intensity effort. For a better understanding and discussion of the results, we have adopted the 3x3+G games as small-sided games, the 6x6+G games as medium-sided games, and the 10x10+G games as large-sided games (Hodgson *et al.*, 2014; Owen, Wong D, Poul, & Dellal, 2013). Unlike the studies of Hill-Hass *et al.*,(2010), who used the rules to intensify the games, we believe that they have a key role in the development of the game model adopted by the coach and, thus, cannot simply be used to obtain physical results. They should establish the work with games, since the mere performance of these games, without the knowledge of the rules, can lead athletes to negative adjustments in the physical, technical and tactical aspects.

The physical, physiological, technical and tactical demands arising from the manipulation of the rules should be in accordance with the objectives proposed by the coaching staff. The stipulated rules must be designed to encourage and emphasize the aims of each training session. Thus, each of the small-sided games can provide different answers (technical, tactical, physical and physiological) due to the handling of certain rules. In addition, the rules often need to be modified during training to keep athletes in high state of concentration to the game, and ensure that the technical, tactical, physical and physiological objectives previously established are achieved.

Through conceptual games, the rules are intended to model the tactical behavior of the players and team. However, when considering the game as a complex environment, those rules will also influence the emergence of different physical and physiological stimuli to the players. Therefore, the coaching staff needs to be aware of the importance of training control leading to achieve all the objectives in an integrated manner.

The importance of the rules in the control of the physical variables could be observed, for example, on the amount of high intensity efforts, in which we can observe a significant difference between the medium-sided games, in which the athletes performed on average 45 high intensity efforts on the control field and only 31 on the experimental field. It is important to highlight that, although no significant difference was found on the interval between the high intensity efforts in the control fields, the interval between these efforts is an important variable in the effort/pause ratio and should be considered, as the smaller the interval time between one effort and another, the greater the physiological intensity of the athletes.

In the literature, it is well described the importance of the games for soccer training, because of their specificity in training, as well as the seamlessly development of the physical, technical and tactical aspects (Dellal *et al.*, 2012; Eniseler, 2005; Impellizzeri *et al.*, 2006). However, for a practical and scientific advancement, it is important to know the intensities in different games. That is why the control of training loads must be conducted individually. Since it is not enough only to know the distances covered, but rather at which intensities they are carried out, as the distance may not change in different games by several factors, but the intensities can be different. In this study, when analyzing the total distance covered in small-, medium- and large-sided games between the control and experimental fields, we did not find significant differences. However, when dividing the total distance covered into intensity ranges, we can note that there is a significant difference in the distances covered at high intensity between the control and experimental fields in the three field sizes studied. These results corroborated with the studies of Hill-Haas *et al.*,(2009); although the author evaluated the influence of the field size. He found no difference in the total distance covered, but the intensity of the efforts was significantly different, since the distances covered above 18 km/h were higher in medium fields in relation to small fields. That is why it is essential to evaluate the intensity of the efforts and not only the distances covered. The author in his experiments used an external rule to intensify the games, in which the whole team needed to walk past the midfield to validate the goal. With this rule, the game automatically becomes more positioned, less individualized and more collective; by becoming a collective team, the athletes remain closer and more compressed and therefore do not need to run long distances to perform an offensive or defensive effort.

The significant difference in the distances covered at low intensity in large-sided games is another important factor that reinforces the greater physiological intensity of fields without external rules. It reinforces that the intensity of the control field is greater than the experimental field, as the athletes covered less at low intensity, which means that they spent less time standing and or walking during the training. Therefore, they performed more moderate and high intensity efforts. This difference in the intensity of the efforts can be explained by the fact that the athletes do not have a game model in the absence of the effort rule, and even in the official field they play less positioned, making the game less structured and with a tactical disorganization. It is important to note that the position of the players on the field and their tactical behavior influence the physical variables (Clemente *et al.*, 2013; Costa, Garganta, Greco, & Mesquita, 2009; Dellal *et al.*, 2011).

The organization of the team is of the utmost importance for energy saving during the match; when observing the distances of the high intensity efforts, we can note that there is a significant increase for the medium- and large-sided games, between the control and experimental fields. Thus, we understand that the rule induces the training of a more organized team, in which the athletes do not need to run long distances or spend energy to carry out an offensive or defensive action. In the studies of Dellal *et al.*,(2012), when comparing 4x4 games with 11x11 games, he noted that the rules of one or two touches on the ball increases the intensity of small-sided games in relation to the official game, precisely because this is a game with a lower amount of athletes and consequently has a greater number of efforts and movements. Unlike the official game with a greater number of athletes, the players remain tactically positioned and organized, therefore moving less.

In this study, by analyzing the maximum velocities reached between the control and experimental fields, we found that there was a statistically significant difference both in small-sided games and medium-sided games. The study of Koklu *et al.*,(2013) corroborates with our study in relation to the higher intensities of the efforts in less sophisticated games. When comparing the physiological responses and the intensity of the efforts in SSG with and without the presence of goalkeepers, the author found that the intensities of the efforts and the physiological responses are significantly higher in the games without the presence of the goalkeepers. Hill-Haas *et al.*(2010), although he found no physiological differences in some changes in rules and field, it was emphasized the importance of the rules on the intensity of efforts and the motivation of players. The motivation of the players is of paramount importance to ensure that the objectives are achieved, and the rules need to be well prepared and often changed during training for this end. Corroborating the importance of the motivation during training with games, Scaglia *et al.*,(2013) use the term "State of play", which means that the athletes are in a state of maximum concentration and complete involvement, because only this way they can be certain that they are offering their maximum in every effort. However, the author points out that the complexity of the rule can withdraw the athlete from the state of play; thus, it is important for the coaches to know the effort rules to not influence negatively the physiological responses, as well as to not generate negative adjustments on the game model of the team.

However, we conclude that the effort rule, with the principle of maintaining ball possession, is able to control directly the intensity of the efforts and the time motion characteristics of the players on the field. We believe that the variables that were not significantly different between the control and experimental fields can be explained by the increase in size and number of players, but other studies need to be conducted to verify the influence of field size and number of players on the intensity of the efforts and the movement of players in training conducted through games.

We believed that this study allows researchers and football coaches to understand the effect of the effort rules on the preparation of games. The elaboration of small-sided games, without the knowledge on the rules – disregarding the periodization of workloads – and also on the game model that is going to be adopted which could lead players to negative adjustments, both in physical variables and in technical and tactical variables. The coaches need to be aware of which game to apply, as well as which rule to use to intensify the training. Another important factor is to check the training intensity individually and not only the total distance covered, since athletes can cover the same distances, but at different intensities. As limitation of the study, we can highlight the use of biochemical or rating of perceived exertion (RPE) to ensure the different intensities of the applied games.

References

Abdel-Aziz, Y.I., & Karara, H.M. (1971). Direct linear transformation from comparator coordinates into object-space coordinates *Synposium Onclosee-Rane Photogrammetrry* (pp. 1-18). Urbana: ASP/UI.

Aguiar, M., Botelho, G., Lago, C., Macas, V., & Sampaio, J. (2012). A review on the effects of soccer small-sided games. *Journal of Human Kinetics, 33*, 103-113. doi: 10.2478/v10078-012-0049-x

Aguiar, M., Botelho, G.M., Goncalves, B.S., & Sampaio, J.E. (2013). Physiological responses and activity profiles of football small-sided games. [Research Support, N.I.H., Extramural Research Support, Non-U.S. Gov't]. The *Journal of Strength & Conditioning Research, 27*(5), 1287-1294. doi: 10.1519/JSC.0b013e318267a35c

Almeida, C. H., Ferreira, A. P., & Volossovitch, A. (2012). Manipulating task constraints in small-sided soccer games: Performance analysis and practical implications. *The Open Sports Sciences Journal, 5*, 174-180.

Bangsbo, J. (1994). The physiology of soccer - with special reference to intense intermittent exercise. [Review]. *Acta Physiologica Scandinavica Supplementum, 619*, 1-155.

Bangsbo, J., Norregaard, L., & Thorso, F. (1991). Activity profile of competition soccer. [Research Support, Non-U.S. Gov't]. *Canadian Journal of Sports Science, 16*(2), 110-116.

Barros, R.M.L. (2007). Analysis of the distances covered by first division Brazilian soccer players obtained with an automatic tracking method. *Journal of Sports Science and Medicine, 6*(2), 233-242.

Bayer, C. (1994). *O ensino dos desportos colectivos*. Lisboa: Dina Livros.

Bloomfield, J., Polman, R., O'Donoghue, P., & McNaughton, L. (2007). Effective speed and agility conditioning methodology for random intermittent dynamic type sports. [Comparative Study Randomized Controlled Trial]. The *Journal of Strength & Conditioning Research, 21*(4), 1093-1100. doi: 10.1519/R-20015.1

Brandes, M., Heitmann, A., & Muller, L. (2012). Physical responses of different small-sided game formats in elite youth soccer players. [Research Support, Non-U.S. Gov't]. The *Journal of Strength & Conditioning Research, 26*(5), 1353-1360. doi: 10.1519/JSC.0b013e318231ab99

Castellano, J., Casamichana, D., & Dellal, A. (2013). Influence of game format and number of players on heart rate responses and physical demands in small-sided soccer games. The *Journal of Strength & Conditioning Research, 27*(5), 1295-1303. doi: 10.1519/JSC.0b013e318267a5d1

Clemente, F.M., Couceiro, M.S., Martins, F.M., Ivanova, M.O., & Mendes, R. (2013). Activity profiles of soccer players during the 2010 world cup. *Journal of Human Kinetics, 38*, 201-211. doi: 10.2478/hukin-2013-0060

Costa, I. T., Garganta, J.M., Greco, P.J., & Mesquita, I. (2009). Princípios táticos do jogo de futebol: conceitos e aplicação. *Revista Motriz, Rio Claro., 15*, 657-668.

Coutts, A.J., & Duffield, R. (2010). Validity and reliability of GPS units for measuring movement demands of team sports. *Journal of Science and Medicine in Sport, 13*, 133-135.

Coutts, A.J., Rampinini, E., Marcora, S.M., Castagna, C., & Impellizzeri, F.M. (2009). Heart rate and blood lactate correlates of perceived exertion during small-sided soccer games. [Validation Studies]. *Journal of Science and Medicine in Sport, 12*(1), 79-84. doi: 10.1016/j.jsams.2007.08.005

Dellal, A., Chamari, K., Pintus, A., Girard, O., Cotte, T., & Keller, D. (2008). Heart rate responses during small-sided games and short intermittent running training in elite soccer players: a comparative study. [Comparative Study]. The *Journal of Strength & Conditioning Research, 22*(5), 1449-1457. doi: 10.1519/JSC.0b013e31817398c6

Dellal, A., Chamari, K., Wong, D., Ahmaidi, S., Keller, D., Barros, R., . . . Carling, C. (2011). Comparison of physical and technical performance in European soccer match-play: FA Premier League and La Liga. *European Journal of Sport Science, 11*, 51- 59.

Dellal, A., Owen, A., Wong, D.P., Krustrup, P., van Exsel, M., & Mallo, J. (2012). Technical and physical demands of small vs. large sided games in relation to playing position in elite soccer. *Human Movement Science, 31*(4), 957-969. doi: 10.1016/j.humov.2011.08.013

Eniseler, N. (2005). Heart rate and blood lactate concentrations as predictors of physiological load on elite soccer players during various soccer training activities. The *Journal of Strength & Conditioning Research, 19*(4), 799-804. doi: 10.1519/R-15774.1

Figueroa, P.J., Leite, N.J., & Barros, R.M. (2003). A flexible software for tracking of markers used in human motion analysis. *Computer Methods and Programs in Biomedicine, 72*(2), 155-165.

Gabbett, T.J., & Mulvey, M.J. (2008). Time-motion analysis of small-sided training games and competition in elite women soccer players. The *Journal of Strength & Conditioning Research,, 22*(2), 543-552. doi: 10.1519/JSC.0b013e3181635597

Harrison, C.B., Gill, N.D., Kinugasa, T., & Kilding, A.E. (2013). Quantification of physiological, movement, and technical outputs during a novel small-sided game in young team sport athletes. The *Journal of Strength & Conditioning Research, 27*(10), 2861-2868. doi: 10.1519/JSC.0b013e318280c98d

Hill-Haas, S.V., Coutts, A.J., Dawson, B.T., & Rowsell, G.J. (2010). Time-motion characteristics and physiological responses of small-sided games in elite youth players: the influence of player number and rule changes. [Research Support, Non-U.S. Gov't]. The *Journal of Strength & Conditioning Research, 24*(8), 2149-2156. doi: 10.1519/JSC.0b013e3181af5265

Hill-Haas, S.V., Coutts, A. J., Rowsell, G.J., & Dawson, B.T. (2009). Generic versus small-sided game training in soccer. [Comparative Study Randomized Controlled Trial]. *International Journal of Sports Medicine, 30*(9), 636-642. doi: 10.1055/s-0029-1220730

Hill-Haas, S.V., Dawson, B., Impellizzeri, F.M., & Coutts, A.J. (2011). Physiology of small-sided games training in football: a systematic review. [Review]. *Sports Medicine, 41*(3), 199-220. doi: 10.2165/11539740-000000000-00000

Hill-Haas, S.V., Dawson, B.T., Coutts, A.J., & Rowsell, G.J. (2009). Physiological responses and time-motion characteristics of various small-sided soccer games in youth players. *Journal of Sports Sciences, 27*(1), 1-8. doi: 10.1080/02640410902761199

Hill-Haas, S.V., Rowsell, G.J., Dawson, B.T., & Coutts, A.J. (2009). Acute physiological responses and time-motion characteristics of two small-sided training regimes in youth soccer players. [Research Support, Non-U.S. Gov't]. The *Journal of Strength & Conditioning Research, 23*(1), 111-115.

Hodgson, C., Akenhead, R., & Thomas, K. (2014). Time-motion analysis of acceleration demands of 4v4 small-sided soccer games played on different pitch sizes. *Human Movement Science, 33*, 25-32. doi: 10.1016/j.humov.2013.12.002

Hoff, J., Wisloff, U., Engen, L. C., Kemi, O.J., & Helgerud, J. (2002). Soccer specific aerobic endurance training. [Clinical Trial Comparative Study]. *British Journal of Sports Medicine, 36*(3), 218-221.

Impellizzeri, F.M., Marcora, S.M., Castagna, C., Reilly, T., Sassi, A., Iaia, F.M., & Rampinini, E. (2006). Physiological and performance effects of generic versus specific aerobic training in soccer players. [Randomized Controlled Trial]. *International Journal of Sports Medicine, 27*(6), 483-492. doi: 10.1055/s-2005-865839

Jackson, A.S., & Pollock, M.L. (1978). Generalized equations for predicting body density of men. *British Journal of Nutrition, 40*(03), 497-504. doi: doi:10.1079/BJN19780152

Johnston, R.J., Watsford, M.L., Pine, M.J., Spurrs, R.W., Murphy, A.J., & Pruyn, E.C. (2012). The validity and reliability of 5-Hz global positioning system units to measure team sport movement demands. The *Journal of Strength & Conditioning Research, 26*(3), 758-765. doi: 10.1519/JSC.0b013e318225f161

Kelly, D.M., Gregson, W., Reilly, T., & Drust, B. (2013). The development of a soccer-specific training drill for elite-level players. [Comparative Study]. The *Journal of Strength & Conditioning Research, 27*(4), 938-943. doi: 10.1519/JSC.0b013e3182610b7d

Kemi, O.J., Hoff, J., Engen, L.C., Helgerud, J., & Wisloff, U. (2003). Soccer specific testing of maximal oxygen uptake. [Comparative Study]. *Journal of Sports Medicine and Physical Fitness, 43*(2), 139-144.

Koklu, Y., Sert, O., Alemdaroglu, U., & Arslan, Y. (2013). Comparison of the Physiological Responses and Time Motion Characteristics of Young Soccer Players in Small Sided Games: The Effect of Goalkeeper. The *Journal of Strength & Conditioning Research.* doi: 10.1519/JSC.0b013e3182a744a1

Lizana, C., J, R., Reverdito, R.S., Brenzikofer, R., Macedo, D.V., Misuta, M.S., & Scaglia, A.J. (2015). Technical and tactical soccer players' performance in conceptual small-sided games. *Motriz, Rio Claro, 21*, 312-320.

Lourenco, T.F., Martins, L.E., Tessutti, L.S., Brenzikofer, R., & Macedo, D.V. (2011). Reproducibility of an incremental treadmill VO(2)max test with gas exchange analysis for runners. [Research Support, Non-U.S. Gov't]. The *Journal of Strength & Conditioning Research, 25*(7), 1994-1999. doi: 10.1519/JSC.0b013e3181e501d6

Misuta, M.S., Menezes, R.P., Figueroa, P.J., Cunha, S.A., & Barros, R.M.L. (2005). Análise de distâncias percorridas e velocidades de jogadores de futebol durante uma partida. João Pessoa, PB.

Owen, A., Wong D, P., Poul, D., & Dellal, A. (2013). Physical and technical comparisons between various-sided games within professional soccer. *International Journal of Sports Medicine, 35*, 386-392.

Rampinini, E., Impellizzeri, F.M., Castagna, C., Abt, G., Chamari, K., Sassi, A., & Marcora, S.M. (2007). Factors influencing physiological responses to small-sided soccer games. *Journal of Sports Sciences, 25*(6), 659-666. doi: 10.1080/02640410600811858

Reilly, T. (2005). An ergonomics model of the soccer training process. [Review]. *J Sports Sci, 23*(6), 561-572. doi: 10.1080/02640410400021245

Scaglia, A.J., Reverdito.R., Leonardo, L., & Lizana, C. (2013). Collective sports games teaching: essential competencies and logic amid the systemic organizational process. *Movimento, 19*(4), 227-249.

Spencer, M., Lawrence, S., Rechichi, C., Bishop, D., Dawson, B., & Goodman, C. (2004). Time-motion analysis of elite field hockey, with special reference to repeated-sprint activity. [Comparative Study Research Support, Non-U.S. Gov't]. *Journal of Sports Sciences, 22*(9), 843-850. doi: 10.1080/02640410410001716715

Stolen, T., Chamari, K., Castagna, C., & Wisloff, U. (2005). Physiology of soccer: an update. [Research Support, Non-U.S. Gov't Review]. *Sports Medicine, 35*(6), 501-536.

Authors' note

Felipe Lovaglio Belozo, Eliel Calazans Ferreira, Cristian J. R. Lizana, Guilherme Grandim and Alcides José Scaglia are affiliated with the Laboratory of Sports Pedagogy Studies, School of Applied Science, University of Campinas (UNICAMP), Campinas, SP, Brazil.

João Claudio Machado is affiliated with the studies Laboratory of Human Development, Federal University of Amazonas, UFAM, Manaus, AM, Brazil.

René Brenzikofer and Milton Shoiti Misuta are affiliated with the studies Laboratory in Biomechanics, Faculty of Applied Sciences, University of Campinas (UNICAMP), Campinas, SP, Brazil.

Denise Vaz Macedo is affiliated with the Biochemistry Laboratory Exercise, Biology Institute, University of Campinas (UNICAMP), Campinas, SP, Brazil.

Corresponding author

Felipe Belozo
Laboratory of Sports Pedagogy Studies, School of Applied Science, University of Campinas, UNICAMP, Campinas, SP, Brazil.
Email: flbelozo@yahoo.com.br

26

Reference index and reduction in physical fitness tests proposed by PROESP-BR

Camila Fernanda Brandão
Núcleo de Aptidão Física, Informática, Metabolismo, Esporte e Saúde da Universidade Federal de Mato Grosso, MT, Brasil
Universidade de São Paulo, Ribeirão Preto, SP, Brasil

José Henrique de Queiróz Fontes
Arturo Alejandro Zavala Zavala
Waléria Christiane Rezende Fett
Roberto Jaime dos Santos
Carlos Alexandre Fett

Núcleo de Aptidão Física, Informática, Metabolismo, Esporte e Saúde da Universidade Federal de Mato Grosso, MT, Brasil

Abstract—The purpose of this study was to create an unifying index of the PROESP-BR tests for school aged teenagers and propose a reduction in the physical fitness tests. A total of 414 adolescents between the ages of 15 and 17 years old, representative of the public school population in the city of Cuiaba were evaluated. The tests include general physical fitness, proposed by PROESP-BR. Multivariate factorial analysis was used, observing the commonality/representativeness of each test with regard to the set, and the index was created for girls and boys. With this analysis we can choose to use the following tests: female - throwing medicine ball, horizontal jump and run 20 meters; male - throwing medicine ball, representing the overall performance. The created index was divided into quintiles and allowed you to view the whole performance of the six tests, as well as their distribution within the group and away from the ideal reference.

Keywords: performance, diagnosis, motor activity, physical exercise, health and physical fitness.

Introduction

There is growing concern about identifying the existent conditions of risk for any change in the development of children and adolescents (Zajons, Muller & Valentini, 2008). Physical capabilities are directly related to health and sporting performance, and evaluating them has helped with the diagnosis and prevention of diseases as well as in detecting sporting talents (Saraiva & Rodrigues, 2010).

Some international surveys that describe the profile of motor performance of youngsters have observed the association between low physical fitness and school performance (Koutedakis & Bouziotas, 2003). In addition, low physical fitness in adolescence has a negative reflection on adult life (Mikkelsson *et al.*, 2006). Silva, Lima, Silva, and Prado (2009) found a prevalence of 83.1% of sedentary adolescents in the Brazilian population whereas other studies have observed variations between 39% and 93.5% of Brazilian students (Tassitano *et al.*, 2007; Silva *et al.*, 2005).

The lack of standardization of instruments for measuring physical activity hampers comparisons between Brazilian regions, with the Mid-Western region being prejudiced by the scarcity of studies (Silva *et al.*, 2009; Hallal *et al.*, 2007), as well as comparisons with other populations in this area. Therefore, it is crucial to establish equivalent normative values and reference parameters for Brazilian population establishing parameters with others studies of other regions and countries (Drews, Cardozo, Corazza, & Flôres, 2013). Thus, to get a representative number of population it is necessary to have a large scale of the samples, the goal of our study was to evaluate the largest possible number of children and adolescents. It would be interesting to have a general evaluation index for all the factors, whether it is with regard to health or to sporting performance. Therefore, the more condensed the evaluations could be, the easier the reproducibility will be.

Thus, the aim of this study was to create a general index of the tests performed by the parameters of Project Sport Brazil (PROESP-BR) and verify the possibility of reducing the number of tests established by PROESP-BR to the lowest possible number and how reliable is.

Methods

Data was analyzed from 414 adolescents representing the study population of 11.006 high school level students of the 28 schools in the state public network. All of them were within the age-range of 15 to 17 years of age for both sexes and residents within the urban perimeter of the municipality of Cuiabá-MT, situated in the Mid-Western region of Brazil. This study was performed using data Fontes (2013), which held sporting diagnosis and health of students using the parameters and classification of PROESP-BR (2011), in the following tests: abdominal resistance, throwing the medicine ball, horizontal jump, 20-meter run (displacement speed), 4x4 meter square (agility) and 9-minute run (Table 1 and 2).

The project was approved by the Research Ethics Committee of " University Hospital Júlio Muller", Protocol No. 658/CEP/HUJM/09 of July 26, 2009.

Table 1. Performance of PROESP-BR tests of 185 female students from 15 to 17 years of age from Public Network state schools in Cuiabá-MT, Brazil.

		Excellent	Very good	Good	Reasonable	Weak
Abdominal Resistance	%	0.00	3.24	15.14	21.62	60.00
Throwing Medicine Ball	%	2.16	17.30	18.92	25.41	36.22
Horizontal Jump	%	3.24	19.46	23.24	17.30	36.76
20-Meter Run	%	1.08	43.78	19.46	13.51	22.16
Square	%	0.00	3.24	16.22	16.22	64.32
9-Minute Run	%	0.00	17.30	17.84	25.41	39.46

N = no. of subjects % = percentage of subjects with regard to sample of 185 students.

Table 2. Performance of PROESP-BR tests of 229 male students from 15 to 17 years of age from Public Network state schools in Cuiabá-MT, Brazil.

		Excellent	Very good	Good	Reasonable	Weak
Abdominal Resistance	%	0.00	9.17	17.03	24.02	49.78
Throwing Medicine Ball	%	1.31	24.02	30.13	21.40	23.14
Horizontal Jump	%	3.06	24.02	25.33	22.71	24.89
20-Meter Run	%	16.16	37.99	31.00	6.55	8.30
Square	%	0.44	8.73	24.02	18.34	48.47
9-Minute Run	%	0.00	19.21	22.27	24.02	34.50

N = no. of subjects % = percentage of subjects with regard to sample of 229 students.

Statistical Analysis

Multivariate factorial analysis was used to detect the factor of correspondence of each test and afterwards create the index. This was performed with the statistical software program Minitab version 15.0 which, by means of the raw data of the variables found the matrix of correlation and determined the number of factors necessary (≥1). We used commonality for the proposed reduction of the variables with the correlation of each variable being explained by all the factors.T herefore, the higher the value of communality (closer to 1.00); the higher the power of explanation of the variable would be. For the creation of the students' rating it was necessary to create a 'gold standard' reference. Arbitrarily a "school best" was developed, which was established from the best outcome of each test for each sex. In short, no individual had the best marks in all tests, so it was necessary to use the best result obtained in each test for different schools.

The index was obtained by multiplying the standardized variables by the factors obtained, thereby we determined the amplitude between the indices obtained and the data were grouped into 05 groups, in which the lowest values corresponded to the greatest proximity to the values of the excellent adolescent students, therefore meaning the best result.

Results

To create the index of each student, it was necessary observe the score of each test on the whole (values of commonality), thus we see the possibility to reduce the amount of testing and the difference between male and female groups. Regarding the proposal for reduction in the tests, there was a variance of 65% and 58% of the importance of each variable for female and male group, respectively. The female group had two tests with high values, three with medium values, and one with a low value and in the male group there was one high, four medium and one low test value. Thus, if we consider values of correspondence above 70% to represent the set, only two tests would be necessary for the female group and one test for the male group (Tables 3 and 4). However, we observed that there was correlation between the tests themselves, and only 01 test in each group had values below 50%.

Table 3. Result of correspondence factors of each physical test stipulated by PROESP-BR of females.

Tests	Factor 1	Factor 2	Commonality
Abdominal Resistance	0.66	-0.35	0.57
Throwing Medicine Ball	0.34	0.84	0.82
Horizontal Jump	0.75	0.38	0.72
20-Meter Run	-0.83	0.03	0.69
Square	-0.81	-0.15	0.69
9-Minute Run	0.64	-0.07	0.42
Variance	2.9052	1.0216	3.9268
% Var.	0.484	0.170	0.654

Rotated Factors - Quartimax. Rotation.

Table 4. Result of correspondence factors of each physical test stipulated by PROESP-BR of males.

Tests	Factor 1	Factor 2	Commonality
Abdominal Resistance	0.40	0.52	0.43
Throwing Medicine Ball	0.75	-0.26	0.64
Horizontal Jump	0.78	-0.22	0.67
20-Meter Run	-0.64	-0.30	0.50
Square	-0.70	0.05	0.50
9-Minute Run	0.16	0.84	0.73
Variance	2.2965	1.1913	3.4878
% Var.	0.383	0.199	0.581

Rotated Factors - Quartimax. Rotation

According to analysis, we obtained the index of adolescent students and with the creation of the excellent female and male students within our own sample; we divided the classification into five groups, stratifying by the amplitude among the data. For the female classification, the amplitude was 19.56 resulting in the interval of 3.85 for each classification; for the male classification the amplitude was 17.49, resulting in the interval of 3.50 between the classifications. The classification of each student was determined by the distance between the school adolescent students from the excellent adolescent student, and the shorter the distance between them, the better the result (Tables 5 and 6, Figures 1 and 2).

Table 5. Index created for classification of females.

Interval		N	%	Group	Classification
0.00	0.01	1	0.5	Excellent	-
0.01	3.85	5	2.7	G1	Excellent
3.86	7.70	39	21.0	G2	Very Good
7.71	11.55	95	51.0	G3	Good
11.56	15.40	43	23.1	G4	Reasonable
15.41	more	3	1.7	G5	Weak
TOTAL		186	100		

Excellent group: excellent student created
N and %: quantity of students in each group.

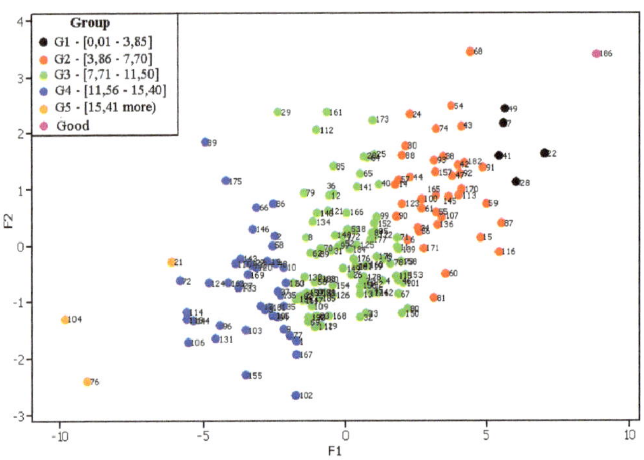

Figure 1. Dispersion graph according to the female group.

Table 6. Index created for classification of males.

Interval		N	%	Group	Classification
0.00	0.01	1	0.4	Excellent	-
0.01	3.50	2	0.8	G1	Excellent
3.51	7.00	16	7.0	G2	Very Good
7.01	10.50	117	51.0	G3	Good
10.51	14.00	83	36.0	G4	Reasonable
14.01	more	11	4.8	G5	Weak
TOTAL		230	100		

Excellent group: excellent student created
N and %: quantity of students in each group.

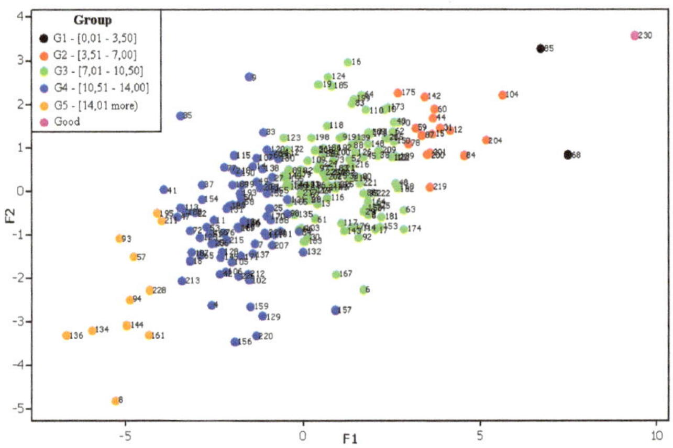

Figure 2. Dispersion graph according to the male group.

Discussion

The present study is a continuation of the work of Fontes (2013) who had identified a low performance of adolescent students in the PROESP-BR tests. Subsequently, we developed a statistical analysis that allowed a different manner of observing the behavior between the genders with regard to the power of the tests. In the female group, two tests were of high importance to represent the overall performance whereas in male group only one test seems high representative. In addition, an index that represents the overall performance of the adolescent students was developed, which provides a spatial view of the distribution of the physical capacity among these adolescent students and in comparison with the excellent adolescent students. This approach shows that these adolescent students had a low physical performance because the best classified among them were equidistant from both the excellent adolescent students and the worst classification. Moreover, it allows an approach to a specific classification for this group, considering that with regard to the original PROESP-BR classification, they are only at the margin of the excellent category.

Studies using multivariate factorial analysis have been explored to a small extent in the field of physical education up to now. In our study, the determination of an index may help future evaluations with the proposal of a smaller number of tests. Thus, we observed that the extraction of two factors was possible, for girls and boys, these representing 65% and 58%, respectively, of the total variance in the results, showing that these tests have greater impact on the entire battery of evaluations performed.

A reduction in the number of tests may facilitate the development of the evaluations, since we observed that if some tests were not performed would not affecting the final score of the overall index. Indeed, Peterson, Alvar & Rhea (2006) stated that the horizontal jump is sufficient in the evaluation of power, speed and agility; while Guedes (2007) reported that the 20-meter run is capable of providing information about the same physical fitness level. One of the main reasons for physical follow-up is related to health; the components of force, resistance, and agility are directly related to the prevention of neuromuscular problems (Welk, Going, Morrow, & Meredith, 2011) since it has been associated with maintaince of the metabolism of some substrates and hormone regulation (Guedes,, Miranda-Neto, Germano, Lopes & Silva, 2012).

Sharkey (1997), demonstrated that performance of physical tests that use greater muscle recruitment are more efficient in the diagnosis of overall physical fitness of youngsters who are not athletes. This corroborates with the finding for the male group in our study, in which the test with greatest score was the 9-minute run. On the other hand, we found that the tests with the greatest score, for the female group, were throwing the medicine ball and horizontal jump. However, in the female group this is not an absolute factor, because the horizontal jump is considered important for overall evaluation. Castro-Pinero *et al.* (2010), observed a strong association between the horizontal jump test and tests of muscle force of the upper and lower limbs. Furthermore, they considered that this test could be used as a general index of muscle aptness in adolescents. Further studies with different populations and biochemical analyses are necessary, in order, to better determine these inter-gender variations.

With the factors of each test, we verified that the female group had more distributed physical performance results, and only two tests were necessary to obtain the same index. Differently, in male group, which was more homogeneous, only one test could be performed providing the same information. With regard to classification, we observed that the female group had better results than the male group. This differs from the classification made by Fontes (2013) and other studies, such as Dumith *et al.*, (2010) and Guedes, Neto & Silva (2011) which analyzed the difference between the genders in some physical fitness tests and found that boys received higher scores than girls in the majority of the tests. Silva, Nahas, Hoefelmann, Lopes and Oliveira (2008) pointed out that male adolescents are more physically active, particularly in the field of leisure and work, due to cultural influences and the strong trend towards self-determination (Viana, Andrade & Matias, 2010).

The index created may facilitate the diagnosis and follow-up of school physical education in the population diagnosed. Persisting with that which the study of Silva, Böhme, Uezu and Massa (2003) considered, the importance of creating indices that provided references for each specific population, with the justification of helping with the follow-up of lessons; and considering that in the present study the adolescent students presented low physical performance. This suggests that they are exposed to a low quality/quantity of motor activities. Similar to our results, Pelegrini, Silva, Petroski, & Glaner (2011) observed that adolescent Brazilian students presented inadequate levels of physical fitness. This situation may be due to cultural changes, as regards exposure to passive leisure, such as electronic games, TV and other entertainment (Dumith *et al.*, 2010). According to Hallal, Knuth, Cruz, Mendes, and Malta (2010), the majority of adolescents in the Mid-Western region of Brazil are insufficiently active.

Physical Education lessons, in turn, which must contribute to improving this situation, are apparently not changing the lack of physical activity. Indeed, other studies have observed that the level of physical effort in the Physical Education lessons are not sufficient to increase physical fitness (Guedes & Guedes, 2001) both in public and private schools (Hallal *et al.*, 2010; Silva, Lima, Silva, & Prado, 2009). Another studied has related that only 49.2% of the adolescents in major Brazilian cities responded to participating in two weekly physical education classes (Hallal, Knuth, Cruz, Mendes & Malta, 2010). Therefore, with the help of school planning, it is necessary for teachers to interact and develop socialization, challenging the processes of upbringing and lifestyles and demonstrating to the adolescent students the importance of physical activity as the opportunity to improve their quality of life (Gallahue & Donnelly, 2008).

Although we created the excellent adolescent students with the best results in our sample, this is not the ideal, because considering the general classification used by PROESP-BR, those students are not within the 98th percentile; so far, obtaining excellent results in at least two tests. The present index is representative for the sample population. Of note, we observed that the studied population lacks specific evaluations, and this instrument is useful for teachers to follow-up the development of their pupils. Furthermore, knowledge of the local reality leads us to the need for formulating public policies and specific interventions with regard to physical education lessons and the promotion of school sports.

Conclusion

With the results of factorial analyses we obtained the score of each test, allowing a reduction in the tests and showing that these tests do not have the same gradet for both sexes, therefore, it is necessary to observe the most characteristic physical qualities of each gender. From the factors analyzed, an index could be created for each pupil, helping with visualization of the overall motor performance of adolescent students, and this can be used by Physical Education teachers for following-up their pupils' performance. This index facilitated visualization of the results of the adolescent students' performance, which pointed out a low level of physical fitness in both genders and demonstrating that the intervention in physical activity may not be adequate for this population.

References

Castro-Pinero, J., Ortega, F.B., Artero, E.G., Girela-Rejon, M.J., Mora, J., Sjostrom, M., & Ruiz, J. (2010). Assessing Muscular Strength In Youth: Usefulness Of Standing Long Jump As A General Index Of Muscular Fitness. *Journal of Strength and Conditioning Research*, 24, 1810-1817.

Drews, R., Cardozo, P.L., Corazza, S.T., & Flôres, F.S. (2013). Análise do desempenho motor de escolares praticantes de futsal e voleibol. *Motricidade*, 9, 105-116.

Dumith, S.C., Ramires, V.V., Souza, M.J.A., Moraes, D.S., Petry, F.G., Oliveira, E.S., Ramires, S.V., & Marques, A.C. (2010). Aptidão física relacionada ao desempenho motor em escolares de sete a 15 anos. *Revista Brasileira Educação* Física e Esporte, 24, 5-14.

Fontes, J.H.Q. (2013). *Diagnóstico do potencial olímpico de alunos de 15 a 17 anos da rede estadual de ensino de Cuiabá-MT*. Dissertação de mestrado.

Gallahue, D.L., & Donnelly, F.C. (2008). Educação Física desenvolvimentista para todas as crianças, 4. ed., São Paulo: Phorte.

Guedes, D.P. (2007). Implicações associadas ao acompanhamento do desempenho motor de crianças e adolescentes. *Revista Brasileira Educação Física e Esporte*, 21, 37-60.

Guedes, D.P., & Guedes, J.E.R.P. (2001). Níveis de prática de atividade física habitual em adolescentes. *Revista Brasileira Medicina do Esporte*, 7, 187-99.

Guedes, D.P., Neto, J.T.M., & Silva, A.J. (2011). Desempenho motor em uma amostra de escolares brasileiros. *Motricidade*, 7, 25-38.

Guedes, D.P., Miranda-Neto, J.T., Germano, J.M., Lopes, V., & Silva, A.J.R.M. (2012). Aptidão física relacionada à saúde de escolares: Programa Fitnessgram. *Revista Brasileira Medicina do Esporte*, 18, 72-76.

Hallal, P.C., Dumith, S.C., Bastos, J.P., Reichert, F.F., Siqueira, F.V., Azevedo, M.R. (2007). Evolução da pesquisa epidemiológica em atividade física no Brasil: revisão sistemática. *Revista de saúde pública*, 41, 453-60.

Hallal, P., Knuth, A.G., Cruz, D.K.A., Mendes, M.I., & Malta, D.C. (2010). Prática de atividade física em adolescentes brasileiros. *Ciência e Saúde Coletiva*, 15, 3035-42.

Koutedakis, Y., & Bouziotas, C. (2003). National physical education curriculum: motor and cardiovascular health related fitness in Greek adolescents. *British Journal of Sports Medicine*, 37, 311-4.

Mikkelsson, L.O., Nupponen, H., Kaprio, J., Kautiainen, H., Mikkelsson, M., & Kujala, U.M. (2006). Adolescent flexibility, endurance strength, and physical activity as predictors of adult tension neck, low back pain, and knee injury: a 25 year follow up study. *British Journal of Sports Medicine*, 40, 107-13.

Pelegrini, A., Silva, D.A.S., Petroski, E.L., & Glaner, M.F. (2011). Aptidão física relacionada a saúde de Escolares brasileiros: dados PROESP-BR. *Revista Brasileira Medicina do Esporte*, 17, 92-96.

Peterson, M.D, Alvar, B.A, & Rhea, MR. (2006). The contribution of maximal force production to explosive movement among young collegiate athletes. *Journal of Strength Conditioning and Research*, 20, 867-73.

Projeto Esporte Brasil (PROESP-BR). (2011). Disponível em: <http://www.proesp.ufrgs.br> Acesso em: 10 jul. 2011.

Saraiva, J.P., & Rodrigues, L.P. (2010). Relações entre atividade física, aptidão física, morfológica e coordenativa na infância e adolescência. *Motricidade*, 6, 35-45.

Sharkey, B.J. (1997). *Fitness and health*. (4 ed.) Champaign: Human Kinetics.

Silva, L.R.R, Böhme, M.T.S, Uezu, R., & Massa, M. (2003). A utilização de variáveis cineantropométricas no processo de detecção, seleção e promoção de talentos no voleibol. *Revista Brasileira Ciência e Movimento*, 11, 69-76.

Silva, M.A., Rivera, I.R., Ferraz, M.R., Pinheiro, A.J, Alves, S.W., Moura, A.A., & Carvalho, A.C. (2005). Prevalência de fatores de risco cardiovascular em crianças e adolescentes da rede de ensino da cidade de Maceió. *Arquivos Brasileiro de Cardiologia*, 84, 387-92.

Silva, K.S., Nahas, M.V., Hoefelmann, L.P., Lopes, A.S., & Oliveira, E.S. (2008) Associações entre atividade física, índice de massa corporal e comportamentos sedentários em adolescentes. *Revista Brasileira Epidemiologia*, 11, 159-168.

Silva, D.A.S., Lima, J.O., Silva, R.J.S., & Prado, R.L. (2009). Nível de atividade física e comportamento sedentário em escolares. *Revista Brasileira Cineantropometria e Desempenho Humano*, 11, 299-306.

Tassitano, R.M., Bezerra, J., Tenorio, M.C.M., Colares, V., Barros, M.V.G., & Hallal, P.C. (2007). Atividade física em adolescentes brasileiros: uma revisão sistemática. *Rev Bras Cineantropom Desempenho Hum*, 9, 55-60.

Viana, M.S., Andrade, A., & Matias, T.S. (2010). Teoria da autodeterminação: Aplicações no contexto da prática de exercícios físicos de adolescentes. *Pensar a Prática*, 13, 1-18.

Welk, G.J., Going, S.B., Morrow, J.R., & Meredith, M.D. (2011). Development of new criterion-referenced fitness standards in the Fitnessgramge program: rationale and conceptual overview. *American Journal of Preventive Medicine*, 41, 63-7.

Zajons, R., Muller, A.B., & Valentini, N.C. (2008). A influência de fatores ambientais no desempenho motor e social de crianças da periferia de Porto Alegre. *Revista Educação Física/UEM*, 19, 159-171.

Authors' note

Camila Fernanda Brandão, master in physical education of Federal University of Mato Grosso and PhD student in the Ribeirão Preto Medical School, University of São Paulo

José Henrique de Queiroz Sources, Master in Biosciences, Federal University of Mato Grosso

Arturo Alejandro Zavala Zavala, PhD in statistics and professor at the Faculty of Economics of the Federal University of Mato Grosso;

Waléria Christiane Rezende Fett, PhD in Medical Sciences and professor at the Faculty of Physical Education, Federal University of Mato Grosso

Roberto Jaime dos Santos, professor at the Faculty of Physical Education, Federal University of Mato Grosso

Carlos Alexandre Fett, PhD Medical Sciences and professor at the Faculty of Physical Education, Federal University of Mato Grosso.

Corresponding author

Camila Fernanda Brandão
Faculdade de Medicina de Ribeirão Preto da Universidade de São Paulo, Anexo A, Bloco B, sala 103 - Avenida Bandeirantes, 3900, Vila Monte Alegre, Ribeirão Preto, SP, Brasil.
Email: camilafbrandao@hotmail.com

PERMISSIONS

All chapters in this book were first published in MREF, by Universidade Estadual Paulista; hereby published with permission under the Creative Commons Attribution License or equivalent. Every chapter published in this book has been scrutinized by our experts. Their significance has been extensively debated. The topics covered herein carry significant findings which will fuel the growth of the discipline. They may even be implemented as practical applications or may be referred to as a beginning point for another development.

The contributors of this book come from diverse backgrounds, making this book a truly international effort. This book will bring forth new frontiers with its revolutionizing research information and detailed analysis of the nascent developments around the world.

We would like to thank all the contributing authors for lending their expertise to make the book truly unique. They have played a crucial role in the development of this book. Without their invaluable contributions this book wouldn't have been possible. They have made vital efforts to compile up to date information on the varied aspects of this subject to make this book a valuable addition to the collection of many professionals and students.

This book was conceptualized with the vision of imparting up-to-date information and advanced data in this field. To ensure the same, a matchless editorial board was set up. Every individual on the board went through rigorous rounds of assessment to prove their worth. After which they invested a large part of their time researching and compiling the most relevant data for our readers.

The editorial board has been involved in producing this book since its inception. They have spent rigorous hours researching and exploring the diverse topics which have resulted in the successful publishing of this book. They have passed on their knowledge of decades through this book. To expedite this challenging task, the publisher supported the team at every step. A small team of assistant editors was also appointed to further simplify the editing procedure and attain best results for the readers.

Apart from the editorial board, the designing team has also invested a significant amount of their time in understanding the subject and creating the most relevant covers. They scrutinized every image to scout for the most suitable representation of the subject and create an appropriate cover for the book.

The publishing team has been an ardent support to the editorial, designing and production team. Their endless efforts to recruit the best for this project, has resulted in the accomplishment of this book. They are a veteran in the field of academics and their pool of knowledge is as vast as their experience in printing. Their expertise and guidance has proved useful at every step. Their uncompromising quality standards have made this book an exceptional effort. Their encouragement from time to time has been an inspiration for everyone.

The publisher and the editorial board hope that this book will prove to be a valuable piece of knowledge for researchers, students, practitioners and scholars across the globe.

LIST OF CONTRIBUTORS

Walan Robert da Silva
Universidade do Estado de Santa Catarina, Florianópolis, SC, Brasil

Elisa Pinheiro Ferrari and Thiago Emannuel Medeiros
Universidade do Estado de Santa Catarina, Florianópolis, SC, Brasil

Kamyla Thais Dias de Freitas
Universidade do Estado de Santa Catarina, Florianópolis, SC, Brasil

Claudio Marcelo Tkac
Pontifícia Universidade Católica do Paraná, Curitiba, PR, Brasil

Fernando Luiz Cardoso
Universidade do Estado de Santa Catarina, Florianópolis, SC, Brasil

Alessandra de Azevedo
Universidade Positivo, Curitiba, PR, Brasil

Lorena Fernanda de Matos
Universidade Federal do Paraná, Curitiba, PR, Brasil

Fábio Yuzo Nakamura
Universidade Estadual de Londrina, Londrina, PR, Brasil

Gleber Pereira
Universidade Federal do Paraná, Curitiba, PR, Brasil

Kamilla Bolonha Gomes, Anselmo José Perez and Luciana Carletti
Universidade Federal do Espírito Santo,Vitória, ES, Brasil

Adilson Marques
Universidade de Lisboa, Portugal

Melissa de Carvalho Souza and Adriana Coutinho de Azevedo Guimarães
Universidade do Estado de Santa Catarina, UDESC, Florianópolis, SC, Brasil

Rodrigo de Rosso Krug, Giovâni Firpo Del Duca, Kelly Samara da Silva and Cecília Bertuol Markus Vinicius Nahas
Universidade Federal de Santa Catarina, Florianópolis, SC, Brasil

Elusa Santina Antunes de Oliveira and Mauro Virgilio Gomes de Barros
Universidade de Pernambuco, Recife, PE, Brasil

Sileno da Silva Santos, Angélica Castilho Alonso and Júlia Maria D'Andréa Greve
Universidade de São Paulo, São Paulo, SP, Brasil

Ronaldo Kobal
Núcleo de alto rendimento esportivo de São Paulo, SP, Brasil

Renato Barroso
Universidade Estadual de Campinas, Campinas, SP, Brasil

Cesar Cavinato Cal Abad and Kátia Kitamura
Núcleo de alto rendimento esportivo de São Paulo, SP, Brasil

Everton Crivoi do Carmo
Centro Universitário Senac, São Paulo, SP, Brasil

Lucas Pereira
Núcleo de alto rendimento esportivo de São Paulo, SP, Brasil

Fábio Yuzo Nakamura
Núcleo de alto rendimento esportivo de São Paulo, SP, Brasil
Universidade Estadual de Londrina, Londrina, PR, Brasil

Irineu Loturco
Núcleo de alto rendimento esportivo de São Paulo, SP, Brasil

Rodrigo Leal de Queiroz Thomaz de Aquino
Universidade do Porto, Porto, Portugal

Luiz Guilherme Cruz Gonçalves, Lucas de Paula Oliveira, Hugo Tourinho Filho and Enrico Fuini Puggina
Universidade de São Paulo, Ribeirão Preto, SP, Brasil

Antonio García-de-Alcaraz
Faculty of Physical Activity and Sport Sciences, Polytechnic University of Madrid, Spain

Enrique Ortega
Faculty of Sport Sciences, University of Murcia, Spain

José M. Palao
University of Wisconsin-Parkside, United States

Eliane Mauerberg-deCastro and Debra Frances Campbell
Universidade Estadual Paulista "Júlio de Mesquita Filho," Rio Claro, SP, Brasil

Carolina Paioli Tavares
Universidade Estadual de Ponta Grossa, Ponta Grossa, PR, Brasil

Raphael N. Pereira, Marcos Fabio R. Abreu and Camila B. Gonçalves
Universidade Metodista de Piracicaba, Piracicaba, Brasil

Wilson Flávio S. Corrêa
Clube dos Deficientes Físicos do Pará – "All Star Rodas", Pará, Brasil

Daniel R. Mizuhira
Associação dos Amigos Paradesportistas de Piracicaba, Piracicaba, Brasil

Marlene A. Moreno
Universidade Metodista de Piracicaba, Piracicaba, Brasil

Isadora Lessa Moreno
Universidade Federal de São Paulo, São Paulo, SP, Brasil

Luiz Carlos Marques Vanderlei, Franciele Marques Vanderlei and Carlos Marcelo Pastre
Universidade Estadual Paulista "Julio de Mesquita Filho", Presidente Prudente, SP, Brasil

Luiz Carlos de Abreu
Faculdade de Medicina do ABC, Santo André, SP, Brasil

Celso Ferreira
Universidade Federal de São Paulo, São Paulo, SP, Brasil

Gabriel Rodrigues Neto
Universidade Federal de Paraíba, João Pessoa, Paraíba, Brasil
Universidade Federal do Rio de Janeiro, Rio de Janeiro, RJ, Brasil

Jefferson da Silva Novaes
Universidade Federal do Rio de Janeiro, Rio de Janeiro, RJ, Brasil

Michel Gonçalves
Universidade Federal do Rio de Janeiro, Rio de Janeiro, RJ, Brasil
Instituto de Pesquisa e Capacitação Física do Exército, Rio de Janeiro, RJ, Brasil

Gilmário Ricarte Batista and Rosa Maria Soares Costa de Mendonça
Universidade Federal da Paraíba, João Pessoa, PB, Brasil

Humberto Miranda
Universidade Federal do Rio de Janeiro, Rio de Janeiro, RJ, Brasil

Giovanni da Silva Novaes
Universidade Castelo Branco, Rio de Janeiro, RJ, Brasil
Centro de Investigação em Esporte, Saúde e Desenvolvimento Humano, Vila Real, Portugal

Maria do Socorro Cirilo-Sousa
Universidade Federal da Paraíba, João Pessoa, PB, Brasil

Ligia Ignêz Engelmann, Giane Veiga Liedtke and Flávio de Souza Castro
Universidade Federal do Rio Grande do Sul, Porto Alegre, RS, Brasil

Johnny Padulo
University e-Campus, Novedrate, Italy
University of Split, Split, Croatia
National Centre of Medicine and Science in Sport, Tunis, Tunisia

Luca Paolo Ardigò
University of Verona, Verona, Italy

Mirjana Milić
University of Split, Split, Croatia

Douglas William Powell
Campbell University, Buies Creek, NC, USA

Juan J. Fernández-Romero
University of A Coruña, Corunã, Spain

Helena Vila Suárez and Jose Mª Cancela
Universidade de Vigo, Vigo, Spain

João Cláudio Machado, Chellsea Alcântara, Carlos Palheta and João Otacílio Libardoni dos Santos
Universidade Federal do Amazonas, Manaus, AM, Brasil

Daniel Barreira
Universidade do Porto, Porto, Portugal

Alcides José Scaglia
Universidade Estadual de Campinas, Limeira, SP, Brasil

Fernando Nazário de Rezende
Universidade Federal do Triângulo Mineiro, Uberaba, MG, Brasil
Universidade Presidente Antônio Carlos, Uberlândia, MG, Brasil

Gustavo Ribeiro da Mota
Universidade Federal do Triângulo Mineiro, Uberaba, MG, Brasil

Charles Ricardo Lopes
Universidade Metodista de Piracicaba, Piracicaba, SP, Brasil
Faculdade Adventista de Hortolândia, Hortolândia, SP, Brasil

Bruno Victor C. da Silva
Centro Universitário de Belo Horizonte, Belo Horizonte, MG, Brasil

Mário A. M. Simim
Universidade Federal de Belo Horizonte, Belo Horizonte, MG, Brasil

Moacir Marocolo
Universidade Federal de Juiz de Fora, Juiz de Fora, MG, Brasil

Adalberto Veronese da Costa
Universidade do Estado do Rio Grande do Norte, Rio Grande do Norte, RN. Brasil
Universidade de Trás-os-Montes e Alto Douro, Vila Real. Portugal

Manoel da Cunha Costa, Jorge Luiz de Brito Gomes and Fernando José de Sá Pereira Guimarães
Universidade de Pernambuco, Recife, PE, Brasil

Tiago Manuel Barbosa
National Institute of Education, Nanyang Technological University, Singapore

Adilson Marques
Universidade de Lisboa, Lisboa, Portugal
Universidade Nova de Lisboa, Lisboa, Portugal

Miguel Peralta
Universidade de Lisboa, Lisboa, Portugal

João Martins
Universidade de Lisboa, Lisboa, Portugal
Universidade Lusófona de Humanidades e Tecnologias, Lisboa, Portugal

Hugo Sarmento
Universidade de Coimbra, Coimbra, Portugal

Ash C. Routen
Loughborough University, Loughborough, United Kingdom

Francisco Carreiro da Costa
Universidade de Lisboa, Lisboa, Portugal
Universidade Lusófona de Humanidades e Tecnologias, Lisboa, Portugal

Raphaelly Machado Felix, Vinicius Martins Farias, Mauren Lúcia de Araújo Bergmann and Gabriel Gustavo Bergmann
Universidade Federal do Pampa, Uruguaiana, RS, Brasil

Sergio Reloba Martínez, Luis Javier Chirosa Ríos and Ignacio Martín Tamayo
Universidad de Granada, Granada, España

Laura Guerrero Almeida
Universidad de Sevilla, Sevilla, España

Miguel Angel López-Gomez
Universidad de Granada, Granada, España

Christian Campos Jara
Universidad Andrés Bello, Santiago, Chile

Marco Correia, António Rosado and Sidónio Serpa
Universidade de Lisboa, Lisboa, Portugal

Danilo de Oliveira Silva, Maira Bergamaschi Coura, Marina Waiteman, Juliana Pradela and Marcella Ferraz Pazzinatto
Universidade Estadual Paulista "Júlio de Mesquita Filho", Presidente Prudente, SP, Brasil

Fernando Henrique Magalhães
Universidade de São Paulo, São Paulo, SP, Brasil

Fábio Mícolis de Azevedo
Universidade Estadual Paulista "Júlio de Mesquita Filho", Presidente Prudente, SP, Brasil

Felipe Lovaglio Belozo, Eliel Calazans Ferreira, Cristian J. R. Lizana and Guilherme Grandim
Universidade de Campinas, UNICAMP, Campinas, SP, Brasil

João Claudio Machado
Universidade Federal do Amazonas, UFAM, Manaus, AM, Brasil

René Brenzikofer, Denise Vaz Macedo, Milton Shoiti Misuta and Alcides José Scaglia
Universidade de Campinas, UNICAMP, Campinas, SP, Brasil

Camila Fernanda Brandão
Núcleo de Aptidão Física, Informática, Metabolismo, Esporte e Saúde da Universidade Federal de Mato Grosso, MT, Brasil
Universidade de São Paulo, Ribeirão Preto, SP, Brasil

José Henrique de Queiróz Fontes, Arturo Alejandro Zavala Zavala, Waléria Christiane Rezende Fett, Roberto Jaime dos Santos and Carlos Alexandre Fett
Núcleo de Aptidão Física, Informática, Metabolismo, Esporte e Saúde da Universidade Federal de Mato Grosso, MT, Brasil

Index